Practical Flow Cytometry in Haematology Diagnosis

This book is dedicated to Dr Norman Lucie, pioneer of flow cytometry in Glasgow.

Practical Flow Cytometry in Haematology Diagnosis

Mike Leach FRCP, FRCPath

Consultant Haematologist and Honorary Senior Lecturer
Haematology Laboratories and West of Scotland Cancer Centre
Gartnavel General Hospital
Glasgow, UK

Mark Drummond PhD, FRCPath

Consultant Haematologist and Honorary Senior Lecturer
Haematology Laboratories and West of Scotland Cancer Centre
Gartnavel General Hospital
Glasgow, UK

Allyson Doig MSc, FIBMS

Haemato-Oncology Laboratory Manager
Haematology Laboratories
Gartnavel General Hospital
Glasgow, UK

(W)WILEY-BLACKWELL

A John Wiley & Sons, Ltd., Publication

This edition first published 2013, © 2013 by John Wiley & Sons, Ltd

Wiley-Blackwell is an imprint of John Wiley & Sons, formed by the merger of Wiley's global Scientific, Technical and Medical business with Blackwell Publishing.

Registered Office
John Wiley & Sons, Ltd, The Atrium, Southern Gate, Chichester, West Sussex, PO19 8SQ, UK

Editorial Offices
9600 Garsington Road, Oxford, OX4 2DQ, UK
The Atrium, Southern Gate, Chichester, West Sussex, PO19 8SQ, UK
111 River Street, Hoboken, NJ 07030-5774, USA

For details of our global editorial offices, for customer services and for information about how to apply for permission to reuse the copyright material in this book please see our website at www.wiley.com/wiley-blackwell

The right of the author to be identified as the author of this work has been asserted in accordance with the UK Copyright, Designs and Patents Act 1988.

Library of Congress Cataloging-in-Publication Data

Leach, Richard M., MD.
Practical flow cytometry in haematology diagnosis / Mike Leach, Mark Drummond, Allyson Doig.
    p. ; cm.
    Includes bibliographical references and index.
Summary: "This book acts as a clinical manual for the diagnostician who cannot turn to reference books when the morphology or immunophenotype are atypical. This volume presents a logical practical approach to the diagnosis of blood disorders, both neoplastic and reactive, and other diagnostic applications of flow cytometry in non-neoplastic haematology diagnosis. Illustrations are provided throughout with worked examples"–Provided by publisher.
    ISBN 978-0-470-67120-7 (hardback : alk. paper) – ISBN 978-1-118-48795-2 (Mobi) – ISBN 978-1-118-48796-9 (obook) – ISBN 978-1-118-48797-6 (epub) – ISBN 978-1-118-48799-0 (ePDF/ebook)
I. Drummond, Mark, PhD.   II. Doig, Allyson.   III. Title.
[DNLM: 1. Hematologic Diseases–diagnosis.   2. Hematologic Neoplasms–diagnosis.
3. Flow Cytometry–methods.   4. Hematology–methods. WH 120]
    616.1'5075–dc23
                                    2012029836
A catalogue record for this book is available from the British Library.

Wiley also publishes its books in a variety of electronic formats. Some content that appears in print may not be available in electronic books.

Cover design by Steve Thompson

Set in 9/12pt Minion by SPi Publisher Services, Pondicherry, India

Contents

Preface

The accurate diagnosis of haematologic malignancies is a complex and challenging task. It routinely involves morphologic, molecular, cyogenetic and flow cytometric expertise; how these results are integrated, interpreted and reported will ultimately determine what treatment protocol will be followed. Flow cytometry is central in this diagnostic pathway.

When the authors began to develop their interest in flow cytometry there were few texts available to assist in the day-to-day interpretation of results from clinical samples. The laboratory texts in most frequent use were technically orientated to assist the cytometrist in providing quality data for subsequent reporting. Excellent morphologic and haematopathology texts were available, but a readable, clinically orientated flow cytometry text was notably absent. Things have certainly changed, with a plethora of textbooks describing the application of flow cytometry in the routine diagnostic laboratory. These have taken a varied approach, with cased-based, pattern-based and traditional pathological entity-based approaches having appeared over the years. However the authors consider something still to be missing, namely the textbook they would have wanted to pick up 15 years ago as enthusiastic but inexperienced flow cytometrists who wanted to better learn how to interpret the data to inform their haematology practice. Two of the authors of this book are practicing haematologists who between them routinely diagnose and treat all the malignancies described herein. There is therefore a clinical emphasis throughout, as to how flow cytometry results should be interpreted and applied to optimize patient care. In the real world samples arrive from a range of body fluids, from both malignant and benign conditions and are of variable quality. We have endeavored to reflect this. This book is therefore not a technical manual, but instead it is aimed at those who instigate, perform, interpret or act upon flow cytometry on patient material. This might include clinical scientists, pathologists, haematologists and research laboratory staff. It has therefore been written to encompass the varied background and knowledge of these individuals. Although it has been written to be read from cover to cover it will be a useful laboratory reference text, and we hope of use to both novice and expert alike.

The approach the authors have taken is to start with the basics in each chapter and 'work up'. We have deliberately kept the number of data plots and histograms on display to a useful minimum to allow the text to flow, and inserted carefully chosen real-life cases in each chapter where relevant. High quality morphological images captured especially for this book are used throughout to illustrate these cases. While there is a necessary emphasis on haematological malignancy, flow cytometry of normal populations is not neglected and somewhat uniquely we emphasize the abnormalities that may be encountered as reactive phenomenon, as well as the challenges encountered across a variety of body fluids. That said, this textbook has a traditional structure in terms of the pathological entities described. This is for the simple reason that in most clinical situations, be it based on clinical features, blood indices or initial morphology the investigating clinician or pathologist will have some idea as to what type of disorder they are likely dealing with from the outset. We hope that the readers of this text will enjoy it as much as we enjoyed writing it.

Mike Leach
Mark Drummond
Allyson Doig
Glasgow

Acknowledgements

The authors wish to thank Linda Knotts, Chief Biomedical Scientist at Haematology Laboratories, Yorkhill Hospital, Glasgow for her contribution to Chapter 9, in particular the role of minimal residual disease assessment in acute lymphoblastic leukaemia.

CHAPTER 1

Introduction

The field of Clinical Haematology is a rapidly evolving specialty. The clinical entities encountered in everyday practice have basically not changed, but our understanding of them and the biological and molecular processes that drive them are undoubtedly much better understood. Our classification of these diseases has been continually refined over the decades, with the WHO classification of tumours of haematopoietic and lymphoid tissues now being firmly established as our current working reference manual [1]. The introduction of the WHO classification of haematological malignancy provides a structure for the development of integrated haematopathology laboratories, with its emphasis on definition of disease entities based on clinical, morphological, phenotypical and molecular features.

The real fascination of diagnostic clinical haematology lies in the diversity of the entities that we encounter. The whole spectrum of abnormal haematological parameters triggered by a variety of reactive and neoplastic processes are studied in the diagnostic laboratory. Flow cytometers are no longer a technical novelty confined to a few highly specialized diagnostic institutions. The flow cytometer methodology is well known, cytometers are readily available and whilst its applications are constantly diversifying its contribution to routine diagnosis is widely appreciated. This technology provides objective, rapid, sensitive and accurate measurement of a broad range of cell characteristics.

Accurate diagnosis is clearly of utmost importance in making decisions on patient management. The cognitive pathways to explain the processes of achieving a diagnosis, have in our opinion, however, been somewhat neglected in the haematological literature. There are many excellent texts which describe the clinical, haematological, immunophenotypic, cytogenetic and molecular char-

acteristics of a wide variety of neoplastic disorders. These texts are ideal reference manuals to study once a diagnosis has been achieved. The missing element, however, is a systematic approach to immunophenotypic diagnosis, taking into account all available clinical and laboratory data. In laboratory diagnostics, we are often left with the chore of finding the missing piece to the jigsaw puzzle. This should not be through a process of aimless searching but should be achieved through a logical carefully considered approach. What this publication aims to achieve is to generate a readable text to clearly explain the principles by which these diagnoses can be achieved, how immunophenotypic data can be analysed in clinical context and how meaningful conclusions can be drawn. We focus on clinical flow cytometry analysis of normal and malignant cells, not just in blood and bone marrow, but also cells in extramedullary sites such as effusions and cerebrospinal fluid. Each of these specimens needs to be handled, analysed and interpreted in a specific way. Of utmost importance is the assessment of features of the clinical history, physical examination, biochemical, immunological and radiological findings of a clinical case in relation to the current haematological parameters. We make no apology for this, as we believe this is of ultimate importance and this principle will be encountered repeatedly throughout this text. This approach, as recommended by the National Institute of Clinical Excellence [2], suggests that the diagnosis of leukaemia and lymphoma should take place in a specialist laboratory and in most cases this should be organized on a regional basis with full access to, and interaction with, diagnostic histopathology, cytogenetic and molecular laboratories with expertise in this field.

Flow cytometry analysis, used to determine the nature, origin and behaviour of cells if carefully directed can be a magnificent diagnostic tool and is exquisite in

Practical Flow Cytometry in Haematology Diagnosis, First Edition. Mike Leach, Mark Drummond and Allyson Doig.
© 2013 John Wiley & Sons, Ltd. Published 2013 by John Wiley & Sons, Ltd.

categorizing cell populations present at low levels through the analysis of cell size, complexity and granularity in relation to the expression of surface, cytoplasmic and nuclear antigens. Many thousands of cells can be so categorized over a short timeframe. It cannot, however, be applied in isolation and flow cytometry, if poorly directed, can lead to erroneous conclusions. For example, identification of the diseased cell population is usually easy in a bone marrow aspirate in a patient presenting with pancytopenia due to acute leukaemia. The disease cells may not be apparent in peripheral blood but are abundant in bone marrow and are identified and categorized using a carefully chosen myeloid panel. In contrast, the disease cells in hairy cell leukaemia may form a minority population in peripheral blood in a second patient with pancytopenia. The bone marrow aspirate is often dry and uninformative. Immunophenotyping using a mature lymphoid panel will provide a diagnosis. Unless the material is carefully scrutinized and the clinical presentation taken into account, then immunophenotyping can be misdirected and the wrong conclusions might be drawn.

We aim to explain from those most basic steps, how to approach clinical flow cytometry analysis of a variety of clinical specimens, to highlight the strengths and pitfalls, and how to safely embark on this fascinating diagnostic process in a variety of clinical circumstances. We aim to cover reactive phenomena, which in our opinion have not been well covered in the world literature. We aim to illustrate to the student that there is clear logic to explain the immunophenotype of any clonal condition and that they should understand this basis and not attempt to remember an immunophenotype as a random set of CD numbers. This latter approach is bound to fail. The former approach will establish a firm understanding and foundation on which to build and will assist in suggesting additional immunophenotypic studies or ancillary investigations in situations where the diagnosis

is not immediately apparent. In addition to the diagnosis of leukaemia and lymphoma we look at flow cytometric applications to response assessment and quantification of minimal residual disease. Finally, we also look at FCM analysis with respect to the diagnosis of red cell, granulocyte and platelet disorders.

This text is written for trainee and practising haematologists, haematopathologists and biomedical scientists with a specific interest. It should assist in preparation for FRCPath UK in Haematology and is intended as a working manual for diagnostic laboratories throughout the world. The chapters are illustrated with morphology images, scatter plots, cytogenetic and molecular data from real clinical cases – often a carefully chosen image will illustrate a principle much more succinctly than a thousand written words.

The authors have done their utmost to ensure the accuracy of data presented in this text. In fact, one of the driving forces in undertaking this exercise was to provide a practical handbook that would assist in the safe and accurate use of flow cytometry as a diagnostic tool. The content is extensively researched and referenced but also relates to personal experience of the authors who interpret flow cytometry on a daily basis in a regional reference centre. We sincerely hope that our readers will find it of interest and of practical value when applied to haematology diagnosis. We cannot, however, accept any responsibility for any error or misinterpretation which might, in any way, arise from its use.

References

1 Swerdlow S. *WHO Classification of Tumours of Haematopoietic and Lymphoid Tissues: International Agency for Research on Cancer.* 2008. World Health Organization, Geneva.

2 Jack A. Organisation of neoplastic haematopathology services: a UK perspective. *Pathology* 2005, **37**(6): 479–92.

2

CHAPTER 2
Principles of Flow Cytometry

Introduction

Over the years, flow cytometry technology, with its multiple applications, has had a significant impact on our understanding of cell biology, immunology and haemopoietic ontogeny, allowing its application to the diagnostic challenges of clinical medicine.

The basic principle of flow cytometry is inherent in the ability to analyse multiple characteristics of a single cell within a heterogenous population, in a short period of time [1, 2]. The term heterogenous is very important. In many clinical scenarios it might be far from clear whether a cellular proliferation is reactive or, indeed, neoplastic. Furthermore, these populations do not exist in isolation but within a milieu of other cell types. The diversity of diseases afflicting the cells of the body compartments is vast. Clinico-pathological correlation is at the very core of accurate diagnosis. Ignore the characteristics of either, at your peril.

Modern flow cytometers have the capability to analyse several thousands of cells per second. Cells in suspension pass through a beam of light (usually a laser beam) in single file; signals generated are related to the size of the cell and the internal complexity or granularity of the cell, enabling the cytometer to identify different cell populations depending on these characteristics. There are a wide range of applications for flow cytometry in a number of different disciplines. However, in haematology it has become an important tool in the identification of haematological disorders from a wide range of diagnostic samples, such as peripheral blood, bone marrow, CSF, pleural effusion, ascitic fluid and lymph node aspirates [1]. For the analysis of solid tissue a cell suspension must first be made.

There are many books and articles available outlining the principles of flow cytometry in great detail [1–7]. This chapter is written with the view of giving a simplified overview of flow cytometry, the gating strategies and data analysis applied in diagnostic flow cytometry applied to haematological disorders. It is aimed at laboratory staff and junior medical staff, and even more senior staff who have not had the privilege to experience clinical flow cytometry in all its diagnostic applications.

Sample preparation

At the outset we begin with a sample, usually of blood or bone marrow. We need to interrogate the cells in the sample as to their nature by determining their surface, cytoplasmic or nuclear immunophenotypic characteristics. As an example (clearly sample management will vary from one institution to another) the following is a simplified version of a sample preparation for flow analysis in our institution.

Direct staining method for surface immunophenotyping of peripheral blood or bone marrow (lyse – no wash method)

1 If sample white cell count is normal, sample may be used undiluted. If white cell count is raised, dilute sample in phosphate-buffered saline (PBS) to within normal value. (For example, if WBC twice normal then dilute 1:2.)
2 Label FACS tubes with sample ID and antibody combinations according to panel being run.
3 Add sample (100 μl) to required number of tubes.

Practical Flow Cytometry in Haematology Diagnosis, First Edition. Mike Leach, Mark Drummond and Allyson Doig.
© 2013 John Wiley & Sons, Ltd. Published 2013 by John Wiley & Sons, Ltd.

4 Add antibody conjugates to sample in volumes as recommended by manufacturer and mix.

5 Incubate at room temperature for 20–30 min in the dark.

6 Add appropriate volume of ammonium chloride RBC lysing solution and vortex.

7 Allow to lyse for 10 min.

8 Analyse on flow cytometer.

Surface immunoglobulin staining

1 Adjust sample white cell count to within normal limits if it is raised.

2 Add 100 µl sample to FACS tube.

3 Wash ×3 in warm (37 °C) PBS to remove excess proteins from the sample.

4 Continue with surface staining as previously described.

Intracellular Staining

1 Carry out surface staining as described in steps 1–5 above, if required.

2 Wash ×1 in warm (37 °C) PBS.

3 Using Fix and Perm* Cell permeabilization reagents add 100 µl Reagent A (fixing reagent) and incubate for 15 min.

4 Wash ×1 in warm (37 °C) PBS, centrifuge for 5 min at 300–500 g.

5 Add 100 µl Reagent B (permeabilizing reagent) and appropriate volume of antibody conjugate.

6 Incubate 20–30 min in the dark

7 Add appropriate volume of ammonium chloride RBC lysing solution and vortex.

8 Allow to lyse for 10 min.

9 Analyse on flow cytometer.

PBS; phosphate buffered saline, RBC; red blood cell solution.

The flow cytometer

There are three main components to the flow cytometer [8]:

1 The Fluidics System

Presentation of the sample to the laser.

2 The Optical System

Gathering information from the scattered light of the analysis.

3 The Computer/Electronic System

Conversion of optical to digital signals for display.

The fluidic system

The aim of the fluidics system is to present cells (or particles) in suspension to the laser interrogation point (the point at which cells pass through the laser light beam) one cell at a time. This is achieved by a process known as 'hydrodynamic focusing' (Figure 2.1). In the flow cell (flow chamber) the sample stream is injected into a faster moving stream of sheath fluid (usually phosphate buffered saline). Differences in the pressure, velocity and density of

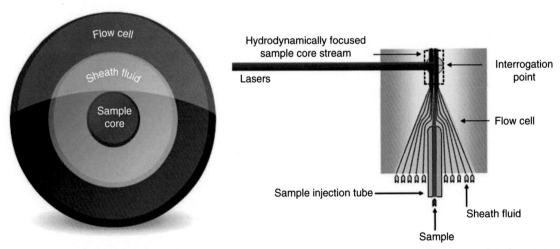

Figure 2.1 Hydrodynamic focusing and interrogation point. The sample core is a narrow coaxial stream (stream within a stream) surrounded by a wider stream of sheath fluid. The shape of the flow cell helps minimize turbulence while ensuring the sample core is focused in the centre of the stream for presentation to the laser. Courtesy of Becton Dickinson.

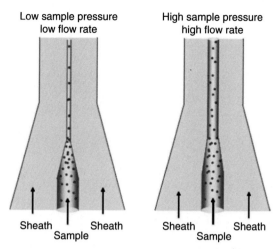

Figure 2.2 Flow rate and sample pressure. Low flow rate=low sample pressure=narrow sample stream=cells pass beam in single file. High flow rate=high sample pressure=wider sample stream=more than one cell passes through the beam at a time. Courtesy of Becton Dickinson.

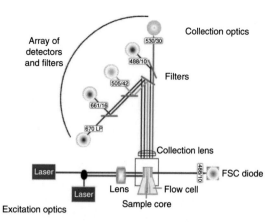

Figure 2.3 Example of the optical bench in the FACSCalibur flow cytometer. Courtesy of Becton Dickinson.

the two fluids prevent them from mixing. The flow cell is designed so that at the laser interrogation point the two streams are under pressure, focusing the sample stream in the centre of the sheath fluid, forcing the cells into single file before passing through the laser beam [3, 5, 6, 8].

Sample pressure is always greater than the sheath pressure. Altering the rate at which the cell suspension is injected into the centre of the sheath fluid will have a direct effect on the width of the sample stream and the number of cells passing through the interrogation point. The higher the sample pressure the wider the coaxial stream, resulting in more cells passing the interrogation point in a less than optimal position. By lowering the sample pressure this narrows the coaxial stream, resulting in cells passing the interrogation point in single file (Figure 2.2).

It is important that the correct flow rate is applied for the application being used. For immunophenotyping, measurements can be acquired quickly and therefore a high flow rate can be applied. DNA analysis, for example, requires a much higher resolution so a narrow sample core is necessary to ensure single cells pass through the laser beam at any given time; here a low flow rate should be applied.

The optical system

The optical system of the flow cytometer comprises excitation optics and collection optics. The excitation optics are made up of the laser with focusing lenses and prisms, whilst the collection optics lenses, mirrors and filters all gather and direct the scattered light to specific optical detectors (Figure 2.3). The intercept point of laser light and cells must be constant so the laser is held in a fixed position.

Light scatter

As a cell passes through the interrogation point, light from the laser beam is scattered in forward and 90° angles. The amount of light scattered is dependent on the physical properties of the cell, such as, cell size, nuclear complexity and cytoplasmic granularity. These light scattering signals are gathered by specific detectors, converted to digital signals and finally displayed as dot plots for analysis.

Light diffracted at narrow angles to the laser beam is called forward scattered light (FSC) or forward angle light scatter (FALS). The amount of FSC is proportional to the surface area or size of the cell. The forward scattered light is collected by a detector placed in line with the laser beam on the opposite side of the sample stream. Some light will pass through the cell membrane and is refracted and reflected by cytoplasmic organelles or nucleus of the cell. This light is collected by a photodiode positioned at approximately 90° to the laser beam and is known as side scattered light (SSC). Side scattered light is proportional to the granularity or internal complexity of the cell (Figure 2.4).

Together, FSC and SSC signals provide information on the physical properties of the cells allowing differentiation of cells within a heterogeneous population, for example the differentiation of white blood cells (Figure 2.5).

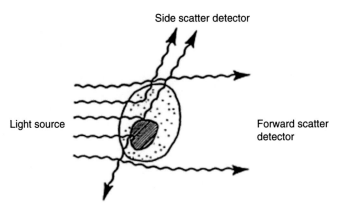

Figure 2.4 Simple illustration of forward and side light scatter properties of a cell. Courtesy of Becton Dickinson.

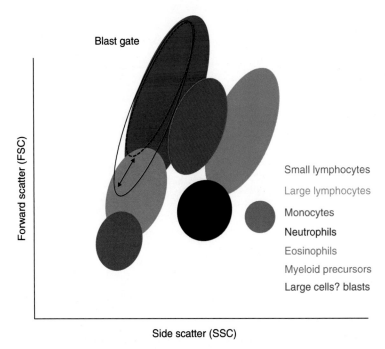

Figure 2.5 Schematic diagram of differentiation of peripheral blood leucocytes according to forward and side scatter characteristics.

Fluorescence

The forward and side scatter light signals are emitted at a 488 nm wavelength and are of the same colour as the laser light [3]. These signals can therefore be determined without the need for a dedicated fluorescent probe.

To determine the specific biochemical properties of a cell, dyes that can bind directly to the cell or fluorochromes that are bound to ligands, for example monoclonal antibodies, are used. The dyes or fluorochromes are excited by light of a wavelength that is characteristic for that molecule. It will absorb the light, gaining energy, resulting in the excitation of electrons within the molecule; on returning to its unexcited state this excess energy is released as photons of light resulting in fluorescence.

The wavelength range at which a fluorochrome absorbs light and becomes excited is known as its excitation (or absorption) wavelength. The wavelength range of the emitted light is termed its emission wavelength. The emitted wavelength range will be longer than that of the absorption wavelength range; this difference is referred to as Stoke's Shift [5] (Figure 2.6). As laser light is of a fixed wavelength, it is essential that the fluorochromes or dyes to be used have excitation wavelengths compatible with the flow cytometer (Table 2.1).

If a fluorochrome or dye can be excited sufficiently by light of a specific wavelength and their emission wavelengths are sufficiently different from one another, more than one fluorescent compound may be used at one time. However, if the flow cytometer uses only a single laser then the absorption spectrum of each fluorochrome would have to be similar.

In the flow cytometer the fluorescent signals are collected by photomultiplier tubes. To optimize these signals, optical filters specific to a wavelength range are placed in front of the photomultiplier, allowing only a narrow range of wavelength to reach the detector. These are as follows: bandpass (BP) filters which transmit light within a specified wavelength range (Figure 2.7)

Figure 2.6 Stoke's shift. Courtesy of Becton Dickinson.

Table 2.1 Maximum excitation and emission wavelengths for some of the common fluorochromes used in flow cytometry.

Fluorochrome	Abbreviation	Excitation max (nm)	Emisson max (nm)
Cascade blue		380, 401	419
Cascade yellow		399	549
Pacific blue		410	455
Alexa 488*		495	519
Fluorescein isothiocyanate*	FITC	494	519
Phycoerythrin*	PE	496, 546	578
Texas red*	ECD	595	615
PE-cyanine 5*	PC5/PE-Cy5	496, 546	667
PE-cyanine 5.5*	PC5.5/PE-Cy5.5	495, 564	696
PE-cyanine 7*	PC7/PE-Cy7	495, 564	767
Peridinin-chlorophyll*	PerCP	482	678
PerCP-cyanine 5.5	PerCP-Cy5.5	482	678
Allophycocyanin*	APC	650	660
APC-cyanine 7	APC-Cy7	650	785

(*most commonly used).

(a)

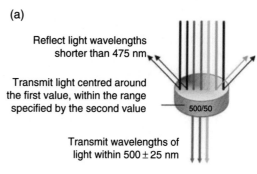

Reflect light wavelengths shorter than 475 nm

Transmit light centred around the first value, within the range specified by the second value

500/50

Transmit wavelengths of light within 500 ± 25 nm

(b)

Reflect light wavelengths shorter than 475 nm

Transmit light that is equal to or shorter than the specified wavelength

500 SP

(c)

Reflect light wavelengths that are not transmitted

Transmit light that is equal to or longer than the specified wavelength

500 LP

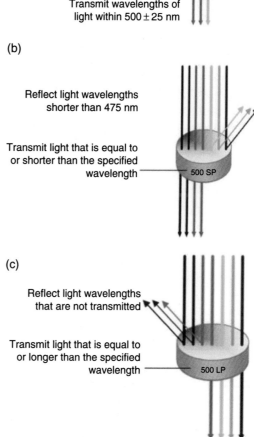

Figure 2.7 Bandpass filters allowing only specific wavelengths of fluorescence to pass through. Courtesy of Becton Dickinson.

(a); shortpass (SP) filters (b) which transmit light with wavelengths equal to or shorter than specified; longpass (LP) filters (c) which transmit light with wavelengths equal to or longer than specified.

Fluorescence intensity

The brightness or fluorescence intensity of any captured event for a particular fluorochrome is recorded by the cytometer for that channel. When many events have been captured it is possible to derive a mean fluorescence value; this is known as the mean fluorescence intensity (MFI) and is a very important characteristic that should be assessed in routine diagnostic practice (Figure 2.8a). It relates to not only the presence of the relevant antigen, but also the strength of expression or integrity of that antigen in a given cell population. It can carry great significance when used in the differentiation of neoplastic from reactive and normal cell populations. Fluorescence intensity can also be used to identify dual populations and allow subsequent directed gating strategies (Figure 2.8b). Some cell populations can show a spectrum of expression of a given antigen, for example CD13 expression in acute myeloid leukaemia, so care has to be used when using MFI data without paying attention to the plot (Figure 2.8c). These patterns of expression can be important in diagnosis.

It is clearly important to maintain consistency in fluorescence intensity data, both on a single cytometer over time and between different cytometers in the same laboratory. The means of achieving this are explained in the calibration section below.

Spectral overlap

Although a detector is designed to collect fluorescence from a specific wavelength, the emission spectra for a given fluorochrome can cover a range of wavelengths, allowing fluorescence spill over to a detector designed for a different fluorochrome. This is referred to as spectral overlap (Figure 2.9). For accurate analysis of data, the spectral overlap between fluorochromes must be corrected. This correction is done by compensation (Figure 2.10). In simple terms, compensation is carried out by correcting for inappropriate signals generated by the fluorochrome responsible for the overlap. With the use of compensation controls, this can be corrected manually and visually set, so minimizing interference from this phenomenon. However, when using multiple

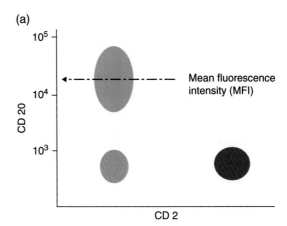

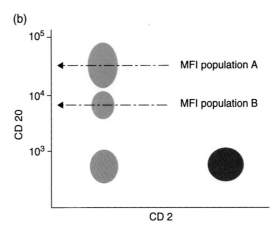

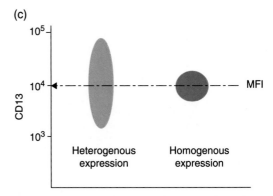

Figure 2.8 (a) Deriving a CD20+ MFI value for a B-cell population in blood. (b) Differences in CD20 MFI values for two different B-cell populations in blood can assist in diagnosis. (c) In addition to MFI, the spectrum of fluorescence intensity for a given antigen is important. Here, although the MFI is the same for the two myeloid populations, the variation in intensity (heterogenous versus homogenous expression) is different and is valuable in diagnosis.

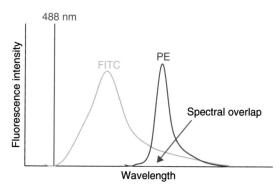

Figure 2.9 Spectral overlap – the emission wavelengths of FITC and PE overlap. In order to ensure accuracy, compensation has to be applied to subtract the overlapping signals. The high wavelength emissions from FITC will be captured by the PE detector and vice versa. If compensation is not applied then inappropriate dual positive events (Q2) will be captured. Courtesy of Becton Dickinson.

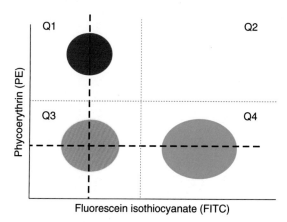

Figure 2.10 Compensation for spectral overlap of fluorochromes. Schematic diagram: this illustrates that the mean fluorescence intensity (MFI) for each fluorochrome should be equivalent for both positive and negative events so compensating for spectral overlap.

fluorochromes in modern flow cytometers this process is much more difficult to carry out manually. Therefore, current four and six colour flow cytometers usually have a software programme to aid with this potentially complex compensation set up process (Figure 2.11).

The electronic system

The electronic system of the flow cytometer allows the light signals to be converted into numerical data for analysis. As light hits the photodetectors, the incoming photons are converted to electrons, resulting in a current [3, 7, 8]. This current passes through an amplifier and a voltage pulse is generated that is proportional to the number of photons detected. The voltage pulse is created as soon as a cell or particle passes through the laser beam, with its highest point achieved when the cell or particle is in the centre of the beam (Figure 2.12).

Two types of photodetectors are used, termed photodiodes and photomultiplier tubes (PMTs). Photodiodes are less efficient with lower sensitivity than PMTs and generally used to collect the forward light scatter which produces a strong signal. Photomultiplier tubes are very efficient and used to collect the weaker side scatter and fluorescent signals. By applying a voltage to the photodetectors the electrical signals can be amplified. For the amplified signals to be displayed by the computer for analysis they require to be digitized. A numerical value is generated for the pulse height, width and area, and assigned a channel number by the analogue-to-digital convertor (ADC). The channel number is then transferred to the computer and displayed as a point on an analysis plot. The signals can be applied linearly or logarithmically for analysis (Figure 2.13).

Threshold

Whenever a particle or cell passes through the laser beam a voltage pulse is generated. To prevent interference from background noise or debris, a threshold can be set. By setting a threshold signal value, processing only occurs when a voltage pulse signal is above this limit. Signals below threshold are not processed (Figure 2.14). It is important to set the threshold limit so that the highest numbers of cells of interest are detected: if the threshold limit is set too low or too high there is the risk that cells of interest are missed [9].

Data display

Once signals have been assigned channel numbers the computer processes and stores these values. Once stored the data is saved in a standard format developed by the Society for Analytical Cytology [10]. These files of raw data are generally referred to as 'listmode files'. The stored data files can then be displayed in a number of ways depending on the analysis software application and reanalysed over and over again. The most common data displays for analysis in immunophenotyping are described below.

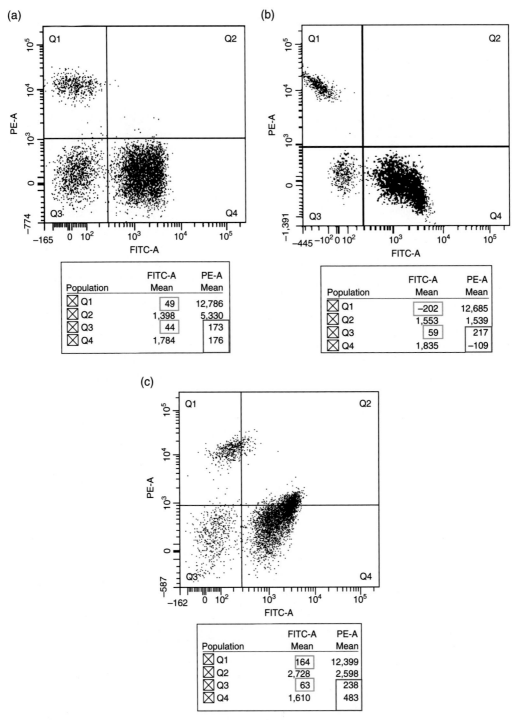

Figure 2.11 Compensation for spectral overlap of fluorochromes: illustrating a worked example.

(a) Correct compensation
Accurate compensation allows for spectral overlap and generates discrete cell populations with equivalent MFI for both FITC (green values) and PE (red values) channels.

(b) Over compensation
This encourages populations to be pulled down the axis for the relevant fluorochrome – too much subtraction collapses/skews the events downward and the MFI values are different. If this is not corrected dual positive population may be missed.

(c) Under compensation
This encourages populations to be pulled up the axis for the opposing fluorochrome – too little subtraction collapses/skews the events upward and the MFI values are different. This may lead to false dual positivity being reported.

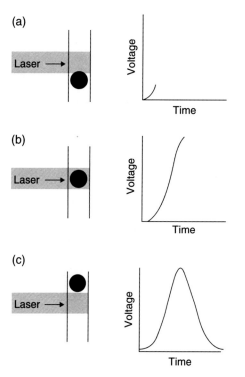

Figure 2.12 (a) The cell enters the laser beam and the voltage pulse is created. (b) The pulse reaches its peak as the cell is in the centre of the beam. (c) The pulse returns to baseline as the cell has left the beam.

Histogram

The histogram represents a single dimension and is used for displaying a single parameter. The Y axis shows the number of events counted and the X axis shows the fluorescence intensity in Figure 2.15(a).

Dot plot

The dot plot is used to display two parameters where each dot represents a cell/particle. The stronger the signal the further along each scale the data is displayed. The forward versus side scatter plot is a frequently used dot plot for peripheral blood analysis and subsequent gating as in Figure 2.15(b). Forward scatter correlates with cell size and nuclear/cytoplasmic complexity, whereas side scatter correlates with cytoplasmic granularity as noted in Figure 2.5.

Other plots for displaying data are density and contour plots but these are less commonly used. Both display two parameters but provide a third dimension and are able to quantify and give a visual representation of multiple events occurring in the same zone of the plot. The contour plot joins x and y coordinates with similar event counts and looks similar to a topographical map. Density and contour plots are not generally used for routine analysis but mainly used for displaying data in publications (Figure 2.15(c)).

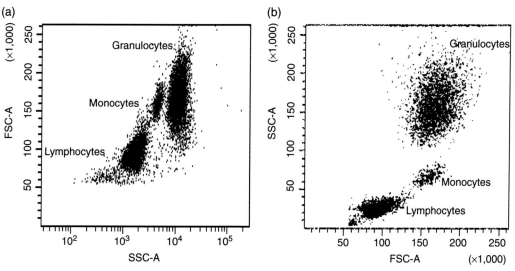

Figure 2.13 Leucocyte differentiation from FSC and SSC signals. (a) Dot plot using logarithmic scale. (b) Display using linear scale. Courtesy of Becton Dickinson.

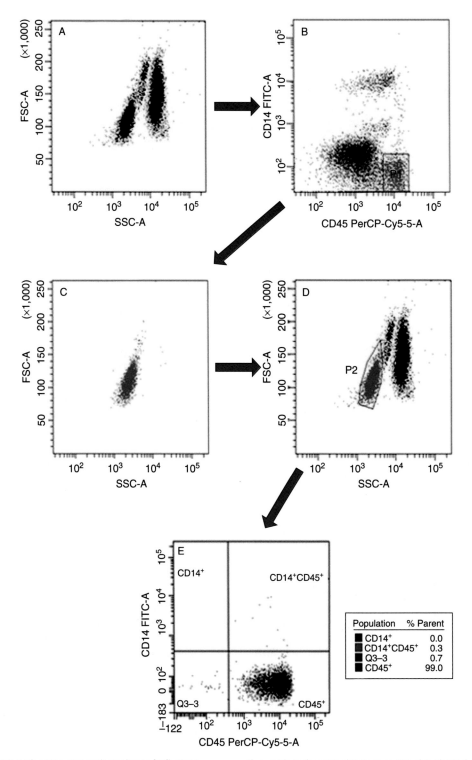

Figure 2.17 Back gating strategy (according to [11]). Plot A shows useful but incomplete separation of peripheral blood leucocytes on the FSC versus SSC plot. Plot B shows the clear identification of lymphocytes in population P1 (CD45bright CD14-). Plot C shows back gating of the P1 lymphocytes indicating where they reside in the original FSC versus SSC plot. Plot D shows subsequent gating on these lymphocytes in population P2. Plot E shows subsequent CD45 and CD14 analysis showing a virtually pure lymphocyte population with minimal monocyte (0.3%) contamination.

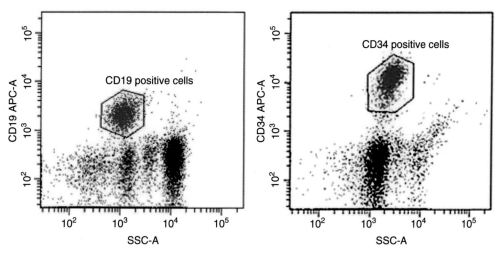

Figure 2.18 Illustration of gating strategy using fluorescence versus SSC to isolate the cells of interest. B lymphocytes are identified using CD19 (left) whilst CD34 (right) is used to identify blasts.

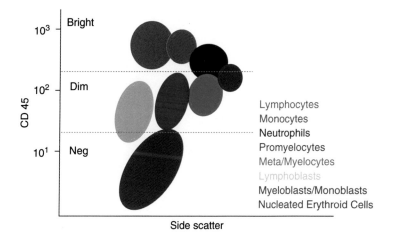

Figure 2.19 CD45 plot leucocyte lineage and maturation.

CD4$^+$ helper T-cell numbers from the total T-lymphocyte population [13, 14] (Figure 2.20).

Instrument set-up and quality control

To ensure the accuracy and precision of the data generated, particularly in the clinical laboratory, the performance of the flow cytometer must be rigorously monitored and controlled. Although most instrument calibration is carried out during installation, it is good laboratory practice for the flow lab to establish a robust internal quality control (IQC) programme. This will ensure that the flow cytometer performs to its expected standard. This can be done through the use of commercial standards and control materials. The term 'standard' usually refers to a suspension of microbeads/particles which do not require further preparation and are generally used to set up or calibrate the instrument. Control material is different in that they are usually analytes, for example fixed whole blood cells that have pre-determined values and require preparation in a similar way to patient samples [15].

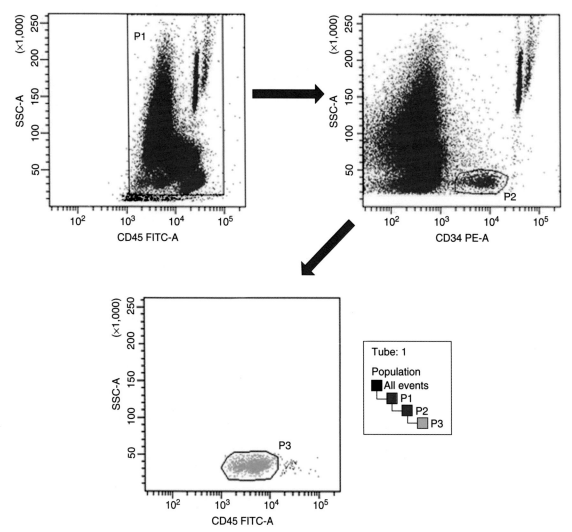

Figure 2.20 Simplified example of sequential gating used in the ISHAGE protocol for absolute CD34 enumeration. A plot displaying SSC versus CD45 FITC fluorescence has a gate P1 drawn around all positive cells excluding noise/debris. Everything within P1 is displayed on a second plot, SSC versus anti-CD34 PE. A gate is drawn around the positive cells in gate P2 which in turn are displayed on another SSC versus CD45 FITC and a gate drawn around the discrete group of cells with moderate FITC fluorescence intensity and low SSC properties, gate P3. By following the population hierarchy the gating sequence can be understood. The cells within the P3 gate are also found in P1 and P2 regions. This sequential gating process effectively purifies the CD34+ population and excludes rogue cells. Gates can be set during acquisition (real time) or post acquisition. Either way since the computer saves the files (listmode data), repeated analysis can be carried out with different gating strategies being applied an infinite number of times without affecting the original file.

The microbead standards can be classified into four categories [15]:

Type 0 (certified blank): these beads are approximately the same size as a lymphocyte, with no added fluorescent dye. They have a fluorescence signal lower than the autofluorescence of unstained peripheral blood lymphocytes, helping to set the threshold level so that there is no interference from noise in the immunophenotyping assay. *Type I (alignment beads)*: these are designed for optical alignment of the flow cytometer. They are subclassified according to size into type Ia (smaller than a lymphocyte)

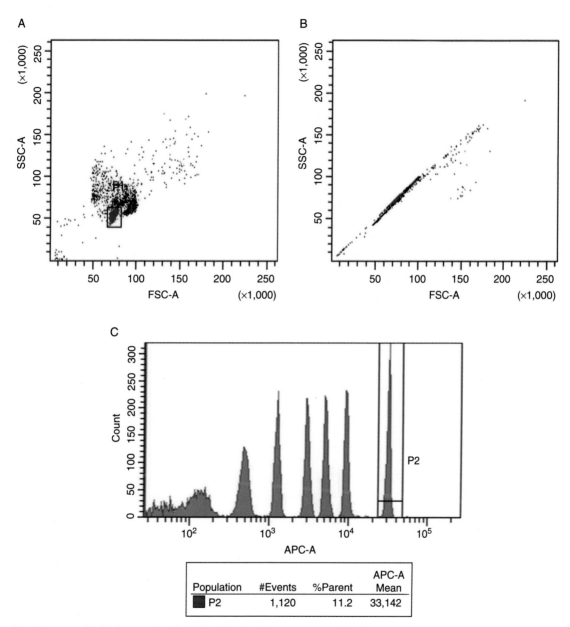

Figure 2.21 Example of daily IQC using eight peak rainbow beads for instrument stability. Plot A: This shows gating on P1 around singlet beads to exclude doublets. Plot B: This indicates that FSC – height versus FSC – area are proportional. Plot C: The brightest peak is gated (P2) and the MFI is displayed. There should be minimal change in MFI between each analysis.

and type Ib (equivalent size to a lymphocyte). Since the optical system of most flow cytometers is fixed it is preferable that the optical alignment is carried out by trained engineers. The use of alignment beads by the user is mainly in the setting up of cell sorters.

Type II (reference beads): these have bright fluorescence intensity and are subclassified into type IIa, IIb and IIc according to their excitation and emission spectra and whether they have antibody binding capacity. Type IIa and IIb beads are labelled with broad spectra or specific fluorochromes respectively. Type IIc beads are unlabelled, allowing binding with the same antibody conjugate used to label the cells.

Type III (calibration beads): these beads are equivalent in size to lymphocytes but have varying fluorescence intensity, ranging from dim to bright. They share the same properties as type IIa, IIb and IIc beads. These beads are used in quantitative flow cytometry where a calibration curve is required to determine the antibody binding capacity of the cell. This analysis provides a measure of the amount of cell surface antigen present on an individual cell [15, 16] and is not normally required for routine diagnostic purposes.

Type IIc and IIIc can be labelled with specific antibody conjugates. As this is the principle applied in immunophenotyping, they are useful for setting spectral overlap or compensation values. However, compensation should be validated using biological samples stained with the specific antibody conjugate of interest.

To ensure unified set up, it is recommended that a window of analysis be determined. This can be achieved using type IIb reference standards and placing beads in specified target channels. Daily monitoring of type IIb reference beads reliably monitors reproducibility of the flow cytometer. If the laboratory has more than one flow cytometer it is important to ensure that all instruments are standardized in the same manner [16].

The IQC protocol for the laboratory should be performed on a daily basis. It is essential that the data generated by the reference beads is recorded and reviewed frequently to verify instrument performance (Figure 2.21).

Values should be plotted on a Levey–Jennings type plot; this provides a means of monitoring the instrument stability and sensitivity over a period of time (Figure 2.22). Most flow cytometers have sophisticated software that plot data from the reference beads automatically [17].

As well as instrument verification it is important that quality control checks are carried out on the reagents and that the laboratory standard operating procedures are assessed regularly. By using biological material both analyst and reagent performance can be assessed. There are a number of commercially available fixed whole blood preparations that have established reference ranges.

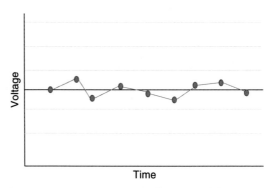

Figure 2.22 Levey–Jennings type plot shows minimal change in voltage over time, confirming stability of the flow cytometer.

These preparations are treated in the same manner as a sample. Another method of competency assessment is the laboratories' participation in an external quality assurance scheme, for example the UK National External Quality Assessment Service (NEQAS), for immunophenotyping or equivalent scheme throughout the world.

The UK NEQAS leucocyte immunophenotyping programme offers flow cytometry based EQA for:
- Immune monitoring
- CD34 stem cell enumeration
- Leukaemia immunophenotyping
- Leukaemia diagnostic interpretation
- Paroxysmal nocturnal haemoglobinuria
- Low level leucocyte enumeration.

These schemes are available to both UK and overseas based organizations. It is good laboratory practice to maintain a log of internal and external quality control with regular reviews to ensure the standards expected are being met.

Flow cytometric immunophenotyping has an important role in the diagnosis of serious haematological malignancies. It is therefore essential for the flow cytometry laboratory to have in place a good training programme with on-going competency assessment as well as regular instrument performance checks [18, 19].

Acknowledgements

We are grateful to Becton Dickinson for permission to reproduce images used in Figures 2.1, 2.2, 2.3, 2.4, 2.6, 2.7, 2.9, 2.13 and 2.14 of this chapter.

References

1 Brown M, Wittwer C. Flow cytometry: principles and clinical applications in hematology. *Clin Chem* 2000, **46**(8 Pt 2): 1221–9.

2 Robinson JP. Flow Cytometry. *Encyclopedia of Biomaterials and Biomedical Engineering*. 2004. pp. 630–40.

3 Givan AL. Principles of flow cytometry: an overview. *Methods Cell Biol* 2001, **63**:19–50.

4 Delude RL. Flow cytometry. *Critical Care Medicine* 2005, **33**(Suppl): S426–S8.

5 McCoy JP, Jr. Basic principles of flow cytometry. *Hematol Oncol Clin North Am* 2002, **16**(2): 229–43.

6 Nunez R. Flow cytometry: principles and instrumentation. *Curr Issues Mol Biol* 2001, **3**(2): 39–45.

7 Shapiro HM. *Practical Flow Cytometry*, 4th edn. 2003. Wiley-Liss, New York.

8 Becton Dickinson Biosciences. *Introduction to Flow Cytometry: A Learning Guide*. 2000. San Jose: Becton Dickinson Biosciences.

9 Wood JC. Principles of gating. *Curr Protoc Cytom* 2001, Chapter 1: Unit 18.

10 Data file standard for flow cytometry. Data File Standards Committee of the Society for Analytical Cytology. *Cytometry* 1990, **11**(3): 323–32.

11 Loken MR, Brosnan JM, Bach BA, Ault KA. Establishing optimal lymphocyte gates for immunophenotyping by flow cytometry. *Cytometry* 1990, **11**(4): 453–9.

12 Stelzer GT, Shults KE, Loken MR. CD45 gating for routine flow cytometric analysis of human bone marrow specimens. *Ann N Y Acad Sci* 1993, **677**: 265–80.

13 Keeney M, Chin-Yee I, Weir K, Popma J, Nayar R, Sutherland DR. Single platform flow cytometric absolute CD34+ cell counts based on the ISHAGE guidelines. International Society of Hematotherapy and Graft Engineering. *Cytometry* 1998, **34**(2): 61–70.

14 Mandy FF, Nicholson JK, McDougal JS. Guidelines for performing single-platform absolute CD4+ T-cell determinations with CD45 gating for persons infected with human immunodeficiency virus. Centers for disease control and prevention. *MMWR Recomm Rep.* 2003, **52**(RR-2): 1–13.

15 Schwartz A, Marti GE, Poon R, Gratama JW, Fernandez-Repollet E. Standardizing flow cytometry: a classification system of fluorescence standards used for flow cytometry. *Cytometry* 1998, **33**(2): 106–14.

16 Stelzer GT, Marti G, Hurley A, McCoy P, Jr., Lovett EJ, Schwartz A. US-Canadian Consensus recommendations on the immunophenotypic analysis of hematologic neoplasia by flow cytometry: standardization and validation of laboratory procedures. *Cytometry* 1997, **30**(5): 214–30.

17 Ormerod MG. *Flow Cytometry: A Practical Approach*, 3rd edn. Oxford University Press, Oxford.

18 Owens MA, Vall HG, Hurley AA, Wormsley SB. Validation and quality control of immunophenotyping in clinical flow cytometry. *J Immunol Methods* 2000, **243**(1–2): 33–50.

19 Greig B, Oldaker T, Warzynski M, Wood B. 2006 Bethesda International Consensus recommendations on the immunophenotypic analysis of hematolymphoid neoplasia by flow cytometry: recommendations for training and education to perform clinical flow cytometry. *Cytometry B Clin Cytom* 2007, **72**(Suppl 1): S23–33.

Limitations

Introduction

Flow cytometric analysis can be effectively applied to the interrogation of a multitude of cell populations from a variety of tissues. We almost take for granted, for example, the ability of flow to assign lineages in acute leukaemias and lymphoproliferative disorders, even when the most experienced morphologist is struggling to define a disorder according to the light microscopic characteristics of cell anatomy. We will see multiple useful applications throughout this text in neoplastic, but also importantly, in non-neoplastic disorders.

Flow cytometry has been described as 'A biomedical platform offering diagnostic diversity'[1]. This diversity of application can only be effectively made in the full knowledge of patient circumstances, however. The design of the referral form and the data supplied is therefore of utmost importance and should gather all relevant clinical information that might direct intelligent use of the flow cytometer. Furthermore, before this fascinating technology can be applied reliably and effectively, it is important to be aware of its limitations. This applies to any technology no matter how incisive its diagnostic capacity. In this chapter we aim to outline such limits and urge readers to consider these caveats at every opportunity.

Clinical context issues

As noted in the introduction, we cannot give adequate emphasis to the importance of some knowledge of the clinical context in which flow might be usefully applied. Most flow laboratories, in addition to serving busy on-site haemato-oncology units, act as reference laboratories and may not have access to important clinical and laboratory background data pertaining to patients from other hospitals. We often receive samples of blood or bone marrow with a request for 'flow cytometry please'. But which cell population might we analyse? Are we looking for blasts in peripheral blood in a pancytopenic patient or should PNH be considered as a possible diagnosis? Are those small compact cells without granules or features of differentiation exfoliating lymphoma cells or M0 type myeloblasts? Should we be gating for blasts using CD45^{dim} or CD34, for lymphocytes using CD2 versus CD19, plasma cells using CD38 and CD138, granulocytes using CD15 and SSC, or even mast cells using CD117? Many of these samples require morphological review and/or a discussion with the referring clinician if flow studies are to be applied cost-effectively and for maximal diagnostic reward. We should not forget that this is expensive technology and to run multiple panels as a process of exclusion is neither desirable nor economically sound.

Sampling issues

Blood

Peripheral blood samples are a perfect medium for flow cytometric analysis and the potential information so acquired will be illustrated in subsequent chapters. It is of utmost importance that samples are delivered fresh to the laboratory. Even with appropriate storage at 4 °C, samples do deteriorate, though much more slowly than if kept at room temperature. Natural cell death of leucocytes becomes particularly evident after 48 hours and appears to be influenced by the nature of anticoagulant used. Blood for FBC analysis, and subsequent flow, is commonly taken into ethylenediamenetetra acetic acid (EDTA) as modern automated analysers are comfortable with this

Practical Flow Cytometry in Haematology Diagnosis, First Edition. Mike Leach, Mark Drummond and Allyson Doig.
© 2013 John Wiley & Sons, Ltd. Published 2013 by John Wiley & Sons, Ltd.

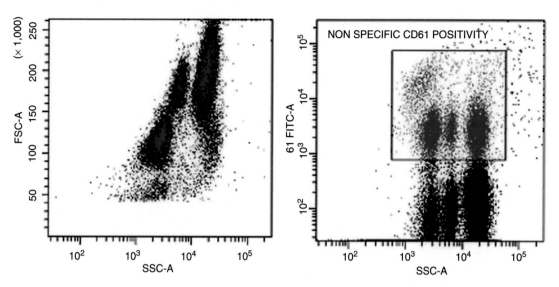

Figure 3.1 Activated platelets adhering to lymphocytes, monocytes and neutrophils (left to right on CD61/SSC plot), which in turn bind anti-CD61 causing apparent positive events. It is important to exclude non-specific platelet adsorption when considering any leucocyte population that might be expressing CD41 or CD61. Back gating confirms that all three lineages are adsorbing platelets (FSC/SSC plot).

anticoagulant. Granulocytes start to show apoptosis at six hours when incubated in EDTA, whilst heparin appears to delay this process significantly and is thus a preferred anticoagulant [2]. Dead and dying cells can lose antigens, change their light scatter properties (see below) and tend to adsorb antibody non-specifically. Paroxysmal nocturnal haemoglobinuria (PNH) screening, for example, is dependent on specimen age. CD16 expression on granulocytes in particular, is progressively lost in ageing pre-apoptotic cells [3]. For this reason old samples (>48 hours, or earlier if not stored at 4 °C) should not be analysed as the results can be misleading. Although sample storage at 4 °C protects from apoptosis, it is still advisable to allow samples to warm to room temperature before analysis, in order to optimize antibody binding.

Changes in cell morphology as a result of ageing and apoptosis also influence their behaviour in terms of FSC/SSC properties. Early apoptotic cells shrink and show reduced FSC/SSC, so moving them toward the lymphocyte zone, whilst late apoptosis causes cell swelling with increased FSC such that they encroach on the monocyte zone [4]. In fact, flow cytometry itself can be a useful tool in the identification of apoptosis by means of identifying cell surface phosphatidyl serine exposure through binding to annexin V (a natural ligand) linked to a fluorochrome.

This is a useful means of assessing cell viability [4], in transported specimens, for example, before definitive diagnostic studies are started.

Debris from dead cells, free nuclei and cytoplasmic stroma need to be identified and gated out as this material has a tendency for non-specific antibody adsorption. Activated platelets like to adhere to neutrophils and monocytes and it is important to be aware of this phenomenon (Figure 3.1). Thorough cell washing prior to analysis is likely to minimize platelet adherence.

Peripheral blood, however, often gives 'clean results' as the sampling difficulties pertaining to bone marrow (discussed below) do not apply. Furthermore there is little or no contamination with nucleated red cell precursors and the normal mature cell populations are very distinct. In pathological states the cells available for analysis in blood are determined by the behaviour of the disease. Endless searches for abnormal populations might be fruitless when the true disease population resides purely in the bone marrow.

Bone marrow aspirates

A good quality aspirate sample is critical to the diagnosis of bone marrow disorders, in particular, the acute leukaemias. The quality of a bone marrow aspirate is undoubtedly operator dependent to some extent, but more importantly the sample quality in terms of available particles and cellularity is clearly influenced by the underlying disease process itself. At the worst extreme the aspirate is dry so yielding no analysable material. We must be alert to disease processes which generate bone marrow fibrosis as this leads to hypoparticulate aspirates and hypocellular specimens. The samples so acquired may not be representative of the bone marrow disease process. Aspirates submitted for flow analysis, therefore, always need morphological review. In some leukaemic disease states with bone marrow fibrosis (such as acute megakaryoblastic leukaemia) the peripheral blood blast count may appear similar to that in the bone marrow due to haemodilution of non-representative acellular marrow aspirates. Furthermore, acute leukaemias should not be discounted on the basis of blood dilute aspirates showing blast populations of less than 20%. The classification and prognosis of the myelodysplastic syndromes, for example, relies on the accurate assessment of bone marrow blasts. Blood dilute aspirates can be misleading in this situation. A good quality bone marrow trephine, with appropriate immunocytochemistry studies, can be very informative in these scenarios and circumvents this problem. This point is also relevant to marrow aspirates submitted for remission status assessment following treatment for acute leukaemia. It is clear that a blood dilute aspirate cannot inform the true marrow remission status of the patient. We also tend to assume, wrongly, that similar hypocellular specimens sent for cytogenetic analysis show encouraging results when the original informative translocation or deletion is no longer evident. Similarly, marrow aspirates taken too early after remission induction for acute leukaemia, are often hypocellular, blood dilute and non-informative unless part of a well-controlled MRD assessment programme (see Chapter 9).

Paradoxically, a packed bone marrow with maximal involvement by acute leukaemia and without significant fibrosis, can also yield hypocellular aspirates. This phenomenon also needs to be considered in the context of flow diagnosis. The relatively few cells acquired, however, are invariably blast cells, a situation that is eminently well-characterized using flow studies.

Some eloquent studies have demonstrated quite clearly that the cellularity, blast proportions and quality of bone marrow aspirates are significantly affected by blood dilution and that this is a common phenomenon [5, 6].

Blood dilution is more evident when large volume aspirates are attempted or when multiple aliquots are taken from the same puncture. In other words, the volume of an aspirate is inversely proportional to its purity and so the best quality aspirate is likely to be acquired in a quick single draw of less than 3 mL. It is also possible to correct an aspirate blast count by accounting for peripheral blood dilution by comparing blood and aspirate populations of CD16[bright] neutrophils. Interestingly, in one study the most representative blast counts were achieved by running flow on disaggregated trephine specimens – these were always higher than the aspirates, which are inevitably affected by blood dilution [5]. It may be useful to develop departmental protocols for flow analysis of disaggregated trephines, particularly in patients with dry or very blood dilute aspirate specimens [7, 8].

A bone marrow aspirate may not be truly representative of bone marrow composition in other situations, particularly where the disease process generates reticulin deposition. Conditions such as Hodgkin and non-Hodgkin lymphoma, mast cell disorders and non-haemopoietic tumours all frequently generate reticulin fibrosis at the sites of disease. Aspiration preferentially removes the interstitial normal cells/particles and tends to leave the diseased cell foci *in situ*. The large B-cell lymphomas can be difficult to identify using flow; they generate marrow fibrosis, appear fragile on aspiration and show frequent apoptosis [9]. The authors have recently encountered a young patient with pancytopenia due to bone marrow involvement by diffuse large B-cell lymphoma. Repeated hypocellular aspirate specimens were submitted but we failed to clearly identify the disease population in any of them. The bone marrow trephine showed almost complete replacement by disease, and immunohistochemistry studies confirmed the diagnosis.

Also of note is that marrow samples are subject to varying degrees of erythrocyte precursor loss during the red cell lysis stage using ammonium chloride. Early red cell precursors sometimes survive this process, whilst later forms are often lost. Morphologically, bone marrow blasts are currently estimated as a percentage of nucleated cells; using flow the assessable cell population is different due to loss of erythroid progenitors, so this is another source of confusion when flow and morphological blast population estimates are compared. Finally, prompt transport of marrow aspirates is always necessary as cells do deteriorate and die. In some cases this cell death

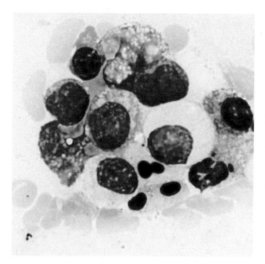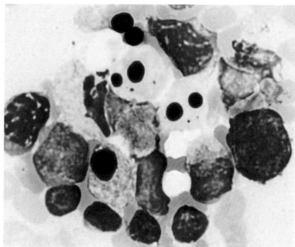

Figure 3.2 Note the prominent apoptosis of cells (likely blasts) within this old marrow specimen.

appears more prominent in the malignant blast population and as non-viable cells are often gated out this can be a further source of error in estimating blasts (Figure 3.2).

Effusions

Pleural, pericardial and peritoneal effusions can all be analysed by flow cytometry and can sometimes be the most easily accessed material for potentially identifying a malignant population [10]. These samples are often highly proteinaceous, with prominent debris from dead cells together with reactive lymphocytic and monocyte populations as well as exfoliating mesothelial cells. In some cases the abnormal cell population is very obvious, but in others it may be less so, with only small numbers of malignant cells present. Furthermore, malignant cells may adhere to serous linings rather than being released into the fluid space. Normal epithelial cells from menstrual shedding can be detected in peritoneal fluid in some situations, and such non-haemopoietic cells should not be misinterpreted as being malignant. In these situations the operator has to look past this 'noise' and be aware of these caveats when searching for a possible clonal population.

A good clinical example highlighting some of the above issues is T-lymphoblastic lymphoma. The cortical subtype in particular often presents with a mediastinal mass and pleural or pericardial effusions due to direct disease involvement. These fluid specimens are a useful diagnostic resource but are subject to early cell death with

the accumulation of cytoplasmic and nuclear debris. Figure 3.3 shows a stained cytospin of pericardial fluid from an eight-year-old female presenting as described above.

Cerebrospinal fluid

Cerebrospinal fluid (CSF) analysis can pose a number of potential pitfalls. Cell numbers in CSF, even in disease states, are relatively low compared to media like blood and bone marrow [11]. This means that large volumes of fluid may need to be processed in order to capture sufficient events to be confident that a disease population is present or absent [12]. In addition, there is no real consensus as to how many cells/events should analysed and particularly how many abnormal events in a cluster are significant. A reasonable postulate is that >25 events is positive, 10–25 events is suspicious and <10 events is negative [13]. In order to capture sufficient events large volumes of CSF (>10 mL) may be necessary [14], but these can be difficult to acquire without access to a reservoir and can generate post-procedure headache. Cerebrospinal fluid samples also need rapid processing in the absence of a fixing procedure as cells deteriorate rapidly; there may also be differential cell loss according to lineage [15]. Furthermore, a negative result does not exclude malignant meningitis and repeat sampling may be necessary in some cases with a high index of suspicion [14]. If the nature of the potential neoplasm is not known it is easy to use up the specimen before the potential disease

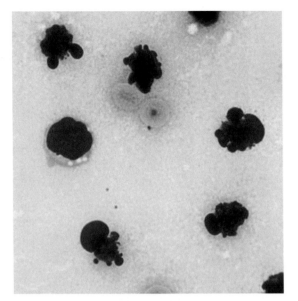
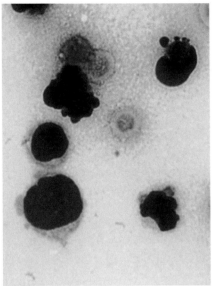

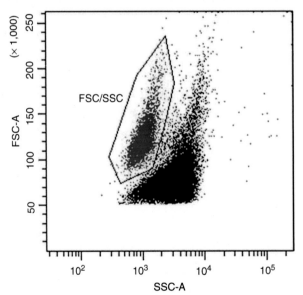

Figure 3.3 Note the background staining in this proteinaceous fluid and the cell debris generated from apoptosis and premature cell death of T-lymphoblastic lymphoma cells in pleural fluid. Flow cytometry generated an unequivocal diagnosis by gating on the red events in the scatter plot. It is important to exclude cell debris and free nuclei (black events) as this material can show non-specific antibody binding and, of course, may fail to bind antibodies directed at membrane antigens. Careful gating is necessary to generate 'clean' results which accurately profile the intact disease cells in such specimens.

population is clearly confirmed. The use of four or six colour flow utilizing multiple antibodies in a single tube is clearly of value in assessing small samples of low cellularity [16–18]. Cytospin preparations cause cell distortion and artefactual changes that may hamper morphologic guidance in this respect (Figure 3.4).

Finally, peripheral blood contamination of CSF due to traumatic taps can lead to potential confusion. The

Malignancy Diagnostic Service (HMDS) in Leeds. From the time a sample enters the laboratory it is tracked by a specialized software system, which generates a multi-disciplinary workflow based on initial morphological scrutiny of the sample. This means testing is appropriate and cost effective. Given the success of this approach it seems very likely that such services will eventually become standard practice.

Conclusion

Flow cytometric immunophenotyping is a remarkable diagnostic technique. This chapter is positioned early in this text to make our readers aware of possible caveats and pitfalls.

'Awareness of these pitfalls comes with experience: experience comes with the awareness of pitfalls.'

References

1 Mandy F, Gratama JW. Flow cytometry: a biomedical platform offering diagnostic diversity. *Cytometry B Clin Cytom* 2009, **76**(6): 365–6.

2 Elghetany MT, Davis BH. Impact of preanalytical variables on granulocytic surface antigen expression: a review. *Cytometry B Clin Cytom* 2005, **65**(1): 1–5.

3 Homburg CH, *et al.* Human neutrophils lose their surface Fc gamma RIII and acquire Annexin V binding sites during apoptosis in vitro. *Blood* 1995, **85**(2): 532–40.

4 Hodge GL, Flower R, Han P. Optimal storage conditions for preserving granulocyte viability as monitored by Annexin V binding in whole blood. *J Immunol Methods* 1999, **225**(1–2): 27–38.

5 Loken MR, *et al.* Normalization of bone marrow aspirates for hemodilution in flow cytometric analyses. *Cytometry B Clin Cytom*, 2008. **76B**(1): 27–36.

6 Brooimans RA, *et al.* Flow cytometric differential of leukocyte populations in normal bone marrow: Influence of peripheral blood contamination. *Cytometry B Clin Cytom* 2008, **76B**(1): 18–26.

7 Novotny JR, *et al.* Failed or inadequate bone marrow aspiration: a fast, simple and cost-effective method to produce a cell suspension from a core biopsy specimen. *Clin Lab Haematol* 2005, **27**(1): 33–40.

8 Vos JA, *et al.* Vortex disaggregation for flow cytometry allows direct histologic correlation: a novel approach for small biopsies and inaspirable bone marrows. *Cytometry B Clin Cytom* 2003, **52**(1): 20–31.

9 Bertram HC, Check IJ, Milano MA. Immunophenotyping large B-cell lymphomas. Flow cytometric pitfalls and pathologic correlation. *Am J Clin Pathol* 2001, **116**(2): 191–203.

10 Risberg B, *et al.* Flow cytometric immunophenotyping of serous effusions and peritoneal washings: comparison with immunocytochemistry and morphological findings. *J Clin Pathol* 2000 **53**(7): 513–7.

11 Subira D, *et al.* Flow cytometric analysis of cerebrospinal fluid samples and its usefulness in routine clinical practice. *Am J Clin Pathol* 2002, **117**(6): 952–8.

12 Kleine TO, Albrecht J, Zofel P. Flow cytometry of cerebrospinal fluid (CSF) lymphocytes: alterations of blood/CSF ratios of lymphocyte subsets in inflammation disorders of human central nervous system (CNS). *Clin Chem Lab Med* 1999, **37**(3): 231–41.

13 Kraan J, *et al.* Flow cytometric immunophenotyping of cerebrospinal fluid. *Curr Protoc Cytom*, 2008. Chapter 6: Unit 6, 25.

14 Glantz MJ, *et al.* Cerebrospinal fluid cytology in patients with cancer: minimizing false-negative results. *Cancer* 1998, **82**(4): 733–9.

15 Windhagen A, Maniak S, Heidenreich F. Analysis of cerebrospinal fluid cells by flow cytometry and immunocytochemistry in inflammatory central nervous system diseases: comparison of low- and high-density cell surface antigen expression. *Diagn Cytopathol* 1999 **21**(5): 313–8.

16 Bommer M, *et al.* Cerebrospinal fluid pleocytosis: pitfalls and benefits of combined analysis using cytomorphology and flow cytometry. *Cancer Cytopathol* 2011, **119**(1): 20–6.

17 Bromberg JEC, *et al.* CSF flow cytometry greatly improves diagnostic accuracy in CNS hematologic malignancies. *Neurology* 2007, **68**(20): 1674–9.

18 Chang A, *et al.* Lineage-specific identification of nonhematopoietic neoplasms by flow cytometry. *Am J Clin Pathol* 2003, **119**(5): 643–55.

19 te Loo DM, *et al.* Prognostic significance of blasts in the cerebrospinal fluid without pleiocytosis or a traumatic lumbar puncture in children with acute lymphoblastic leukemia: experience of the Dutch Childhood Oncology Group. *J Clin Oncol* 2006, **24**(15): 2332–6.

20 Greig B, *et al.* 2006 Bethesda International Consensus recommendations on the immunophenotypic analysis of hematolymphoid neoplasia by flow cytometry: recommendations for training and education to perform clinical flow cytometry. *Cytometry B Clin Cytom* 2007, **72**(1): S23–33.

21 Roederer M. Spectral compensation for flow cytometry: visualization artifacts, limitations, and caveats. *Cytometry* 2001, **45**(3): 194–205.

22 Hulspas R, *et al.* Considerations for the control of background fluorescence in clinical flow cytometry. *Cytometry B Clin Cytom* 2009, **76**(6): 355–64.

23 Perfetto SP, Roederer M. Increased immunofluorescence sensitivity using 532 nm laser excitation. *Cytometry A* 2007, **71**(2): 73–9.

24 Monici M. Cell and tissue autofluorescence research and diagnostic applications. *Biotechnol Annu Rev* 2005, **11**: 227–56.

CHAPTER 4
Normal Blood and Bone Marrow Populations

It is essential to have a sound understanding of the nature and immunophenotypic characteristics of the normal cell populations encountered in bone marrow and peripheral blood. It is also important to have some understanding of lymphoid cellular interactions in the normal lymph node and thymus. This process is necessary if we are to understand the origin of the myeloid and lymphoid neoplasms encountered in routine diagnostic immunophenotyping and helps us understand why certain neoplasms carry a particular repertoire of antigens. It not only helps in the diagnosis of neoplastic disorders but equally gives support to the recognition of reactive phenomena.

The populations of cells which inhabit the bone marrow are constantly changing throughout the life of a normal individual. When this environment is challenged by infection, drugs, intercurrent medical disease and, of course, primary haematological disease, the populations change or can respond and react in a variety of ways. We need to be aware of these reactions such that we do not over or under interpret the findings. This chapter is set out as a framework or foundation of normal myeloid and lymphoid ontogeny. Our understanding of this process is still incomplete but we can only safely recognize abnormal situations once we are fully familiar with the normal resting blood and bone marrow cellular environment.

Normal stem and precursor cell populations

Haematopoietic progenitor cells

Recognition of the immunophenotypic patterns of maturation in normal bone marrow facilitates the identification of acute leukaemia (AL) blast cells, even if they occur at low frequencies. The sequential expression of antigens during normal marrow cell maturation and differentiation from a common stem cell population is well described in the literature but needs to be fully understood.

Normal haematopoietic stem cells (HSC) are CD34$^+$ (conversely not all leukaemic blasts are CD34$^+$, a common source of confusion) [1]. In normal steady state marrow the total CD34$^+$ fraction comprises HSC (early progenitor cells; that is, uncommitted cells that can produce multiple lineages), myelomonocytic (also CD123$^+$), erythroid (CD71$^+$) and B-cell (CD19$^+$) precursor cells [2]. Other antigens expressed by uncommitted HSC include HLA-DR^{dim} and CD133, with the latter broadly correlating with CD34 expression. As the HSC population differentiates, they gain CD38 expression, a so-called 'activation marker' in conjunction with the early lineage commitment antigens detailed above.

By definition, true HSC lack lineage commitment antigens (i.e. markers of lymphoid or myeloid differentiation), a situation often abbreviated to lin$^-$. Furthermore, many primitive haematopoietic stem cells are quiescent (out of cell cycle), with absence of both activation markers and markers of cell division, such as Ki67. These cells comprise only a very small fraction of total marrow CD34$^+$ cells, however, as this antigen continues to be expressed into the early-committed myeloid and lymphoid progenitor compartments before it is lost during further maturation. Despite this caveat, CD34 is a very useful surrogate marker for the normal HSC compartment, and it is routinely used for assessment of stem cell harvests in the transplantation setting, for example, as well as in stem cell research. CD34$^+$lin$^+$ cells are therefore committed progenitors and represent the first

Practical Flow Cytometry in Haematology Diagnosis, First Edition. Mike Leach, Mark Drummond and Allyson Doig.
© 2013 John Wiley & Sons, Ltd. Published 2013 by John Wiley & Sons, Ltd.

identifiable stage through which cells mature sequentially down a particular differentiation pathway.

Normal precursor cell populations in the marrow may occasionally cause confusion in the diagnosis and monitoring of acute leukaemias. This is largely because they share many antigens of immaturity in common with leukaemic blast cells as well as morphological similarities. One of the most obvious differences is that AL blasts are usually much more numerous than normal precursors; for the most part, progenitor cells in normal steady-state marrow samples are present at low levels. CD34+ cells are generally no more than 1–2% of all marrow cells, while CD117+ cells, an antigen that is expressed beyond CD34 in myeloid progenitor cell populations, are generally no more than 2–4% [3–5]. Approximately 25% of CD34+ cells are CD117+ [6]. However, regenerating marrows often express proportionally higher levels of progenitor cell antigens than marrows in steady state, particularly in the case of normal B-cell precursors (haematogones) after chemotherapy or stem cell transplantation for example [7, 8]. In general, for practical purposes, the authors consider a CD34+ population of ≥3% or a CD117 population ≥5% as significant and worthy of full characterization, although this is dependent on the clinical scenario and assessing lower levels than this may be relevant in some circumstances (e.g. post induction therapy in AL or distinguishing MDS from aplastic anaemia in a hypoplastic marrow). Particularly at low levels of blast numbers, demonstration of an abnormal phenotype is of more significance than accurate quantification in most circumstances, particularly when the potential pitfalls in blast enumeration are taken into account (see below). One

further complication is that aberrant or asynchronous maturation can be observed in normal situations, for example expression of CD56 on granulocyte and monocyte precursor cells in regenerating marrows both with and without G-CSF administration. Furthermore, unusually synchronous maturation may be observed in this situation (e.g. accumulation of promyelocytes as the regenerating cells expand and pass through maturational stages together) requiring meticulous attention to flow, morphology, genetics as well as the clinical history to avoid erroneous interpretation. These situations are little mentioned in the literature but should be recognized relatively easily by an experienced cytometrist.

CD45 (a pan-leucocyte antigen) is generally dimly expressed on marrow precursor cells, including myeloblasts, monoblasts, precursor B-cells and erythroblasts [9]. It is, by comparison, bright on mature cells such as monocytes, neutrophils and lymphocytes, although it is lost altogether by later erythroid precursors. CD45dim is therefore a useful feature to allow gating on blast cells of many AL, and it is commonly used in conjunction with the low SSC that is also seen in precursor cells [10], redrawn schematically in Figure 4.1.

By incorporating CD13, an early marker of myeloid differentiation, the following progenitor populations can therefore be easily defined in normal marrow:
1 A CD34+CD117+CD45dimCD13+ pattern, which defines the normal myeloid/monocytic progenitor population.
2 A CD34+CD117-CD45dimCD13- pattern, which defines the normal precursor B-cell population. These cells would in addition express B-cell antigens.

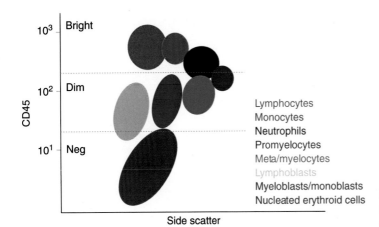

Figure 4.1 Distribution of normal bone marrow populations according to CD45 expression and side scatter properties.

For the purposes of further discussion of normal maturation patterns we will define two major populations:

1 Myeloid (neutrophils, eosinophils, basophils, monocytes, erythroid, megakaryocytes, mast cells and dendritic cells)

2 Lymphoid (B and T-cells)

It is worth drawing attention to two excellent resources with regards precursor cells and normal marrow maturation that are freely available. First, there exist useful consensus descriptions of cytology in normal and abnormal myelopoiesis which have recently been produced by the International Working Group on Morphology of Myelodysplastic Syndrome (IWGM-MDS) [11, 12]. Second, is the most recent of several attempts to accurately document the maturation patterns of precursor cells in normal marrow. The most comprehensive study to date has been performed on behalf of the European Leukaemia Net (ELN) [13]. This study exhaustively documents scatter plot patterns of antigen expression using predefined standard antibody panels, and provides a normal framework upon which abnormal populations can be identified.

Myeloid maturation

As well as being present on pluripotent stem cells, CD34 remains brightly and consistently expressed by committed normal lymphoid and granulocyte – monocyte progenitors, but rapidly reduces in intensity as further differentiation occurs. Along with HLA-DR, it is lost as normal myeloblasts mature into promyelocytes. CD117, the c-kit receptor, is, however, expressed beyond CD34 (including promyelocytes), and is only lost as the cells mature towards the myelocyte stage [14]. As a consequence CD117 therefore describes a larger and slightly more mature myeloid progenitor population than CD34 (as well as being a hallmark of mature mast cells, although these are present at very low frequency in normal marrow). Note that this typical immunophenotype of normal promyelocytes (i.e. $CD34^-HLA-DR^-CD117^+$) is partly 'preserved' in the leukaemic process, and is of use in identifying typical acute promyelocytic leukaemia (APL). However, as with almost all situations where AL may be seen to mirror a particular maturational stage, there are notable differences in antigen expression; malignant promyelocytes are therefore 'similar but different' to their normal counterparts. Knowledge of these differences is important in identifying such cells as leukaemic.

Variations in antigen intensity also occur during maturation; for example CD13 and CD33 expression on myeloblasts progressively increase in intensity up to and including the promyelocyte stage. This $CD33^{bright}$ population then loses intensity (but remains positive) as maturation to neutrophils takes place. This is in contrast to monocyte maturation which is characterized by a continual increase in CD13 and CD33 intensity as cells mature. Late antigens appearing during the myelocyte-neutrophil stages include CD15 (which first appears at a late promyelocyte stage) and CD11b [14]; CD16 and CD10 are expressed from the metamyelocyte/band-form stage onwards. Mature neutrophils therefore have a $CD45^+$, $CD13^+$, $CD33^+$, $CD11b^+$, $CD15^+$, $CD16^+$ phenotype. CD64 may be expressed on early myeloblasts, but disappears beyond this stage. It may be re-expressed by activated neutrophils, where bright CD64 expression can be indicative of sepsis [15]. A graphic summary of myeloid maturation is shown in Figure 4.2.

Monocyte maturation follows a similar course (Figure 4.3). Very early monoblasts are $CD34^+CD117^+$ (and are largely indistinguishable from normal myeloblasts), both of which diminish and disappear with evolution to a promonocyte stage [9]. HLA-DR, in contrast to the situation with granulocytic maturation where it disappears at the promyelocyte stage, remains expressed throughout monocyte maturation. Further differences include the acquisition of CD4 at the promonocyte stage (with normal monocytes remaining $CD4^{dim}$), followed closely by CD64 and CD11c. CD14 becomes brightly expressed at the mature monocyte stage. CD4, CD64 and CD14 are therefore useful markers to identify populations of monocytic lineage. CD14 is specific to monocytes. However, CD4 and CD64 may be found on other normal populations (i.e. CD4 on T-cells and CD64 on myeloblasts, dendritic cells and activated neutrophils). CD15 is expressed on both neutrophils and monocytes. Overall frequency of monocytes is variable in normal steady-state marrow samples, but is in the region of 1–8% [9]. This can increase in reactive conditions and neoplastic processes involving the monocyte lineage.

Eosinophils are present in small numbers in normal bone marrow but their acknowledgement is important in that they should not be mis-identified in circumstances where they are increased, for example myeloid

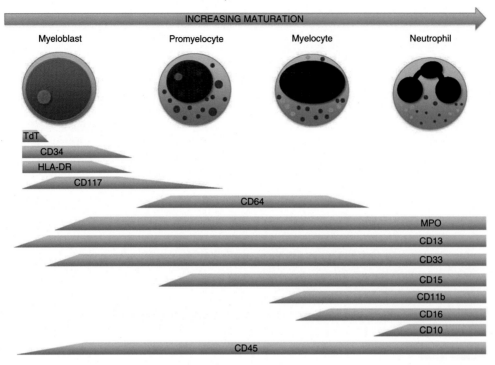

Figure 4.2 Sequential bone marrow maturational stages of the myeloid lineage.

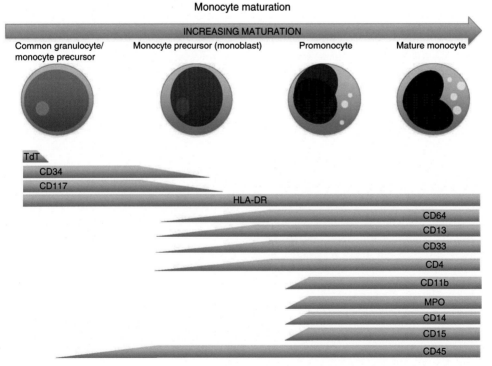

Figure 4.3 Sequential bone marrow maturational stages of monocyte lineage. Note the immunophenotypic characteristics of monocyte precursors on the maturational pathway to mature monocytes and macrophages encountered in blood and tissues, respectively. The characteristics noted here are important in understanding the immunophenotypic profile of monocytic neoplasms.

disorders, especially chronic myeloid leukaemia (CML) and reactive conditions such as allergy, inflammation and vasculitis. On the FSC/SSC plot eosinophils show high side scatter due to their intense granularity and appear slightly smaller on FSC than neutrophils. They express $CD45^{mod}$, CD13, CD11b, CD66 and $CD16^{dim}$.

Basophils are also present at low levels in normal blood and marrow, but are increased in CML and some subtypes of AML; they have a low side scatter compared to other myeloid cells and are difficult to distinguish from lymphocytes and monocytes based on light scatter characteristics. They express $CD45^{mod}$, CD13, CD33 and CD38. Interestingly, they also express CD123, $CD25^{dim}$, CD9 and CD22 [16], the latter in the absence of any other B-cell associated antigens. They can also show an aberrant phenotype in clonal disease states [17].

Erythroid maturation

Primitive erythroblasts have a generic early myeloid precursor phenotype, namely $CD34^+$ $CD117^+$ $CD45^{dim}$ $CD38^+$. As with the other lineages these markers of immaturity are rapidly lost during maturation through the pro-erythroblast to basophilic erythroblast phases, and expression of CD71 and CD235a (glycophorin) becomes established. Later forms express CD36 as CD45 is progressively lost. Note that CD71, the transferrin receptor, is detectable on most actively proliferating cells (i.e. it is another 'activation marker') and is not lineage specific. Expression is, however, at its brightest on the erythroid series, presumably due to the need for large amounts of iron. CD71 is then lost as reticulocytes become mature red cells.

Megakaryocytic maturation

These mature from the generic normal myeloid precursor phenotype (as above) with progressive loss of precursor markers, as lineage-specific CD41, CD42 and CD61 are gained. Platelets maintain expression of these antigens (discussed in more detail in Chapter 10) but are $CD45^-$.

Lymphoid maturation

Early B-cells are produced in the marrow, where they also undergo the first stages of maturation. The antigen expression patterns of maturing B-cells have been described in meticulous detail by several groups [7, 18, 19]. While this process occurs as a physiological continuum, particular stages of antigen expression are seen and can be broadly correlated with the maturation arrest stages typical for B-ALL [4]. An understanding of these patterns can, for example, prevent misidentification of Burkitt's leukaemia/lymphoma as a precursor cell neoplasm.

Mature circulating B-cells express CD19, CD20, CD79a and surface immunoglobulin, but lack CD10 and precursor cell markers. They are therefore easy to separate from the earliest B-cell precursors identifiable in the marrow, which are $CD34^+$ TdT^+ $CD10^{bright}$ $CD19^{dim}$ $CD22^{dim}$ $CD79b^+$ $CD20^-$ [7, 18]. No cytoplasmic or surface immunoglobulin is present in these cells. As these cells mature CD20 becomes positive and steadily more intense as does CD22 (brightly expressed on mature B-cells). Note, though, that this does not imply that CD20 is only expressed in mature B-cell malignancies; again this is a common misconception amongst trainees, perhaps reinforced by the use of anti-CD20 antibody therapy (largely) in the setting of mature B-cell disorders. This therapy is currently being tested in precursor cell ALL within clinical trials (UKALL14 trial protocol), precisely because these disorders are often found to express it (perhaps only 20% at diagnosis, but some experimental data suggest that steroids may promote expression and hence susceptibility to anti-CD20 [20]). As B-cells mature cytoplasmic immunoglobulin heavy chains (μ) are expressed and markers of immaturity (CD34, TdT and CD10) are steadily lost as surface immunoglobulin is gained (Figure 4.4).

The proportions of these maturational stages in bone marrow may differ significantly. In normal paediatric marrow specimens B-cell precursors may comprise up to 40% of all mononuclear cells, even in steady state conditions. When marrow recovery post- chemotherapy is analysed there is a marked left shift to favour the most immature precursors (see dedicated section on haematogones below). Conversely, during ageing there is a steady reduction of immature B-cell progenitor activity in the marrow, with similar levels of the more mature forms preserved throughout life. The presence of these normal populations must be borne in mind when assessing for possible B-cell progenitor neoplasms. As a general rule, normal maturation is characterized by *gradual* gain or loss of relevant antigens, producing a smear of expression from low

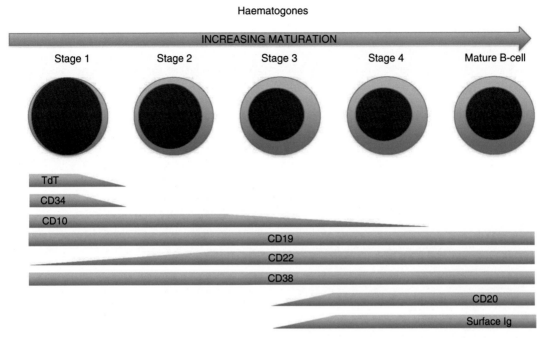

Haematogones

Figure 4.4 Sequential bone marrow maturational stages of B-cell precursors. The progressive maturation from primitive B precursor cells to mature circulating B-cells is illustrated above. Note the gradual and sequential changes in antigen expression, which contrasts with the maturational arrest picture of a B lymphoblastic leukaemia. Note that the earliest stage is typified by TdT, CD34 and CD10^{bright} expression. CD10$^+$ subpopulations predominate in children, whilst in adults the CD10$^-$CD20$^+$ population is the most common [9]. This figure is adapted from data presented in work by McKenna et al. [21].

to high or vice versa. This can be contrasted with a much more homogenous expression, often of abnormal intensity (i.e. too bright or too dim for the relevant normal maturational stage) in lymphoid malignancy.

T-cell development in contrast does not normally occur in the BM, but is initially confined to the thymus. In a manner similar to B-cell development several stages of T-cell development can be described, which bear some resemblance to the maturational stages of T-cell lymphoblastic leukaemia. These stages are summarized in Figure 4.5.

In parallel to this process the T-cell receptor is progressively rearranged and finally expressed on the cell surface in a complex with surface (s) CD3. The majority (>95%) of circulating T-cells express a receptor containing chains designated alpha and beta (TCR alpha/beta). The remainder express receptors for gamma and delta chains (TCR gamma/delta). Alpha-beta and gamma-delta T-cell development diverge at an early stage of development within the thymus and these subclasses differ in their tissue distribution, function and role in the immune response.

Restricted surface expression of alpha-beta or gamma-delta receptors is an indicator of clonality and to some extent helps classify the neoplastic T-cell disorders. Finally, T-regulatory cells (Tregs) express a transcription factor FoxP3 which appears integral to the function of these CD4$^+$, CD25$^+$ cells. Tregs are important in countering inappropriate immune responses to external or internal antigens, in the form of allergy and autoimmunity, respectively. Depletion of these regulatory cells by treatment, for example purine analogues, may be one of the factors which allow autoimmune phenomena to develop.

Haematogones

It is important to pay particular attention to a population of normal bone marrow cells called haematogones. These are normal B-lymphocyte progenitor cells which are prominent in the bone marrow in infants and children and in adults recovering from chemotherapy. They do not cause problems in the assessment of remission status in myeloid leukaemias but they can be easily mistaken

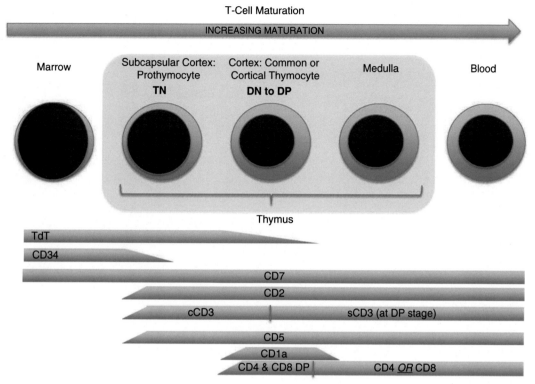

Figure 4.5 Sequential thymic maturation of T-cell precursor cells. T-cell maturation takes place largely within the thymus (over a period of three weeks or so), arising from a common lymphoid progenitor cell in the marrow. The earliest T-cell precursor is known as a triple negative (TN) due to lack of expression of CD3, CD4 and CD8. Note that they express CD34, nuclear TdT and bright CD7. Cortical thymocytes have lost CD34, gained CD1a and then mature from double negative (DN, CD4$^-$ and CD8$^-$) to double positive cells (DP, CD4$^+$ and CD8$^+$). As surface CD3 (sCD3) is expressed, TdT is lost. The final stage of maturation, in the thymic medulla, is characterized by the selection of either CD4 (T-helper cell) or CD8 (T-cytotoxic/suppressor cell) phenotypes.

for low level residual disease in precursor B acute lymphoblastic leukaemia. As the latter entity is the commonest malignancy in children and as paediatric marrow often shows prominent haematogones, it is clear why this issue is important.

Haematologists have been aware of haematogones for over 70 years, but their nature has only been adequately studied with the introduction of flow cytometry. These studies have allowed the characterization of haematogones as a distinct normal bone marrow constituent and their immunophenotypic characteristics are now well characterized.

Morphologically, not surprisingly, haematogones show a spectrum of features. Very early type I haematogones are medium to large cells with a B lymphoblast type appearance showing heterogenous chromatin, sparse agranular cytoplasm and possibly nucleoli (Figure 4.6). Later type II and type III haematogones show increasing morphological maturity with condensation of nuclear chromatin, loss of nucleoli and decreasing size [22]. These later cells are difficult to differentiate on microscopy from normal mature marrow B-cells. Haematogones can be detected in small numbers in most bone marrow specimens and constitute up to 1% of nucleated cells in adults [23], or a mean of 7.15% of nucleated cells in children [18]. They are present at extremely low levels in peripheral blood except in neonates and cord blood [24].

Haematogones have a B-cell precursor type immunophenotype. It is important to recognize, however, that they show a changing surface antigen profile according to their

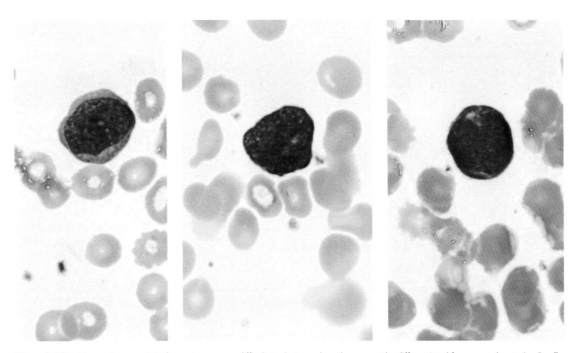

Figure 4.6 Type I haematogones. Later haematogones are difficult to photograph as they cannot be differentiated from normal maturing B-cells.

Table 4.1 The stages of haematogone maturation in contrast to mature B-cells.

Antigen	Stage I	Stage II	Stage III	Mature B-cells
TdT	Pos	Neg	Neg	Neg
CD34	Pos	Neg	Neg	Neg
CD10	Pos^bright	Pos	Pos	Neg
CD19	Pos^dim	Pos	Pos	Pos
CD38	Pos	Pos	Pos	Pos/neg
CD20	Neg	Pos^dim	Pos	Pos
Cyt IgM	Neg	Neg	Pos	Pos

stage of maturity. The early forms express CD34, TdT, DR, CD19 and CD10, whilst later maturing haematogones start to lose CD34 and TdT and acquire CD20. The intensity of antigen expression also changes as these cells progress through stages of maturation [18, 21, 25]. The immunophenotypic maturation of haematogones in relation to mature B-cells is summarized in Table 4.1 above.

Each stage of haematogone maturation is normally present in different proportions. Stage II haematogones, the intermediate stage, normally constitute about two-thirds of the total, whilst the remainder is equally made up by stages I and III. Bone marrows recovering post chemotherapy often show a significant increase in haematogones, particularly in the stage I population (left shift). Similar increases can be seen in autoimmune cytopenias and in bone marrows recovering after viral infection. Reduced numbers are seen in bone marrow infiltration, bone marrow hypoplasia and myelodysplasia. In many respects they are reflective of the degree of potential bone marrow reserve. In bone marrow failure syndromes a bone marrow transplant can successfully regenerate normal haematogone populations [22].

Precursor B lymphoblasts have a variable immunophenotype according to the maturity of the cell of origin and this explains why it is not possible to arrange a straight comparison. The individual patient precursor B-ALL phenotype has to be considered in relation to haematogones in the context of assessing remission status. For example, a pro B-ALL with absent CD10 and aberrant myeloid antigen expression can easily be identified in low numbers in bone marrow (discussed in greater detail in the next chapter). Similarly, a pre B-ALL expressing uniform CD20, with absent CD34/ TdT may be more easily discerned from haematogones. The common ALL immunophenotype CD34+, TdT+, CD19+, CD10+ is the most frequently seen lymphoblastic

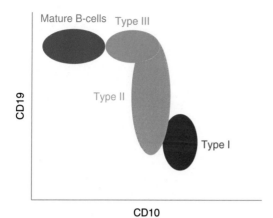

Figure 4.7 A schematic scatter plot showing the distribution of haematogones and normal B-cells according to CD19/CD10 expression (the inverted S pattern).

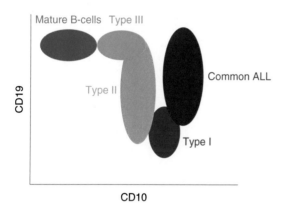

Figure 4.8 As per Figure 4.6, with common ALL blasts superimposed.

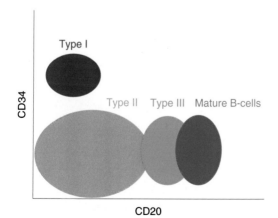

Figure 4.9 A schematic scatter plot showing the distribution of haematogones and normal B-cells according to CD34/CD20 expression.

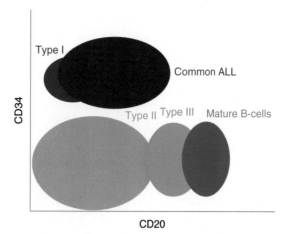

Figure 4.10 As per Figure 4.9, with common ALL blasts superimposed.

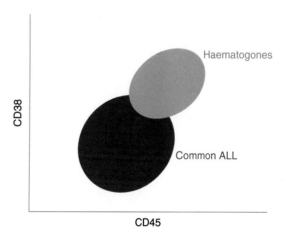

Figure 4.11 Expected distribution of haematogones and ALL blasts according to CD38 and CD45 expression.

leukaemia in adult, and particularly paediatric, haematology practice. When assessing remission here, it is of utmost importance to compare the diagnostic ALL immunophenotype, including fluorescence intensity for each antigen, with the immunophenotype of any coexistent haematogone population. It is low levels of common ALL which can cause most difficulty, particularly as CD19+, CD10+ haematogone populations are normally increased in bone marrow samples taken during recovering from chemotherapy. A schematic comparison of immunophenotypic characteristics of haematogones with mature B-cells and common ALL blasts is shown in Figures 4.7, 4.8, 4.9, 4.10, 4.11 and is derived from a

WORKED EXAMPLE 4.1

Illustrated below are a series of plots from a bone marrow analysis of a patient with a residual population of common ALL blasts alongside haematogones. First, note the separation of lymphoblasts (red, 25% events) from haematogones (blue, 75% events) according to the CD45^{dim} gate: haematogones appear less dim than blasts. The blasts have a CD34$^+$ TdT$^+$ CD79a$^+$ CD10^{bright} CD20$^-$ phenotype whilst the haematogones (which are predominantly type II) are CD34$^-$ TdT$^-$ CD79a$^+$ CD10^{mod}. Second, note the particular characteristic of the haematogones in terms of the smeared acquisition of CD20 (CD10/CD20 plot) unlike the blasts which have a 'fixed' phenotype. Finally, note the difference in strength of CD10 expression between the two populations.

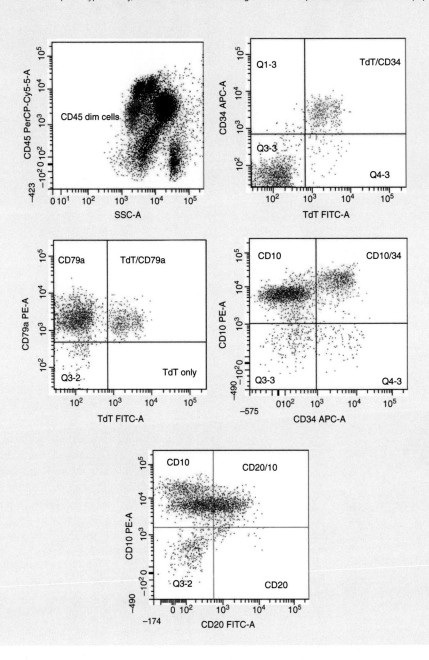

condensation of a number of important publications [18, 19, 21–23, 25, 26]. It is clear that it is not just the nature, but also the intensity of antigen expression, which is important. Haematogones demonstrate a consistent reproducible maturational pattern and should not show a discordant or aberrant immunophenotype. One exception to the rule might be following anti-CD20 monoclonal antibody therapy as this can cause diminished or blocked CD20 expression not only in neoplastic cells but also in marrow type II/III haematogones [22] .

So the template is set and the standard immunophenotypic profiles of the normal blood and bone marrow populations have been described. Proceed to work through the subsequent chapters where the wide spectrum of disorders encountered in the diagnostic immunophenotyping laboratory will be considered.

References

1 Macedo A, et al. Phenotypic analysis of CD34 subpopulations in normal human bone marrow and its application for the detection of minimal residual disease. Leukemia 1995, 9(11): 1896–901.

2 Wood BL, et al. 2006 Bethesda International Consensus recommendations on the immunophenotypic analysis of hematolymphoid neoplasia by flow cytometry: optimal reagents and reporting for the flow cytometric diagnosis of hematopoietic neoplasia. Cytometry B Clin Cytom 2007, 72(1): S14–22.

3 Ashman RI, et al. The mast cell-committed progenitor. In vitro generation of committed progenitors from bone marrow. J Immunol 1991, 146(1): 211–6.

4 Strobl H, et al. Antigenic analysis of human haemopoietic progenitor cells expressing the growth factor receptor c-kit. Br J Haematol 1992, 82(2): 287–94.

5 Bain BJ, et al. Revised guideline on immunophenotyping in acute leukaemias and chronic lymphoproliferative disorders. Clin Lab Haematol 2002, 24(1): 1–13.

6 Kuci S, et al. Phenotypic and functional characterization of mobilized peripheral blood CD34+ cells coexpressing different levels of c-Kit. Leuk Res 1998, 22(4): 355–63.

7 Dworzak MN, et al. Multiparameter phenotype mapping of normal and post-chemotherapy B lymphopoiesis in pediatric bone marrow. Leukemia 1997, 11(8): 1266–73.

8 van Lochem EG, et al. Regeneration pattern of precursor-B-cells in bone marrow of acute lymphoblastic leukemia patients depends on the type of preceding chemotherapy. Leukemia 2000, 14(4): 688–95.

9 van Lochem EG, et al. Immunophenotypic differentiation patterns of normal hematopoiesis in human bone marrow: reference patterns for age-related changes and disease-induced shifts. Cytometry B Clin Cytom 2004, 60(1): 1–13.

10 Stelzer GT, Shults KE, Loken MR. CD45 gating for routine flow cytometric analysis of human bone marrow specimens. Ann N Y Acad Sci 1993, 677: 265–80.

11 Mufti GJ, et al. Diagnosis and classification of myelodysplastic syndrome: International Working Group on Morphology of myelodysplastic syndrome (IWGM-MDS) consensus proposals for the definition and enumeration of myeloblasts and ring sideroblasts. Haematologica 2008, 93(11): 1712–7.

12 Goasguen JE, et al. Morphological evaluation of monocytes and their precursors. Haematologica 2009, 94(7): 994–7.

13 Bene MC, et al. Immunophenotyping of acute leukemia and lymphoproliferative disorders: a consensus proposal of the European LeukemiaNet Work Package 10. Leukemia 2011, 25(4): 567–74.

14 Arnoulet C, et al. Four- and five-color flow cytometry analysis of leukocyte differentiation pathways in normal bone marrow: a reference document based on a systematic approach by the GTLLF and GEIL. Cytometry B Clin Cytom 2010, 78(1): 4–10.

15 Hoffmann JJ. Neutrophil CD64: a diagnostic marker for infection and sepsis. Clin Chem Lab Med 2009, 47(8): 903–16.

16 Han X, et al. Immunophenotypic study of basophils by multiparameter flow cytometry. Arch Pathol Lab Med 2008, 132(5): 813–9.

17 Lichtman MA, Segel GB. Uncommon phenotypes of acute myelogenous leukemia: basophilic, mast cell, eosinophilic, and myeloid dendritic cell subtypes: a review. Blood Cells Mol Dis 2005 35(3): 370–83.

18 Lucio P, et al. Flow cytometric analysis of normal B cell differentiation: a frame of reference for the detection of minimal residual disease in precursor-B-ALL. Leukemia 1999, 13(3): 419–27.

19 Rimsza LM, et al. Benign hematogone-rich lymphoid proliferations can be distinguished from B-lineage acute lymphoblastic leukemia by integration of morphology, immunophenotype, adhesion molecule expression, and architectural features. Am J Clin Pathol 2000, 114(1): 66–75.

20 Dworzak MN, et al. CD20 up-regulation in pediatric B-cell precursor acute lymphoblastic leukemia during induction treatment: setting the stage for anti-CD20 directed immunotherapy. Blood 2008, 112(10): 3982–8.

21 McKenna RW, et al. Immunophenotypic analysis of hematogones (B-lymphocyte precursors) in 662 consecutive bone marrow specimens by 4-color flow cytometry. Blood 2001, 98(8): 2498–507.

22 Sevilla DW, et al. Hematogones: a review and update. Leuk Lymphoma 2010, 51(1): 10–19.

23 Kroft SH, et al. Haematogones in the peripheral blood of adults: a four-colour flow cytometry study of 102 patients. *Br J Haematol* 2004, **126**(2): 209–12.

24 Motley D, et al. Determination of lymphocyte immunophenotypic values for normal full-term cord blood. *Am J Clin Pathol* 1996, **105**(1): 38–43.

25 McKenna RW, Asplund SL, Kroft SH. Immunophenotypic analysis of hematogones (B-lymphocyte precursors) and neoplastic lymphoblasts by 4-color flow cytometry. *Leuk Lymphoma* 2004, **45**(2): 277–85.

26 Babusikova O, et al. Hematogones in acute leukemia during and after therapy. *Leuk Lymphoma* 2008, **49**(10): 1935–44.

CHAPTER 5
Acute Leukaemia

Introduction

Acute leukaemia: definition and classification

Acute leukaemia (AL) is generally understood to be a neoplastic process that exerts a maturational block at a haematopoietic precursor cell level, accompanied by a proliferative drive of varying degree. The resulting accumulation of cells, most frequently in the marrow, causes the typical clinical picture, which includes marrow failure, tissue infiltration, organomegaly and on occasion, tumour masses. Often the disease is obvious in the peripheral blood, where blast cells may be present in extreme numbers, but in some cases peripheral blasts may not be seen or blood counts may even be normal. Acute leukaemia is traditionally deemed as a primary disorder of the bone marrow, requiring marrow aspiration for diagnosis. Detection of an abnormal precursor cell population from another site may also be diagnostic, such as in the case of granulocytic sarcoma or lymphoblastic lymphoma. These are now recognized to be tissue-based equivalents of AL, and demand similar treatment approaches.

Acute leukaemia is most frequently diagnosed from marrow specimens which by definition exhibit ≥20% blasts, the 'cut-off' established by the WHO [1]. This allows clear distinction from the pre-leukaemic conditions of myelodysplasia (MDS), myeloproliferative neoplasms (MPN) and chronic myeloid leukaemia (CML), all of which demonstrate <20% blasts. Classification of AL was first attempted in 1976 when a panel of experts from France, the USA and the UK developed the so-called FAB morphology-based criteria [2]. This was followed by the European Group for Immunophenotyping of Leukaemias (EGIL) criteria in 1995 (which included

flow cytometric assessment [3]) and has culminated in the 2008 WHO Classification, which further incorporates results from cytogenetic and molecular testing [1]. These classification systems are summarized in Table 5.1. Some knowledge of the early systems is useful as many texts continue to use some aspects of these.

Flow cytometry is central to the diagnosis, classification and monitoring of AL. Together with a thorough morphological assessment, flow allows the identification of a maturational stage and lineage, which are the first steps on the diagnostic pathway leading to full characterization of the disorder (Figure 5.1). Integration of these results with karyotypic analysis can facilitate targeted molecular testing, followed by assignation of a WHO 2008 diagnosis [1].

This approach, however, has practical implications with regards to immediate communication of results to clinicians; genetic testing takes some days or even weeks, therefore full WHO 2008 subclassification is often unavailable over this period. Instead a pragmatic, clinically relevant 'temporary' classification may be used, such as simply defining precursor cell B-ALL, T-ALL and AML (including identifying probable APL) to guide initial therapy including entry into clinical trials. Some labs may initially utilize the widely understood FAB-based terminology incorporating morphology plus flow data. This facilitates timely diagnosis and treatment; early recognition of APL can be life saving and a recent large retrospective study suggests that younger patients with AML do significantly better when treated early after presentation [4].

Initial flow profiling can rapidly identify the immunological subtype and direct downstream genetic testing in a cost-effective and timely manner. The production of a complete, comprehensive report detailing the exact diagnosis with relevant prognostic information is an

Practical Flow Cytometry in Haematology Diagnosis, First Edition. Mike Leach, Mark Drummond and Allyson Doig.
© 2013 John Wiley & Sons, Ltd. Published 2013 by John Wiley & Sons, Ltd.

Table 5.1 The major classification systems for acute leukaemia. These continue to evolve as more knowledge, particularly with regards genetic abnormalities, is gained. Thus there has been a move away from a simple morphological classification (namely AML M0-M7 and L1-L3 ALL) to one where genetic results are incorporated in a diagnostically and prognostically valid way.

Classification system	Modalities of testing	Broad subtypes
French-American-British (FAB) Classification, 1976	Morphology Cytochemistry AL defined as ≥30% myeloblasts/monoblasts/lymphoblasts in blood or marrow Erythroleukaemia: ≥50% erythroid cells, ≥30% myeloblasts in non-erythroid cells	Eight subtypes of AML (M0-M7): M0 – AML minimal differentiation M1 – AML without maturation M2 – AML with maturation M3 – acute promyelocytic leukaemia M4 – acute myelomonocytic leukaemia M5 – acute monoblastic (M5a) or monocytic (M5b) leukaemia M6 – acute erythroleukaemia or pure erythroid leukaemia M7 – acute megakaryoblastic leukaemia Three subtypes of ALL based on morphology: L1, L2, L3
European Group for Immunologoical Classification of Leukaemias (EGIL), 1995	Morphology Cytochemistry Immunophenotyping	AML: introduced immunological definitions for AML M0, M6 and M7 Immunological subclassification of B and T precursor ALL Biphenotypic and undifferentiated AL defined
WHO 2008	Morphology Cytochemistry Immunophenotyping Cytogenetics Molecular testing Blast threshold reduced to ≥20% blood or marrow cells	Three main categories: AML, AL of ambiguous lineage and precursor lymphoid neoplasms Subclassified on presence or absence of recurring genetic abnormalities

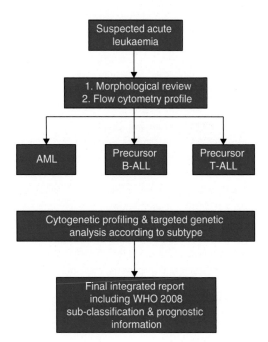

Figure 5.1 Flow cytometry in the diagnosis of acute leukaemia.

essential final stage, to allow clear communication with clinicians. To facilitate this process the optimal arrangement involves all disciplines operating in an integrated laboratory environment. An overview of this integrated approach can be found in reference [5].

Clinical presentation and sampling for flow cytometry

For most cases of AL, the diagnosis is straightforward; bone marrow sampling is initiated based on peripheral blood indices and morphology. For others, marrow sampling is normal and cells may be identified in other fluid (e.g. pleural, pericardial or CSF) or tissue samples. There are important pitfalls to be aware of with all these approaches, which are discussed in detail in Chapter 3. Of the utmost importance is that the final interpretation of results must always be in the context of the clinical situation, which acts as a final 'validation' step for laboratory results. Likewise, the integration of morphologic and genetic results; an incongruous clinical or laboratory picture must prompt a rethink.

Identification of neoplastic precursor cells

The blast population

The term 'blast cell' is in common use as a morphological descriptor for cells of an immature or primitive appearance, mainly in the setting of haematological neoplasms, but also in normal marrow. It has morphological (e.g. high nuclear to cytoplasmic ratio, immature chromatin, often visible nucleoli), immunophenotypic (precursor cell antigen positive, a lack of maturity-associated antigens) and functional (stem or precursor cell) definitions. The hallmark of AL is an abnormal accumulation of blasts in marrow, peripheral blood and/or other tissues. Light microscopy appearances cannot always be relied upon, however; leukaemic-phase lymphomas, normal precursor cells and even some non-haemic neoplasms may display blast cell characteristics and be a trap for the unwary. Likewise this term is often used to define a primitive population identified by flow cytometric means. The flow defined equivalents of morphologic blasts in normal marrow will incorporate early progenitor cells, more committed myelomonocytic progenitor cells, promyelocytes, promonocytes and B-cell progenitors [6]. Correlating flow data with what is interpreted down the microscope as a blast population can therefore be challenging, particularly when other confounding factors are involved as described below.

It is vital to have a working knowledge or 'framework' of antigen expression during normal myeloid and lymphoid maturation, to allow identification of abnormal populations. This has been discussed in some detail in the previous chapter. It is also useful to emphasize at the outset that none of the antibodies currently in routine use for flow cytometry of AL are specific to neoplastic precursor cells. For example the common precursor-cell (such as CD34, CD117 and TdT) and cell activation antigens (such as HLA-DR and CD38) are expressed on normal stem and precursor cells as well as in many cases of AL. Furthermore, some mature cell types may express these antigens (e.g. HLA-DR on B-cells, activated T-cells and monocytes and CD38 on plasma cells). Note that CD34, CD117 and TdT are not expressed on mature cells under normal circumstances (with the exception of CD117 expression on mature mast cells). There is often an initial misconception amongst laboratory trainees that

particular antigens in isolation can be used to define an AL with absolute certainty, which is not the case. Rather, it is the 'company that these antigens keep' which is of paramount importance, allowing a profile of the cells in question to be constructed in terms of their maturational stage and lineage. In other words, it is the whole pattern of expression, sometimes termed the 'leukaemia associated phenotype' or LAP, that is relevant. Identification of a leukaemic cell population, as for any malignancy, therefore depends upon the recognition of non-random patterns of antigen expression as different from that of the tightly regulated normal situation. These non-random antigen patterns on AL cells include:

1 Abnormal expression of foreign-lineage antigens (termed *aberrant* expression, for example lymphoid markers present in AML).

2 Abnormal co-expression of markers of both maturity and immaturity not seen normally (*asynchronous* antigen expression (e.g. the stem/precursor cell antigen CD34 co-expressed with CD15, a marker of myeloid maturity).

3 Abnormally increased or decreased expression of an antigen, or unusually homogeneous expression of an antigen more usually associated with heterogeneous expression.

Blast populations are heterogeneous

An additional complication for the cytometrist is the fact that AL populations are heterogeneous. Some, if not all, AL is likely arranged in a hierarchical fashion (in a parody of normal haematopoiesis) ranging from a rare, primitive leukaemic stem cell population through to the 'bulk' population of leukaemic blasts which may display a profile akin to a 'maturation arrest' of an equivalent normal precursor cell [7]. Outside the research setting, diagnostic flow cytometry concerns itself with the analysis of this bulk population and it is on this basis that the disease is classified. In general terms precursor B and T-acute lymphoblastic leukaemia/lymphoma (B-ALL or T-ALL) present a much more homogenous picture of cell maturation and antigen expression than acute myeloid leukaemia (AML). For example, compare the morphological appearance and cell marker expression of precursor B-ALL to that of acute myelomonocytic leukaemia. The former usually exhibits a uniform population of lymphoblasts with relatively homogeneous antigen expression (thus easily distinguishing it from the normal 'spread' of antigen expression in normal maturing B-cell

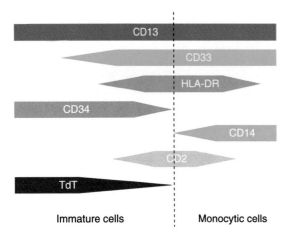

Figure 5.2 Schematic diagram of the immunophenotypic profile of the various leukaemic cell populations in AML M4Eo. Not the strikingly different phenotypes of the primitive myeloid and monocytic populations. The choice of gating strategy is clearly important here. Figure adapted from data presented in Adriaansen *et al.* [9].

progenitors), while the latter demonstrates a mixed population of myeloblasts, immature and maturing monocytes, immature myeloid cells and perhaps a clonal eosinophilic population. As a consequence the marker profile is complex and dependent on what particular subpopulation is being analysed (Figure 5.2). From a technical standpoint, flow cytometry is therefore very easy on the former in terms of identifying the blast population (usually the majority of marrow cells), but potentially more challenging on the latter as a variety of cell populations, including residual normal cells, are present. A separate LAP would be apparent for each of these populations and this heterogeneity must be taken into account to allow a comprehensive diagnostic profile and facilitate accurate analysis of follow-up specimens [8]. An MRD analysis of B and T-ALL is therefore generally much more straightforward than in AML, as is identifying a maturational-arrest stage.

Correlating the immunophenotype with genetic analysis

It might be argued that there is little to be gained by subclassifying AL on the basis of maturational stage of the precursor blast cells, particularly in the context of B and T-ALL where such stages are best defined. Certainly the 2008 WHO Classification groups these entities together (as either B or T-lineage ALL) and subclassifies

the former on the basis of genetic abnormalities [1]. Furthermore, modern treatment protocols stratify therapy of both AML and ALL on the basis of genetic abnormalities rather than immunophenotype, with the *individual* prognostic significance of CD antigens largely unproven in the AL setting. Within flow based maturational and/ or phenotypic subgroups, however, there exist some well-recognized genotypic-phenotypic entities of disease. By identifying the immunophenotype and correlating with subsequent genetic results an element of internal quality assurance is built in; if the data agree then it greatly strengthens the diagnostic process and can robustly inform clinical practice. For example, flow may support morphological suspicion of APL and guide initial therapy pending urgent genetic confirmation. Furthermore, having a system which recognizes different maturational stages of precursor cell AL allows ready detection of conditions which sit outside it; for example the identification of a mature B-cell phenotype in a suspected B-ALL often indicates a Burkitt leukaemia/lymphoma, which segregates closely with the presence of a *MYC* translocation and dictates a short intensive treatment approach very different to that of precursor B-ALL.

In precursor neoplasms some correlations between phenotype and genotype are strong, and these are covered later in this chapter. For most situations the genetic data is prioritized, however, as these relationships are often not absolute. New correlations continue to be described; for example using microarray technology a recent study extensively genotyped childhood T-ALL and identified a particularly poor prognostic group with a consistent and readily identifiable immunophenotype indicative of a very primitive T-cell maturational stage [10]. Microarray-profiling remains expensive and currently unavailable to most routine haematology laboratories, but treatment for these genetically distinct patients can be altered based on their identification by flow cytometry. Furthermore, as discussed later in the chapter, the rapid development of flow cytometric detection of genetic lesions (usually via the expressed protein) may ultimately allow full characterization of AL (both phenotypic and genetic) using a single technique.

Blast cell characteristics

An overview of blast gating strategies are given in Figure 5.3. Morphology is likely to give the first clue to the presence of a precursor cell neoplasm, with visual

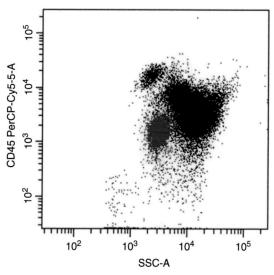

Figure 5.3a Gating on CD45 dim cells in a CD45 versus SSC analysis.

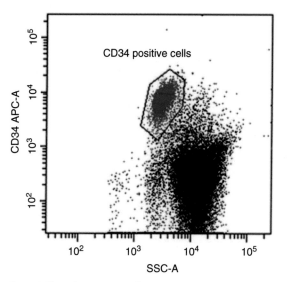

CD34 positive cells

Figure 5.3b Gating on CD34⁺ cells in a CD34 versus SSC analysis.

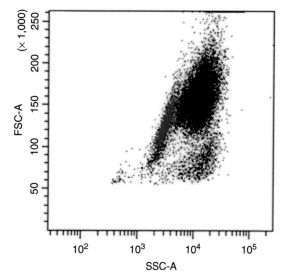

Figure 5.3c Gating on potential blasts (large cells, low side scatter) in an FSC versus SSC analysis.

identification of blast cells. However, some acute leukaemias might display some considerable degree of morphological maturation by definition, such as acute promyelocytic or acute monocytic leukaemias. That said, for a majority of AL the expression of precursor-cell markers and absence (or asynchronous expression) of maturation antigens, allows a straightforward identification of a primitive population. Aside from the SSC/

CD45^{dim} strategy (Figure 5.3a) it is also useful to assess CD34/SSC (Figure 5.3b) or simply analyse the blast gate (Figure 5.3c) when identifying precursor cells. A CD45 versus SSC analysis is normally favoured as this will potentially identify a primitive cell population regardless of lineage. A recent study quantified the median proportion of SSC/CD45dim cells and CD34⁺ cells in normal marrow as 4.7% and 1.4%, respectively [11].

The main expression patterns of the important precursor cell antigens are shown in Table 5.2. Note that CD34 is expressed across the spectrum of ALL and AML, but by no means in all cases. TdT is most frequently seen in ALL, but it should be noted that it may also be expressed in some cases of primitive AML (such as FAB subtype AML M0) and is therefore not lineage specific. This can be a common misconception amongst laboratory trainees. However, TdT is much more intensely expressed in ALL as opposed to TdT⁺ AML [12]. CD117 is the most 'lineage specific' of the precursor cell antigens, being largely confined to AML (although <5% of ALL cases were positive in a large study often in conjunction with CD13 and/or CD33 in primitive T-ALL [13]). Note, however, that CD117 is surpassed by MPO in terms of myeloid lineage assignment (discussed in detail later), and CD117 should not be solely relied upon as a specific marker for AML (note its promiscuous expression in a range of cell types and tumours).

Table 5.2 Antigens useful in identification of a precursor cell neoplasm. This table lists the most useful antigens in common use. In addition to the expression patterns of those antigens listed, the absence of antigens associated with a mature phenotype is important. For AML, absence of maturation markers may be noted (most notably CD10, CD11b, CD15, CD16 and CD65), although these can be seen asynchronously expressed with precursor cell antigens. Expression patterns on non-haemic tissues and neoplasms are included, if only to emphasize the point that many of these antigens are not unique to haematological conditions. Unless otherwise specified summarized from [18–21]. GIST, gastro-intestinal stromal tumours; MHC, major histocompatibility complex.

Antigen	Physiological role	Normal expression pattern	AL and other haematological malignancy expression patterns	Other disease expression
CD34	Cell surface glycoprotein and adhesion molecule	Haematopoietic stem cells Myelomonocytic precursor cells Haematogones and T-cell precursors Endothelial cells Some marrow fibroblasts	AML (approx 70%) MDS blast cells (50–100%) B-ALL (67–80%) [14] T-ALL (30–50%) [15]	Vascular tumours including Kaposi's sarcoma Dermatofibrosarcoma protruberans GIST
CD117	Stem cell factor receptor, also known as c-kit	Myeloblasts and promyelocytes Monoblasts and promonocytes Megakaryoblasts Erythroblasts Mature mast cells Some plasma cells	AML (60–70%) Clonal Mast cells (mastocytosis) ALL (very rarely, <5%) (note: occasionally positive in CD8+ T-PLL) Some myeloma	GIST and other stromal tumours Small cell carcinoma
TdT	Terminal deoxynucleotydil transferase; catalyses the addition of nucleotides to the 3' terminus of a DNA molecule	Primitive lymphoid and some myeloid precursors (mainly haematogones and thymocytes)	ALL (>90%, stronger in B-ALL than T-ALL [12]) AML (dimly in approx 50% of AML M0, occasionally other subtypes)	
CD1a	Involved in antigen presentation by dendritic cells	Cortical thymocytes Langerhans cells Immature dendritic cells	T-ALL (approx 40–60%, indicative of a cortical phenotype).	Thymomas Langerhans cell histiocytosis PEComas
CD45	A tyrosine phosphatase, which helps regulate B and T-cell antigen receptor-mediated activation	All leucocytes. Brighter expression on mature cells, particularly lymphocytes and monocytes. (note mature erythrocytes and platelets are negative)	Dim expression on precursor cell neoplasms, occasionally negative in B-ALL Note: may be more strongly expressed on blasts of monocytic lineage.	expression of CD45 can be used to confirm a haemic origin for a tumour
HLA-DR	Antigen presentation (an MHC class II surface receptor)	HSC and precursor cells B-cells Monocytes and macrophages Activated T-cells, NK cells and basophils Dendritic cells	B-ALL (100%) and mature B-cell neoplasms including myeloma. T-ALL (10–20%) and some mature T-cell malignancies AML (85%, not AML M3, AML with 'cup-like' blasts or NPM1 mutated AML[16])	Interdigitating dendritic cell sarcoma Small round cell tumours
CD38	An 'ectoenzyme' regulating intracellular calcium Also involved in cell-cell interactions and transmembrane signal transduction	Immature T-cells and activated mature T-cells Haematogones and mature circulating B-cells (up to 50% in adults, higher in children), germinal centre B-cells and plasma cells Monocytes (subset) [17] HSC and myeloid precursors Mature myeloid cells (dim, including neutrophils, eosinophils and basophils; it is brightest on the latter)	B-ALL (60–90%) T-ALL (100%) AML (75%, not expressed in M0 or M7). Many mature B-cell malignancies (in particular myeloma). Subset of B-CLL (poor prognostic marker) Many mature T/NK malignancies	

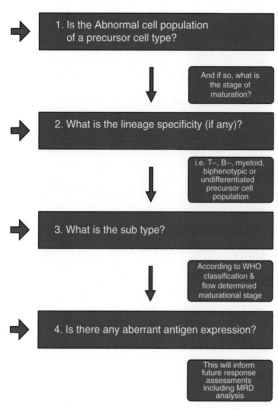

1. Is the Abnormal cell population of a precursor cell type?

And if so, what is the stage of maturation?

2. What is the lineage specificity (if any)?

i.e. T−, B−, myeloid, biphenotypic or undifferentiated precursor cell population

3. What is the sub type?

According to WHO classification & flow determined maturational stage

4. Is there any aberrant antigen expression?

This will inform future response assessments including MRD analysis

Figure 5.4 Summary of approach to flow cytometry data interpretation in acute leukaemia. This is an illustration of the key questions that need to be answered during the flow cytometric analysis of an acute leukaemia.

How these antigens may be incorporated into a gating strategy to reliably identify blast cells demands some further explanation. With four-colour flow cytometry in general use, a common approach is to incorporate 'anchor' antigens in each tube, such as CD34 and CD45. Using these antigens, in conjunction with SSC, an SSC^{low} CD45^{dim}, CD34^{+} or CD34^{-} population of blast cells can be consistently identified in each tube, with other antigens (including TdT, CD117 and a comprehensive panel of lineage markers) added in sequential combination to further characterize the population (Figure 5.4). Thus, the same precursor population is consistently identified in each 'tube' and a complete picture of antigen expression gradually built up. Appropriately applied back-gating strategies using these precursor related antigens, can be used to better define the blast population. Once negative control antibodies are included, upwards of

12 tubes or more can be required to do a standard acute leukaemia panel.

A typical acute panel is highlighted below with each line representing a separate tube:

CD45, CD34, FITC NEG/PE NEG CONTROL1
CD45, CD34, CD15, CD117
CD45, CD34, CD7, CD33
CD45, CD34, HLA-DR, CD13
CD45, CD34, CD14, CD64
CD45, CD34, FITC NEG, PE NEG CONTROL2
CD45, CD34, CD2, CD19
CD45, CD34, CD20, CD10
CD45, CD34, CD38, CD56

Cytoplasmic:

CD45, CD34, FITC NEG, PE NEG CONTROL
CD45, CD34, TdT, CD79a
CD45, CD34, MPO, CD3

Failure to express maturation-associated antigens is the other common characteristic of AL cells. Examples here would include:

1 Lack of cytoplasmic or surface immunoglobulin in B-cell ALL (although cytoplasmic IgM heavy chains may be expressed in a subgroup exhibiting a later maturational stage). Note that CD20 (an antigen often associated with a mature B-cell phenotype) may be positive in approximately 40% [22, 23] and should not be misinterpreted as indicative of a mature B-cell disorder. A lack of surface (s) CD3 in T-ALL. CD3 is a component of the T-cell receptor, although cytoplasmic (c) CD3 is detectable and is lineage specific. Additionally, lack of CD4 or CD8 restriction is indicative of a precursor cell phenotype (most cases are CD4^{-}/CD8^{-} or CD4^{+}/CD8^{+}, with only very occasional cases displaying single antigen expression).

2 For AML, absence of maturation markers (most notably CD10, CD11b, CD15, CD16 and CD65) are also noted in some precursor cell neoplasms [18], although their asynchronous expression with precursor antigens is commonly seen also.

Determination of Antigen Positivity in Acute Leukaemia

It is worth digressing briefly at this juncture to discuss what it means for an antigen to be 'positive' in the context of AL. It has traditionally been accepted that a cell population is deemed positive for an antigen when 20%

or more of cells express it, as compared to a proposed threshold of 30% in the chronic lymphoproliferative disorders [24]. The reason for these thresholds is to facilitate standardization, classification of disease and communication of results, but they are underpinned by little evidence. Furthermore they often originate from a period when two-colour flow cytometers were standard, which made accurate characterization of abnormal subpopulations much more challenging than with four-colour. This likely resulted in thresholds of positivity being set at a level which could incorporate some 'background' positivity in other cell types. In recognition of these issues, recent guidelines suggest that for the critical precursor cell related antigens (specifically TdT, CD34 and CD117) the threshold for positivity be accepted as 10% [3, 25]. The slavish adherence to strict thresholds of single antigen positivity must, however, be tempered by a full appraisal of the morphological, genetic and clinical characteristics of the disorder in the clinic, allowing a final clinical assessment to take priority.

Analysis of follow-up specimens

Using the approaches described above, for most AL marrow samples the identification of the blast population is very easy, as even on a simple FSC/SSC plot it is apparent that the sample is comprised mostly of blast cells. When analysis of follow-up marrow samples is performed, for example after induction chemotherapy, the use of an identical gating strategy as that performed on the first sample can facilitate detection of small numbers of blast cells with the diagnostic LAP. One caveat to this is in *relapsed* cases, where antigen expression patterns may change, and prior blast characteristics cannot always be relied upon. In one study almost 25% of AML cases demonstrated a complete immunophenotypic shift at relapse [26]. Whether this is due to a shift in proportions of blast cells within a heterogeneous 'hierarchy' or a genuine alteration in antigen expression is unknown. A full re-analysis of such cases should therefore be completed at the time of relapse, which should not only include immunophenotype but also molecular and cytogenetic analysis as these parameters can also change [26].

Patterns of precursor antigen expression in acute leukaemia

For AML, 76% of cases will be CD34$^+$ CD117$^+$ or CD34$^-$ CD117$^-$, and the remainder (24%) will express either one

of these antigens [13]. Overall, approximately 67–92% of AML expresses CD117, with 67% expressing CD34 [27]. While CD117 is apparently more specific for the myeloid lineage than either CD13 or CD33 [28], it may very rarely be found on T and B-ALL (4% of ALL cases overall in one study) [13]. These observations remain controversial, however, with Hans *et al.* speculating that the particular antibody clone used in these studies was contributory and noting that only rarely is CD117 mRNA identified in alleged CD117$^+$ cases [28]. The authors have only seen a single case of CD117$^+$ ALL (unpublished observations). Immunocytochemistry on histological specimens can also be used to study these antigens; there is a good correlation between CD34 expression when ICC on marrow trephines and flow on marrow aspirate are compared. CD117, on the other hand, is optimally detected by flow, which is the more sensitive technique. For AL displaying a degree of morphologic maturation (e.g. the presence of granules, Auer rods, granulocytic and monocytic precursors) flow is generally confirmatory, although patterns of antigen expression differ widely from normal cell counterparts (discussed later in chapter).

Precursor lymphoid neoplasms are identified using the same principles as above, namely the presence of precursor cell markers (most frequently CD34, TdT and additionally in T-cell entities CD1a) and absence of markers of maturity. The presence or absence of surface immunoglobulin (Ig) is a good example, where by definition detectable Ig is an indicator of a mature pathology (i.e. a lymphoma or lymphoproliferative disorder). Note that the converse is not always true, that is, the absence of surface Ig does not always dictate a precursor cell neoplasm. Examples of surface Ig negative mature B-cell malignancies include rare cases of Burkitt leukaemia/lymphoma (all exhibiting a typical *MYC* translocation) [29], CLL and occasional cases of other lymphoma subtypes (mainly diffuse large B-cell or follicular non-Hodgkin lymphoma [30]). This is a good example of one of the central themes of this book, namely the need to interpret such aberrancies in the context of the other markers, morphology and genetic analysis. In the latter cases appropriate genetic analysis would pick up the typical abnormalities associated with these mature malignances, effectively 'trumping' equivocal flow results.

Occasional cases of AL lack any expression of lineage commitment markers (acute undifferentiated leukaemia, AUL) and only express precursor related antigens. These cases are usually characterized as CD34$^+$ CD45^{dim}, which confirms their haemic origins.

Considerable research effort continues to be invested in attempts to identify leukaemia specific antigens, particularly in the LSC compartment. Thus far, several antigens that are *preferentially* expressed (i.e. found more commonly on LSC than their normal counterparts) rather than specifically expressed, have been described. These include CD25, CD32, CD47, CD44, CD96, CD123 and CLL-1 [31]. They are found on AML LSC (in 25–100% of cases) as well as normal tissues (in particular normal haematopoietic cells). Some of these antibodies may enter routine diagnostic use in this setting (some are of course already used routinely in other conditions such as CD123 in B-cell LPDs), particularly if attempts to target these molecules with monoclonal antibodies are clinically successful (reviewed in Majeti [31]).

Enumeration of blast cells

An apparently simple parameter, determination of the proportion of blast cells in a sample is important for a number of reasons:

1 It facilitates a diagnosis of AL, due to the diagnostic threshold of 20% marrow /blood blasts or more.
2 It helps establish remission status in follow-up samples.
3 The accurate enumeration of residual blast numbers can establish the degree of residual disease for prognostic studies and can allow adapted treatment approaches (so-called minimal residual disease, or MRD analysis).

When a diagnostic sample is composed mainly of blasts most of the cells passing through the instrument, and hence most of the data 'events' captured, are blast cells. For most AL at the time of diagnosis, the leukaemic blast population dominates the marrow, often with marked suppression of residual polyclonal haematopoiesis. When small populations are present, however (e.g. in MDS at presentation, or in follow-up of treated AL), it requires a particular strategy to separate out (or 'gate' on) the blasts to reduce the 'contamination' of the population of interest by cells of other lineages. This is seen at its most extreme in measuring MRD, where an exact knowledge of the blast characteristics at diagnosis is a prerequisite to allow precise enumeration of very small numbers of blast cells (often on a background of a normal or regenerating marrow).

Furthermore, in certain circumstances, particularly in regenerating marrows, it can sometimes be difficult to discern what represents a genuine phenotypically abnormal population as compared to shifts in the relative proportions of haematopoietic precursor cells (often termed a 'left-shift' due to prominence of more immature cells). One obvious example is an increase in CD34$^+$ cells as compared to normal in a recovering marrow post chemotherapy comprising regenerating HSC, myelomonocytic precursors and, particularly in younger patients, haematogones.

Furthermore, unusual phenotypes can be detected by flow in this setting (such as low level CD56 expression on G-CSF stimulated granulocytes and monocytes [6] and increased HLA-DR and CD64 on granulocytes). To reduce the possibility of confusion, attention needs to be paid to both the timing of marrow specimens and the clinical situation in question. The author's practice is, where possible, to allow peripheral count recovery prior to sampling and to avoid performing marrows on G-CSF treated, or very recently treated, patients.

It is very tempting to utilize the 'automated' blast count from flow data as accurately representative. However, outside of the protocol-led and strictly controlled scenario of MRD analysis, accurate quantification of leukaemic blasts by flow (as a percentage of marrow cells), should be interpreted with a degree of caution for a number of reasons, including:

1 The marrow aspirate may be haemodilute (a frequent problem in light of the sampling demands for genetic analysis and clinical trials) or technically difficult (e.g. in marrow fibrosis or with packed marrows) and therefore non-representative. In general terms, the larger the aspirate volume, the greater the peripheral blood contamination and the lower the proportion of blast cells [11].
2 The blast hierarchy may be immunophenotypically heterogeneous. For example, not all blast cells in a sample will be CD34$^+$, as some cell types such as monoblasts, promonocytes and promyelocytes will have lost this antigen, as will some more mature myeloblasts. Furthermore, many AMLs and ALLs are comprised entirely of CD34$^-$ blast cells (approximately 30% of AML, 30–40% of B-ALL and up to 90% of T-ALL in some studies). It is therefore important not to rely on expression of a single antigen to characterize these disorders. Accepting the percentage of CD34$^+$ cells as an accurate indication of blast numbers is a common pitfall for the unwary.
3 The denominators for calculating blast percentage with flow cytometry or morphology are different as red

cells are deliberately lysed during sample preparation and some nucleated red cells are inevitably lost. As blast cells are usually counted as a proportion of all nucleated cells morphologically, discrepancies may arise between the two techniques.

4 The morphologist and the cytometrist may be unwittingly analysing different populations. One drawback of flow cytometry is that there is no way to be completely sure that the abnormal population as identified by light microscopy is identical to that described by flow. Morphological assessment of blast cell numbers should therefore still be taken as the 'gold standard' [32]. The caveats above are of particular importance during diagnostic work-up of myelodysplastic syndromes (MDS) or lymphoblastic lymphoma, where marrow blast percentages of greater than 20% or 25% respectively will allow a diagnosis of acute leukaemia to be made. Likewise, the diagnosis of erythroleukaemia demands ≥50% erythroid precursors and ≥20% myeloblasts within the remaining population; such data are not best gleaned by flow cytometry, but rather by morphology. To facilitate an accurate morphological count it is recommended that a minimum of 200 leucocytes on blood smears or 500 nucleated cells on a particulate marrow smear be counted [32, 33]. Note that erythroblasts should not be counted as blast cells, with the exception of pure erythroid leukaemia.

Phenotypic heterogeneity is increasingly recognized within the leukaemic CD34+ compartment. For example, in many AML cases, an immunophenotypic hierarchy of CD34+ cells exists with true leukaemic stem cells (LSC) appearing to reside in the CD34+CD38−lin− minority population [34]. Patients who expressed >3.5% LSC in this study (based upon CD34+CD38− population expressed as a percentage of the total CD34+ population) had a median relapse free survival of 5.6 months compared to 16 months for those with a low LSC frequency (≤3.5%). Targeting this primitive subpopulation of blasts is currently a major thrust of research.

Lineage assignment of acute leukaemia

Morphological assessment remains important for lineage classification, which is often fairly straightforward for cases exhibiting maturation. In other cases it is, however, extremely difficult, for example in AML M0 blasts are

1. MPO
2. CD117
3. CD13
4. CD33

Decreasing specificity for AML

Figure 5.5 Hierarchy of myeloid specific antigen expression in acute leukaemia. This illustrates the hierarchy of commonly used myeloid antigens in terms of their myeloid specificity [36–38]. MPO is never positive in ALL, but note that occasional cases of AML may not express MPO – such as very primitive AML and some monocytic cases. Some reported MPO-negative cases might reflect the ongoing uncertainty as to the cut-off threshold for MPO positivity [39].

often small with nucleoli and scant agranular cytoplasm. They give few anatomical clues to lineage and can be difficult to differentiate morphologically from lymphoblasts. Therefore, in conjunction with the 'anchor' markers for precursor cells described above, an AL immunophenotyping panel will include an extensive panel of antibodies designed to allow lineage assignment and identify expression of those recognized antigens 'foreign' to the lineage in question (aberrant markers). It is this propensity for aberrant antigen expression in haematological malignancy that imparts a note of caution to the idea of 'lineage-specific' antigens.

Each lineage marker has a recognizable pattern of expression typical for normal and pathological states, and it is vital that the reporting lab staff have a good knowledge of these patterns. Some, such as MPO, are exquisitely lineage specific; it is a reliably specific marker of myeloid differentiation, as it is not detected in ALL. Others, such as CD2 and CD7 (pan T-cell markers), which are lineage-specific in normal circumstances, are much less so in disease states as they may be expressed aberrantly in AML, for example.

Lineage assignment in acute myeloid leukaemia

For the myeloid leukaemias a 'hierarchy' of lineage determining antigens is recognized (Figure 5.5 and Table 5.3), although only MPO is reliable enough to incorporate into strict lineage assignment criteria. In one study CD33 was the most frequently expressed antigen in AML (but the least specific given its propensity for expression in ALL) at 88% of cases, with CD13, CD117 and MPO each being expressed in up to 75% of cases [14]. Overall, more than 95% of AML cases will express at least one of these antigens [35]. The variable and arbitrary threshold used for

Table 5.3 WHO 2008 criteria for lineage assignation in acute leukaemia.

Lineage	Relevant antigen
Myeloid	MPO positive Monocytic antigens (at least two of CD11c, CD14 or CD64)
T-lineage	Cytoplasmic CD3 or surface CD3 (rare in mixed phenotype AL)
B-lineage	*Strong* CD19 with at least one of: CD79a, cCD22, CD10 strongly expressed *Weak* CD19 with at least two of: CD79a, cCD22, CD10 strongly expressed

The weighting of antigens with regards to lineage specificity allows identification of cases with a mixed phenotype (MPAL) such as B/myeloid or T/myeloid, the diagnosis of which is dependent on the demonstration of myeloid and lymphoid specific antigens as detailed, to be present on the same cell (previously termed biphenotypic AL) or on different populations within the same patient (previously termed bilineage AL). Note that CD117, CD13 and CD33 are not specific enough myeloid antigens to be useful here. Also, the lack of a single truly B-cell specific antigen necessitates the use of multiple B-cell related antigens. It is worth emphasizing that genetic results must also be taken into account here; the identification of AML specific lesions such as t(8;21), t(5;17) or inv(16) would determine a case to be AML. Genetic abnormalities are reported in MPAL, including BCR-ABL and MLL gene rearrangements, but these are clearly not specific. Modified from Swerdlow et al. [1] with permission from Wiley.

describing an antigen as positive in any given population (i.e. percentage of cells expressing it) may contribute to some AMLs being described as MPO negative (discussed further below). This is recognized particularly in AML M0 which is not uncommonly MPO negative (over 80% of cases in one study using a cytochemical approach [14]); in such circumstances CD13, CD33 and CD117 are the most useful antigens for confirming myeloid lineage. For AML exhibiting monocytic differentiation, expression of two or more monocytic antigens indicates myelomonocytic lineage (Table 5.3). It can be seen from these classification rules that AML is easily diagnosed when there is myeloid specific antigen expression (MPO, and/or at least two monocytic markers) *and* without significant T or B-cell lineage specific antigen expression (i.e. lacking cCD3 or B-lineage criteria). Note that many lymphoid associated antigens may be *aberrantly* expressed in AML (and of course *vice versa*), most often in isolation. Care must therefore be taken to avoid erroneous lineage

assignation based upon failure to recognize aberrant antigen expression.

Lineage assignment in acute lymphoblastic leukaemia

In contrast to AML, B lymphoid malignancies do not express any strict B-lineage specific antigens (e.g. CD19, amongst the earliest expressed B-lineage associated antigens, may be found in some cases of AML, often M2 alongside CD56). Emphasis is therefore placed upon the *co-expression* of other B-cell associated antigens alongside CD19 (Table 5.3). Conversely, T-lineage assignment is based upon the detection of CD3, a T-cell specific component of the T-cell receptor brightly expressed in the cytoplasm (termed cCD3) but very occasionally on the cell surface. T or B-ALL is therefore diagnosed when T or B-lineage is established and the absence of myeloid *specific* antigens is confirmed. Note that the term 'specific' here, relates to MPO or monocytic lineage criteria. Non-specific myeloid related antigens include CD13 and CD33, both of which may be aberrantly expressed on B or T-ALL and which do not impact on lineage assignment.

Acute leukaemia of ambiguous lineage

It should be self-evident that the lineage criteria described above may allow assignation of more than one lineage to a blast population; where both myeloid and lymphoid lineage specific antigens are co-expressed on the same cells (historically termed *biphenotypic* AL) or two separate blast populations (i.e. myeloid and B or T-lymphoid) co-exist (historically termed *bilineage* AL). These entities are now described as mixed phenotype acute leukaemia (MPAL) in the most recent WHO classification. Furthermore, by their absence, lineage markers allow identification of rare cases where no differentiation is apparent, classified by the WHO as acute undifferentiated leukaemia (AUL, usually CD34+ HLA-DR+ CD45$^{dim/+}$lin−). Note that the latter diagnosis requires careful exclusion of other rare leukaemias and also non-haemic tumours. The nomenclature can be confusing in this setting, and the most recent WHO classification has sensibly combined these entities under the umbrella term acute leukaemias of ambiguous lineage (which includes AUL and MPAL, summarized in Table 5.4). Readers are referred to the most recent WHO

Table 5.4 Acute leukaemia of ambiguous lineage. The most clearly defined of these rare malignancies are described below. Note that where recurring genetic lesions are described, these have a central role in the classification. Their rarity makes accurate outcome data difficult but it is generally felt that these entities have a poor prognosis. MLL, mixed lineage leukaemia gene.

Diagnosis	Subclassification/description
Acute undifferentiated leukaemia (AUL)	Often CD34+, HLA-DR+. TdT and/or CD38 may be positive. No expression of lymphoid or myeloid specific markers. Exclude megakaryocytic, basophilic, NK- or plasmacytoid dendritic cell tumours. Non-haemic infiltrates should also be excluded.
Mixed phenotype acute leukaemia (MPAL)	MPAL with t(9;22)/BCR-ABL: Meets the strict criteria for MPAL [1]. BCR-ABL is the commonest genetic lesion seen in MPAL, but other genetic abnormalities (sometimes complex) may be seen. Caution required to avoid confusion with lymphoblastic crisis of CML. MPAL with t(v;11q23); MLL rearranged: Meets strict criteria for MPAL [1]. Caution required to avoid confusion with ALL plus MLL rearrangements with aberrant myeloid antigen expression, or even AML with monocytic differentiation plus MLL. These cases most often display a primitive precursor B-cell blast population (often CD15 positive) plus a separate myeloid (often monoblastic) population. MPAL T/myeloid or B/myeloid: These meet the strict criteria for MPAL(1). Myeloid markers (MPO, and often others) co-exist with either B or T-lymphoid specific antigens. By definition they lack the genetic lesions described above.

Adapted from Swerdlow et al. [1], with permission from Wiley.

classification for a full discussion of these rare leukaemias, which is outside the scope of this text [1].

By following these fairly simple rules and being aware of the common pitfalls, lineage assignment in AL should be relatively straightforward. With previous classification systems [40, 41] biphenotypic AL comprised 5.8% of cases in one large series of over 500 AML patients; using current WHO 2008 criteria [32] this figure has now fallen to 1.5% being classified as MPAL [42]. Thus, a majority of these cases are now able to be classified as either ALL or AML (but with aberrant antigen expression). This supports the authors' experience that inappropriate lineage assignment is most commonly as a result of failure to recognize antigen expression as aberrant. This may culminate in treatment failure due to misclassification of AL; for example treatment of an assumed mixed phenotype leukaemia with AML type therapy when in fact the leukaemia was pro-B-ALL with aberrant myeloid expression.

Thus far, the reader should now be able to comfortably distinguish an AL case as either AML, ALL or of ambiguous lineage. These entities will now be further discussed separately and in greater detail.

Acute myeloid leukaemia

The flow cytometric profiles of the WHO-recognized subtypes of AML are summarized in Table 5.5. Note that the pattern of antigen expression generally parodies that of the equivalent normal precursor population, in large part supporting the long-established FAB morphology and cytochemistry-based classification system. Some subtypes have flow cytometric profiles that are better described than others (e.g. compare the large body of literature on the genetically defined APL to that of the rarer and less easily defined AML with erythroid or megakaryoblastic differentiation). In almost all flow cytometry texts considerable weight is given to patterns of aberrant antigen expression in AML subgroups, which can in some cases be relatively specific to the disorder in question (e.g. co-expression of CD19 and CD56 in AML with t(8;21)), but less so in others (e.g. CD2 expression in both inv(16) and t(15;17)). The significance of these aberrancies and their diagnostic and prognostic significance are detailed in Table 5.5.

WORKED EXAMPLE 5.1

The flow plots below show an example of mixed phenotype acute leukaemia (B-ALL/myeloid). The cells are CD34+, MPO+, TdT+, cCD79a+, CD10+, CD20+. MPO positivity indicates a mixed phenotype acute leukaemia according to WHO criteria for a blast population which otherwise has the phenotype of common ALL. The patient achieved remission with an ALL type induction with added cytarabine but relapsed early and was refractory to further therapy.

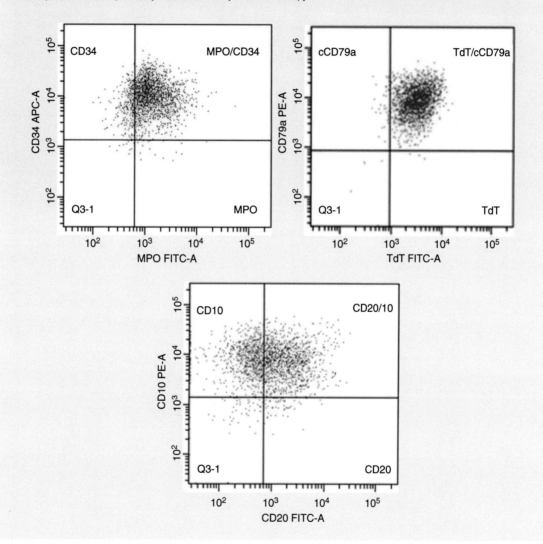

Aberrant and asynchronous antigen expression in acute myeloid leukaemia

Understanding the principle of lineage assignment allows easy identification of *aberrant* antigen expression which is defined as: 'Expression of an antigen that is unexpected on the lineage in question (i.e. is not present during normal maturation), but which does not alter the lineage assignation.'

These patterns are of critical importance; misinterpretation may result in inappropriate lineage assignment and incorrect treatment as noted above. In addition, some

Table 5.5 Summary of immunophenotypic patterns of WHO (2008) Defined AML and related precursor neoplasms. This table provides a reference for the typical immunophenotypic patterns of the WHO AML subtypes. Where appropriate the related FAB subtype is defined, as many published studies on flow in AML predated the WHO classification. Note that where present, specific genetic abnormalities take precedence over flow results in terms of classification (and treatment). Unless otherwise specified the data here are summarized from references [1, 20, 46]. The phenotypes that are most tightly linked to specific genetic abnormalities (namely t(8;21) and t(15;17)) are described in greater detail in the text.

WHO 2008 subtype	Corresponding FAB subtype (where applicable)	Typical antigen expression	Notable negative antigens	Notable and aberrant antigens
AML with t(8;21)(q22;q22); RUNX1-RUNX1T1	AML M2 (occasionally myeloid sarcoma, M1 or M4)	CD34, HLA-DR, MPO, CD117 (all in >95% of cases) CD13, CD33 (weak); some CD11b, CD15 and CD65		CD19 (weak) and CD56 in most cases (approx 80%); note TdT and CD79a may also be expressed [27]
AML with inv(16)(p13.1q22) or t(16;16)(p13.1;q22); CBFB-MYH11	AML M4 (eo) (occasionally M1, M2, M2 (eo) or M4/5 morphology)	CD34, HLA-DR, CD117 on primitive blasts, with heterogeneous subpopulations of CD13, CD33, CD65, MPO (myeloblasts) and CD4, CD14, CD64 (monoblasts); CD11b pos	MPO may be negative in monoblastic population	CD2 is often observed [9], but is not specific for this subtype Occasional TdT expression reported
APL with t(15;17)(q22;q12); PML-RARA	AML M3	High SSC, CD117 (occasionally weak), CD13 (heterogenous), CD33 (bright), and typically CD64	HLA-DR and CD34 typically negative CD11b and CD11c absent (specific for APL) [43] CD15 and CD65 usually negative (or weak)	CD56 (20%) of cases (possible poor prognostic marker) Microgranular variant more likely to express CD2 (and CD34)
AML with t(9;11)(p22;q23); MLLT3-MLL	Most typically AML M4 and M5; most cases are M5a	Some (rarely all) monocytic or monoblastic markers expressed; CD4, CD11b, CD11c, CD14, CD36, CD64; variable CD34 and CD117 expression. CD33, CD15 and HLA-DR usually +; CD13 variable	Note that CD14 is frequently negative, particularly in monoblastic (M5a) cases	CD7 and/or CD56 may be expressed
AML with t(6;9)(p23;q34); DEK-NUP214	Most typically AML M2 or M4 (with basophilia)	'Generic AML' phenotype, namely CD13, CD33, HLA-DR; usually CD117, CD34, CD15+; some CD64+		Some TdT positive cases reported
AML with inv(3)(q21q26.2) or t(3;3)(q21;q26.2); RPN1-EVI1	Any FAB category (not M3); cases of M7 well recognized.	'Generic AML' phenotype, CD13, CD33, usually CD34; some cases express CD41 and CD61		CD7 expression reported
AML (megakaryoblastic) with t(1;22)(p13;q13); RBM15-MKL1	AML M7, restricted to infants and young children	CD13, CD33, CD36, CD41 and CD61 usually positive.	Note CD34, CD45 and HLA-DR may be negative MPO negative; CD11b and CD15 usually negative	CD7 expression reported

Entity	FAB correlation	Immunophenotype		Other notes
AML with mutated NPM1	Usually AML M4 and M5, other FAB subtypes seen (not M3)	CD13, CD33, MPO+; most HLA-DR+; some monocytic markers, notably CD11b, CD14 and CD68	Typically associated with lack of CD34, independent of cell maturational stage	Occasional CD7; note that cytoplasmic (as opposed to nuclear) NPM1 as detected by flow, is a useful surrogate for the mutation [44]
AML with mutated CEBPA	Mainly AML M1, other categories reported	CD13, CD33, CD11b, CD15, CD34 and HLA-DR most frequently		CD7 in 50–75%
AML with MDS-related changes	Any FAB criteria (not M3), often AML M6	Very variable, non-specific; blasts usually CD13, CD33, CD34+		CD7, CD56 and TdT reported
Therapy-related myeloid neoplasms		Very variable, non-specific; blasts usually CD13, CD33, CD34+		CD7 and CD56 reported
AML with minimal differentiation	AML M0	CD34, HLA-DR, CD38 usually positive; CD13 and CD117 often positive, CD33 positive in 60%	Lack of granulocytic or monocytic differentiation antigens such as CD11b, CD14, CD15, CD14, CD65; MPO negative on cytochemistry; some cases positive by flow	TdT frequently [45], CD7 in 40%
AML without maturation	AML M1	Similar to above but MPO positive in at least a subpopulation of cells	Lack of granulocytic or monocytic differentiation antigens as above	CD7 in 30% of cases; CD2, CD4, CD19 and CD56 are reported as occasionally positive in 10–20%
AML with maturation	AML M2	CD13, CD33 positive; CD34, CD117, HLA-DR may be positive, sometimes only on a proportion of blasts; presence of granulocytic differentiation antigens; often positive for, CD11b, CD15, CD65	Lack of monocytic antigens	CD7 in up to 30% of cases; CD2, CD4, CD19, CD56 very occasionally positive
Acute myelomonocytic leukaemia	AML M4	CD34, HLA-DR, CD117 on primitive blasts, with subpopulations of CD13, CD33, CD65 MPO (granulocytic) and CD4, CD14, CD64 (monocytic) blasts; CD11b pos; co-expression of CD64 (bright) and CD15 is typical of monocytic differentiation		Up to 30% may express CD7 Other lymphoid markers are rare
Acute monoblastic and monocytic leukaemia	AML M5	CD34 in 30% of case; CD117 more frequent HLA-DR positive almost always. CD13, CD33 (may be bright), CD15 and CD65; usually at least two monocytic markers present; CD11b, CD11c, CD14, CD64, CD68	MPO most likely negative in monoblasts, often positive in promonocytes and monocytes	CD7 and/or CD56 found in approx 25–50% of cases

(Continued)

Table 5.5 (cont'd).

WHO 2008 subtype	Corresponding FAB subtype (where applicable)	Typical antigen expression	Notable negative antigens	Notable and aberrant antigens
Acute erythroid leukaemia	AML M6	Erythroid/myeloid leukaemia: myeloblast population similar to M0/M1 description above; erythroblasts may be GPA pos and CD71 (dim) and/or CD117 pos; pure erythroid leukaemia; no myeloblast component, all erythroblasts	Erythroblasts lack myeloid/ monocytic antigens (including MPO); primitive ones may be GPA neg; often lack CD34 and HLA-DR	CD41 and CD61 have been reported in some cases of pure erythroid leukaemia
Acute megakaryoblastic leukaemia	AML M7	CD13 and CD33 often positive. CD41 and/or CD61 (cytoplasmic staining may be most specific); CD36 positive	CD34, HLA-DR and CD45 can be negative (particularly childhood cases); MPO negative; granulocytic and monocytic markers negative	CD7 reported
Acute basophilic leukaemia		CD13 and/or CD33. CD123, CD203c and CD11b usually positive; CD34 and HLA-DR often positive; CD9 is often positive (not specific)	MPO negative	
Acute panmyelosis with myelofibrosis		Usually CD34, CD117, CD13 and CD33 positive	MPO often negative	
Myeloid sarcoma		Flow of cell suspension; CD13, CD33, CD117 and MPO usually positive in those with myeloid differentiation; CD11c and CD14 may be positive in those with monocytic differentiation		
Myeloid proliferations related to Down's syndrome: transient abnormal myelopoiesis (TAM)		Typically, CD34, CD117, CD13 and CD33. CD41 and CD61 are positive; HLA-DR in approx 30% of cases	MPO, CD14, CD15 and GPA negative	CD7 and CD56 common; CD4 (dim) common
Myeloid proliferations related to Down's syndrome: myeloid leukaemia		Similar to TAM as above, but CD34 and CD41 often negative		Similar to TAM, but CD56 often negative

significance and several segregate closely with particular genetic abnormalities. Aberrant antigen patterns are therefore discussed in some detail in this section.

It is important to recognize that aberrant antigen expression may only be present on a subpopulation of blast cells; a useful but arbitrary practical definition of aberrancy is where the antigen combination in question is found on ≤0.1% of normal marrow cells, but ≥10% of leukaemic blasts [47]. In this particular study of AML, aberrant T-lymphoid, B-lymphoid and NK-cell markers were expressed in 38%, 13% and 21% of AML respectively. The most commonly expressed aberrant antigens on AML include: CD2, CD7, CD19 and CD56. Note that very occasional (i.e. very small) normal myeloid progenitor subpopulations may co-express CD4, CD5, CD7 or occasionally CD56 (particularly in the context of regenerating marrows) [6]. Some steady state myeloid populations may even express these antigens in normal circumstances, most notably $CD4^{dim}$ on monocytes. Conversely, for precursor B or T-ALL commonly expressed aberrant antigens include CD13 and/or CD33 and CD15.

Asynchronous antigen expression is defined as: 'The situation where antigens that are expressed sequentially (but separately) during normal haematopoiesis are found simultaneously on the malignant cells.'

The quantitative threshold described above for aberrant antigen expression has also been used in this setting [47]. Generally this involves antigens associated with an early cell stage being co-expressed with those of a late cell stage, for example CD117 with CD15 in AML or MDS (Figure 5.6).

CD2 positive acute myeloid leukaemia

In normal circumstances CD2 is a pan T and NK-cell marker [48]. However, CD2 is aberrantly expressed on around 5–16% of all AML [8, 47, 49], being most frequently found in APL (approximately 25%) [50, 51] and AML M4Eo. In APL its expression appears to segregate most closely with the microgranular variant (M3v) as compared to the classical hypergranular type (56–80% versus 3–12% respectively) [19, 51]. Its prognostic significance remains uncertain: one recent study suggested that CD2 expression is independently associated with a shorter duration of CR [51]. However, a previous larger study detected significantly better outcomes [50]. Acute myeloid leukaemia with inv(16) and eosinophilia (AML

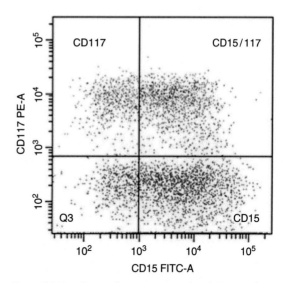

Figure 5.6 Note the asynchronous co-expression of CD117 and CD15 in populations of myeloblasts (blue), but not monoblasts (red) in a case of M4 AML.

M4Eo), a disorder that exhibits particularly heterogeneous blast populations [9], regularly expresses CD2 on a subpopulation of myeloblasts. This entity also has fairly typical morphology, with myeloid and monocytic blasts alongside abnormal basophilic granulated eosinophils.

Outwith these two well-described situations, CD2 may be detected in other cases of AML, such as acute or chronic monocytic leukaemias (<10%) [52, 53]. A handful of CD2 positive AML M0 cases (AML with minimal differentiation) have been described in a number of small studies [36, 45, 54]. In systemic mastocytosis (SM, described in more detail in Chapter 7) CD2 is aberrantly expressed on the surface of neoplastic mast cells; however, as the spectrum of mast cell disease proceeds from indolent SM to aggressive mast cell leukaemia, CD2 expression is frequently lost [55].

CD4 positive acute myeloid leukaemia

CD4 is most commonly recognized as a marker of T-helper cells; however, it is expressed (generally dimly) on normal monocytes [56], eosinophils [57], dendritic cells and subsets of $CD34^+$ precursor cells, including both a phenotypically primitive population as well as a more committed myelomonocytic precursor [58]. Thus, its expression on AML is not true aberrancy; it is included here for completeness and due to the fact that it

WORKED EXAMPLE 5.2

A 36-year-old female presented with anaemia and thrombocytopenia, with circulating myeloblasts and monoblasts in peripheral blood. Bone marrow examination showed dual populations of myeloblasts and monoblasts and prominent eosinophils and eosinophilic precursors, some of which showed aberrant basophilic granulation.

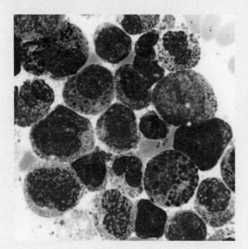 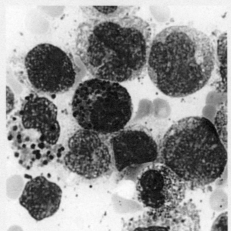

In the immunophenotyping studies note the differential behaviour of the myeloblasts (blue) and monoblasts (red), particularly in terms of their light scatter properties and expression of CD34, CD14/CD64 and MPO. Note both populations express CD2. If gating was performed purely using CD34 positive cells then the monoblasts would be neglected and the true blast proportion underestimated.

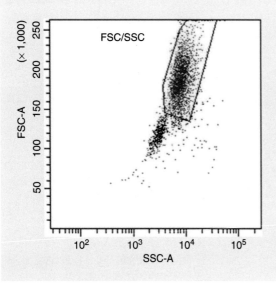 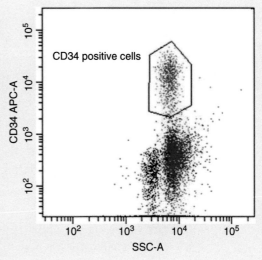

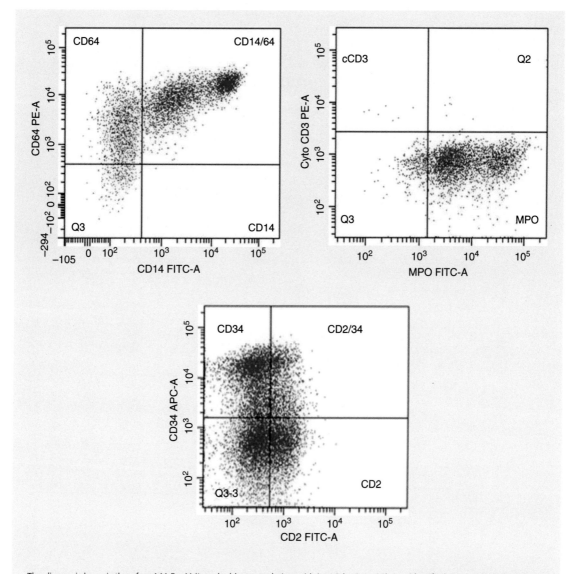

The diagnosis here, is therefore M4 Eo AML and a blast population with inv16 (p13.1;q22) was identified on cytogenetic studies.

can be erroneously assumed to be synonymous with a T-cell phenotype (perhaps through its common recognition as the receptor for HIV). It is worth noting that CD4+ restricted T-ALL is very rare, with by far the majority of cases being CD4+/CD8+ or CD4-/CD8-. CD4 is found relatively frequently in AML ([59] most often on those of monoblastic/monocytic lineage from 50% [36] to >90% [19]) and in occasional cases, dimly expressed, of APL. It is also a frequent finding in histiocytic tumours and CMML. One other important situation in which it is found is in conjunction with CD56 on blastic plasmacytoid dendritic cell neoplasm. This rare and aggressive tumour can resemble acute leukaemia morphologically [1]. It is further discussed in detail later in this chapter.

WORKED EXAMPLE 5.3

A 26-year-old male presented with pancytopenia. The peripheral blood smear showed a number of nucleolated agranular blast cells without features of differentiation. Marrow examination showed 70% blasts with similar morphology.

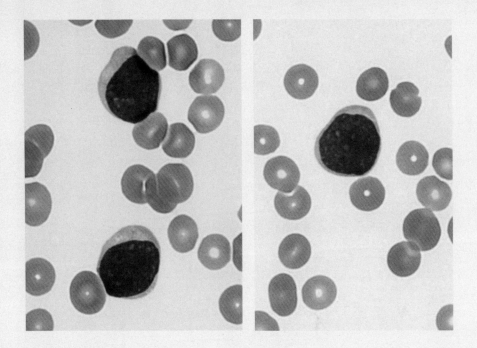

Flow cytometry identified a primitive MPO⁻ myeloblast population expressing CD34, TdT, CD38 (and a subpopulation expressing CD56) together with aberrant CD7. This is a typical example of M0 AML.

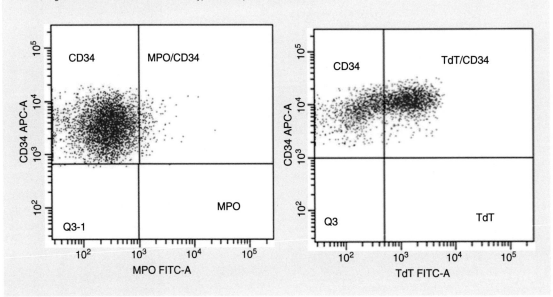

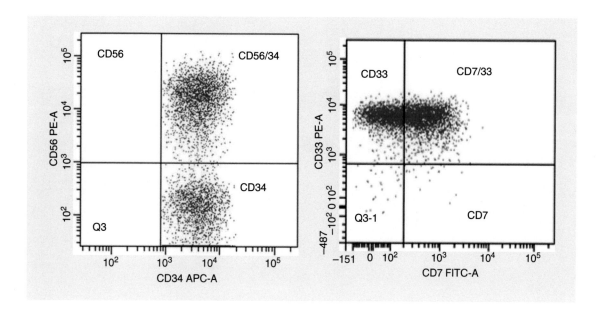

CD7 positive acute myeloid leukaemia

CD7, a surface glycoprotein, is a pan-T cell marker also found on thymocytes and NK cells. It is expressed very early on during T-lineage commitment and on occasional primitive normal myeloid precursors [60]. It is the most commonly detected aberrant lymphoid marker on AML, being found on 25–37% of cases [37, 61]. Its expression is not restricted to any particular subtype of AML (but it is typically absent from APL), although it's frequent association with markers of primitive myeloblasts (i.e. CD34 and TdT) have led some to associate it with more primitive disease [62]. In keeping with this observation Kaleem et al. described it in almost 50% of AML M0, compared with 25% of AML M1 and M2 disease [36]. Although included in small numbers, 50% of AML M7 also expressed CD7. Many, but not all studies, have identified it as a marker of poor outcome with reduced CR rates reported (reviewed in [62]). CD7 was a frequent finding in high risk MDS and secondary AML in one study, while not being detected on the blasts of lower risk disease [63]. Its association with CD56 in MPO negative cases led Suzuki et al. to propose a novel 'myeloid/NK' precursor acute leukaemia [64], an aggressive disorder with a poor outcome. The WHO does not draw a distinction between these cases and primitive AML, however [1], and currently recommends they should be regarded as such.

M0 type AML blasts are often small with nucleoli and scant agranular cytoplasm. They give few anatomical clues to lineage and can be difficult to differentiate morphologically from lymphoblasts.

CD19 positive acute myeloid leukaemia

CD19 expression (generally dim) is well recognized in AML, particularly in cases associated with the t(8;21) (q22;q22) translocation (although it is not specific for this feature) [47, 65]. Rare CML myeloid blast crisis cases with t(8;21) may also express CD19 [66]. Two large studies identified CD19 in approximately 75% of t(8;21) AML (usually in conjunction with CD56 [27]) in comparison to only 12% of other AML cases [27, 65]. Its expression is, however, considerably less intense than is found on typical progenitor B-ALL [65] and it can easily be missed. This unusual phenotype (CD19+, CD34+, CD56+) is hardly present in normal bone marrow (<0.01% of cells [67]) and is now regarded as predictive for t(8;21). Interestingly, the mechanism for its expression has recently been explained and would appear to be due to PAX5, a transcriptional activator of B-cell differentiation, which is also detectable in such cases [68]. PAX5 binds specifically to the promoter and enhancer region of the CD19 gene, thereby allowing its expression. The morphology in t(8;21) M2 AML is also fairly characteristic,

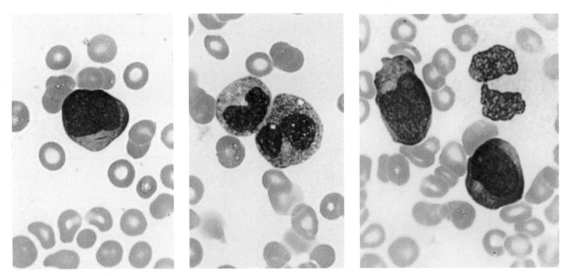

Figure 5.7 Typical morphology of blasts and neutrophils in t(8;21) M2 AML.

with large granular blasts showing frequent Auer rods alongside maturation to granular but dysplastic neutrophils (Figure 5.7).

TdT positive acute myeloid leukaemia

TdT is expressed transiently in cell nuclei during early T- and B-lymphocyte development and its nuclear location necessitates a cell permeabilization step to optimize staining for flow cytometric analysis. TdT⁺ myeloid cells in normal marrow are extremely rare (<0.03% of cells) [69]. Outwith the B and T-ALL setting (where it is expressed in >90% of cases) it is occasionally expressed in AML, with overall estimates of its frequency at around 10% of cases [20]. TdT is therefore clearly *not* lineage specific (*but is precursor-cell specific*), and its presence does not therefore automatically imply a diagnosis of ALL. In AML, TdT is most commonly reported in AML with minimal differentiation (AML M0), where it is found in approximately 50% of cases, albeit usually at a low intensity (certainly less so than is usual in ALL) [36]. It may also be found (infrequently) in AML M1 and M2 with t(8;21), often in conjunction with CD19 and CD56 as described above [70]. An interesting study detailing the heterogeneity of the blast population of AML M4Eo documented frequent TdT expression in the primitive (CD34⁺) myeloblast compartment, although overall this often represented only a small proportion of all leukaemic cells [9] (Figure 5.2). This group also described small CD34⁺ TdT⁺ myeloid

subpopulations in other cases of AML, again reflecting the cellular heterogeneity of this disorder [69]. It has also been reported in occasional cases of AUL [71].

CD56 positive acute myeloid leukaemia

Detection of CD56 in any malignancy should give rise to some careful thought, due to the well-recognized promiscuity of this antigen. It is otherwise known as neural cell adhesion molecule (N-CAM), which in normal circumstances is expressed on NK cells [72] and small subsets of T cells, including a cytotoxic CD8⁺ population [73]. Because of the latter it cannot simply be regarded as an NK-specific antigen.

CD56 expression has been reported at low level on the surface of granulocytes and monocytes in G-CSF driven marrows [6], reactive monocytosis [74] and on a probable functionally distinct subpopulation of normal monocytes at steady-state (approximately 1–2% of total monocytes) [75, 76]. Intensity and extent of expression are therefore important factors to take into account to differentiate true aberrant CD56⁺ abnormal populations from reactive or rare normal cells. It is expressed on a wide variety of tumour cells, both in haematological and solid cancers and a good working knowledge of this range of expression is useful to allow accurate interpretation and, more importantly, avoid misdiagnosis. Expression of CD56 on AML blasts occurs in approximately 10–30% of cases and it has been variously associated with drug-resistance, extramedullary disease and poor out-come. Its expression is well described in several AML subtypes, as well as related myeloid disorders, as follows:

1 It is found on a subset of cases of myeloid sarcoma (10–15%), which together with expression of CD68, MPO and CD117 (and occasionally CD34 and TdT) on paraffin section should avoid confusion with either another 'solid' haematological malignancy (e.g. lymphoma) or a solid tumour [77].

2 A subgroup of AML M0, described by some authors as myeloid/NK precursor AL. This rare entity remains unrecognized by the WHO classification, but displays a typical immunophenotype akin to AML M0 (CD34+, HLA-DR+, MPO+/- CD33+) as well as aberrant CD7 and CD56 [64]. Clinically it presents with extramedullary disease (including lymphadenopathy and/or mediastinal masses) and would seem to have a particularly poor prognosis. It remains classified as likely primitive AML by the WHO [1].

3 In AML M2 its co-expression with CD19 is tightly associated with the presence of the t(8;21) translocation, where CD56 expression is reported in a majority of cases and seems to predict for relapse and reduced overall survival in this otherwise good prognostic group [27, 78, 79].

4 It is detectable on 10–20% of AML M3, where it is reported to predict for short remission duration and extramedullary relapse [80, 81].

5 AML M5: up to 50% of acute monoblastic (AML M5a) and acute monocytic (AML M5b) leukaemias may be positive for CD56, again often in association with CD7 [52].

6 AML and transient abnormal myelopoiesis (TAM) in Down's syndrome, where a majority of cases express aberrant CD56 and CD7 and frequently the megakaryocytic markers CD41 and CD61 [82].

7 MDS blasts not infrequently express CD56, as do cases of AML with MDS-related changes [63] and therapy-related MDS/AML often in conjunction with CD7 [1]. It is also expressed on up to 80% of CMML monocyte populations [74], where in conjunction with other aberrancies it is useful to distinguish from reactive mono-cytosis (see Chapter 7).

Due to the promiscuity of CD56 expression it is important to recognize the other situations (outside of AML and related myeloid disorders) where it may be found. For completeness, these are highlighted in this section and are as follows:

1 ALL: it is detected on T-ALL (approximately 10–15%), where it has been noted to be associated with frequent aberrant myeloid marker co-expression (CD13 and/or CD33), CD34 and HLA-DR positivity a non-thymic phenotype and reduced CR rates [83]. Overall, survival was, however, no different in CD56+ as compared with CD56− cases within the risk-adapted treatment trial population in which this was described. The presence of TCR rearrangements and lack of other NK markers described in this study precludes such cases arising from a common NK/T precursor cell. Its expression in B-ALL is rare, but recognized in very occasional cases [84, 85].

2 Mature T-cell disorders: it can be detected in a range of mature T and NK-cell malignancies. These are discussed in Chapter 6.

3 Myeloma: it is expressed on neoplastic plasma cells in most cases of multiple myeloma, discussed in Chapter 8.

4 Blastic plasmacytoid dendritic cell neoplasm.

5 Non-haemopoietic tumours: it is co-expressed with CD117 in small cell/neuroendocrine tumours and neuro-blastoma which often involve marrow and might lead to confusion with AML (these tumours are of course CD45 and MPO negative and positive for other non-haemic antigens) [86].

Other non-myeloid antigens in acute myeloid leukaemia

CD3 and CD8 are generally not reported in AML [1]. However, a recent study reported an occasional case as positive [87], although in the authors' experience and others [36] this is particularly rare. Few studies have reported on the presence or absence of CD10, a surface molecule present on B and T-cell precursors, follicle (germinal) centre B-cells and mature granulocytes. Note the latter; CD10 is not a true lymphoid specific antigen but is included here for completeness. It is generally considered to be absent from AML (but is of course common on B and less so T-precursor ALL), although two studies have identified its expression in very occasional cases (<3% [36, 88]). Its presence on a precursor cell neoplasm should therefore demand careful scrutiny of all relevant lymphoid markers. CD5, a co-stimulatory molecule involved in the regulation of immune tolerance, is expressed on the surface of some normal B and most T-lymphoid cells [48]. It has been described on the surface of 16% of AML cases in one recent small study [87], considerably more than in previous larger series (5–6%) [47, 88]. It has also been described as more frequent on acute monoblastic leukaemia [88]. These observations are, however, inconsistent, with at least one large study detecting no CD5$^+$ AML cases [36]. Its prognostic significance, if any, is unknown. CD25 is regarded as an activation antigen, being a component of the surface receptor for IL-2. While not detected on normal marrow myeloid cells, it can be induced via incubation with IL-3 [89] and has been detected on up to 12% of AML [47] including LSC where it might present a legitimate target for antibody therapy [90]. It is also expressed on normal basophils [91], the rare acute basophilic leukaemia [92], as well as mast cell leukaemia. Note that while CD2 would appear to decrease in expression with more aggressive mast cell disease, CD25 continues to be expressed (reviewed in Valent *et al.* [93]). One additional situation where it may be expressed in conjunction with (aberrant) myeloid antigens is in *BCR-ABL*$^+$ progenitor B-ALL which should be easy to distinguish from AML [94].

Antigenic patterns of particular significance in acute myeloid leukaemia

Certain recurring patterns of antigen expression in AML are worthy of separate consideration, particularly with regards to failure of expression. Their recognition and interpretation are of importance in correct classification. These are:

1 MPO negative AML
2 CD34 and HLA-DR negative AML

These are discussed in further detail below.

Myeloperoxidase negative acute myeloid leukaemia

Myeloperoxidase is a lysozyme enzyme expressed in the cytoplasm of myeloid cells (particularly the azurophilic granules of neutrophils, but also CD34$^+$ and CD34$^-$ myeloid precursor cells, promonocytes and monocytes). Its intracellular location requires a cell permeabilization step prior to its detection by flow cytometry. Myeloperoxidase is a critical lineage associated antigen and recent guidelines have suggested using 10% of cells as a threshold for positivity [25] in a similar fashion to TdT, CD34 and CD117. Published studies where a high cut-off was used (such as 20%) have unsurprisingly shown a high frequency of MPO negative AML by flow, particularly in cases with minimal differentiation (in a study by Kaleem *et al.* almost 30% of AML M0 was negative for MPO by flow cytometry [36]). Further confusing this picture is

that conventional cytochemistry has historically used 3% as a cut-off. A recent study proposed such a cut-off for flow cytometric detection of MPO, where at this level sensitivity of flow was found to be superior to cytochemistry [39]. A very few cases in this study were MPO positive by cytochemistry alone. Although cytochemistry continues to receive considerable mention in the literature, in the authors' experience many UK diagnostic laboratories have largely abandoned it, as it is cumbersome to prepare as compared to flow. Further studies (likely correlating flow data with genetic lineage profiling) are needed to determine what should be the optimal cut-off for critical antigens such as MPO.

As a result of these inconsistencies it is therefore remarkably difficult to establish the incidence of true MPO-negative AML. Myeloperoxidase is, however, detectable in the vast majority of AML (approximately 70–95% in numerous studies), in particular being positive in AML M1, M2, M3 and M4 and often detectable in M5b (i.e. those subtypes exhibiting some degree of myeloid or monocytic differentiation). Its expression is particularly strong in AML M3 [95]. The situations where MPO may be negative or only very weakly expressed are:

1 Acute monoblastic leukaemia where the monoblastic population is likely to be negative. Promonocytes generally show some MPO positivity and monocytes (normal and leukaemic) are often positive [1].
2 Acute erythroid leukaemia [96], although any myeloblastic component is generally MPO$^+$.
3 Acute megakaryoblastic leukaemia [1].
4 Acute basophilic leukaemia (approximately 80% of cases) [97].
5 Acute mast cell leukaemia [92].

Thus, although MPO is indicative of myeloid differentiation, its absence does not preclude the diagnosis of AML and the latter entities should be considered in MPO-negative cases.

CD34-negative HLA-DR-negative acute myeloid leukaemia

Dual negativity for these antigens in AML is an important finding in clinical practice, as this combination, alongside morphological assessment showing granular blasts with Auer rods, should always raise the possibility of M3 AML (discussed below). The latter represents a haematological emergency and requires very specific early management. Many of these cases will be confirmed as M3 using cytogenetics, FISH or PCR for *PML/RARA*. In a large study comprising 800 cases of all subtypes of AML, a total of 15% of cases were HLA-DR negative [15]. Half of these cases were confirmed as APL, but the remainder were non-APL, a proportion in line with previous studies. Only 16% of the latter were CD34+, so the antigen combination HLA-DR⁻ CD34⁻ is clearly not uncommon outside the APL setting. These cases also demonstrated a not infrequent lack of one or more of CD13, CD33, CD117 or MPO. In contrast, expression of all of these antigens (a 'pan-myeloid' phenotype) was almost always seen in APL. Acute myeloid leukaemia subtypes commonly displaying a CD34⁻ HLA-DR⁻ immunophenotype are discussed in turn below:

Acute promyelocytic leukaemia (APL): APL comprises 10–15% of AML cases. Typical (hypergranular) APL is recognized using a combination of typical morphology (granular promyelocytes, Auer rods, faggotcells and bilobed overlapping reniform nuclei) alongside high SSC, CD34 and HLA-DR negativity and CD117 positivity. Note the latter: while normal promyelocytes lack CD117 APL cells express it, although sometimes at low level [103]. This occurs in the context of a CD13+ (heterogenous), CD33+ (strong homogenous) and MPO+ picture. These antigen patterns lack specificity, however, with only 75% of cases exhibiting a typical CD34⁻, HLA-DR⁻, CD117+ phenotype in one recent study [43]. However, by incorporating antibodies to the adhesion molecules CD11b and CD11c this study was able to identify a specific immunophenotype in 100% of cases of APL, namely CD11b⁻ and CD11c⁻, with >96% of cases also HLA-DR⁻. CD11b and CD11c were consistently negative (the former in the maturing myeloid/granulocytic compartment and the latter in all cells including myeloblasts), irrespective of CD34 status, and allowed easy differentiation from residual normal CD11b+ CD11c+ myeloid cells and blasts of other AML subtypes. Complicating this well-defined picture, however, is the microgranular variant of APL (AML M3v), which often expresses CD2, CD34 and HLA-DR (at least on a fraction of cells) and the typical immunophenotype described above is often absent. Interestingly, this phenotype correlates closely with the expression of a particular *PML-RARA* molecular variant (the so-called S-form) [104]. In recognition of this some authors suggest that the detection of CD2+ AML should prompt PCR for *PML-RARA* (particularly in hypogran-

ular cases) [103]. The aberrant expression of CD56 in APL has been discussed above, where it may be indicative of a poorer outcome [84].

6 Acute leukaemia with NPM 1 and/or FLT 3 ITD mutation: NPM1 mutations are detected in 86% of CD34⁻ HLA-DR⁻ AML cases. These mutations were also found in 72% of CD34⁻HLA DR+ AML, but are much less common in CD34+ cases (11–40%) [15]. Interestingly 'Cup-like' cytomorphology and pseudo-Chediak granulation is particularly associated with the CD34⁻ HLA-DR⁻ AML phenotype [101], with both flt-3 internal tandem duplication (flt3-ITD) and NPM1 mutations being commonly detected.

7 Acute leukaemia NOS: we have encountered a series of other CD34⁻ HLA-DR⁻ AML cases, which also had granular blasts with Auer rods such that they might have been mistaken for APL (unpublished observation). Unlike APL, however, the blasts were often small, with nuclear pleomorphism and clefts and showed some differentiation to dysplastic neutrophils. These cases have had normal cytogenetics and without a recurring molecular abnormality. Immunophenotypically they are similar but often show weak or absent CD13 and are positive for CD56. It remains to be determined whether these cases represent a distinct biological entity. Series of similar cases have been reported and have been described as myeloid/natural killer cell acute leukaemias.

8 Erythroleukaemia and megakaryoblastic leukaemia: these two entities have clinical and morphological characteristics that should allow easy differentiation from APL as well as a distinctive immunophenotypic profile (Table 5.4).

Finally we should mention basophils, which in normal circumstances are typically CD34⁻ HLA-DR⁻, and when in excess may occasionally cause some diagnostic confusion (reviewed in Lichtman and Segel [92]) particularly as they often fall into the blast gate on CD45/SSC plots due to loss of granules during processing [18]. In contrast, clonal basophilia associated with haematological disorders (e.g. in CML) and true acute basophilic leukaemia would appear to be HLA-DR+ [91, 98].

Identifying particular acute myeloid leukaemia subtypes by flow

The WHO and FAB defined AML subtypes are summarized in Table 5.4 with regards to flow characteristics.

WORKED EXAMPLE 5.4

A 39-year-old male presented with a short history of lethargy and bruising with almost continuous bleeding from his gums and nose. The FBC showed Hb 80 g/L, WBC 1.0×10^9/L (neutrophils 0.3) and platelets 40×10^9/L. Coagulation studies showed PT 12 sec (NR 12–14), APTT 28 (NR 30–34), Fibrinogen 0.8 g/L (NR 2–4.5) and D dimer 25,000 units (NR < 230). The peripheral blood smear showed occasional hypergranular promyelocytes with a proportion containing Auer rods. The bone marrow aspirate showed a large population of malignant hypergranular promyelocytes including faggot cells with multiple Auer rods.

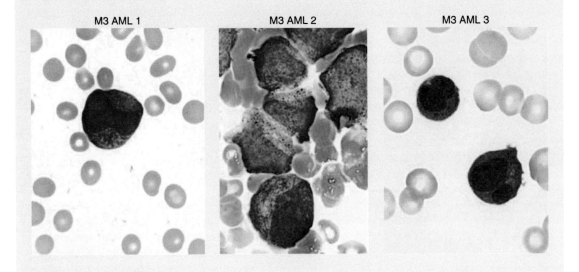

M3 AML 1   M3 AML 2   M3 AML 3

Immunophenotyping studies on bone marrow, using a blast gate, are shown below.

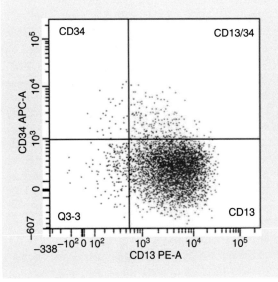

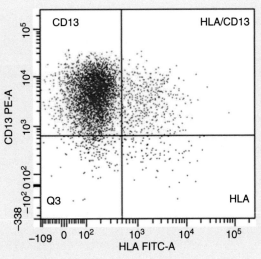

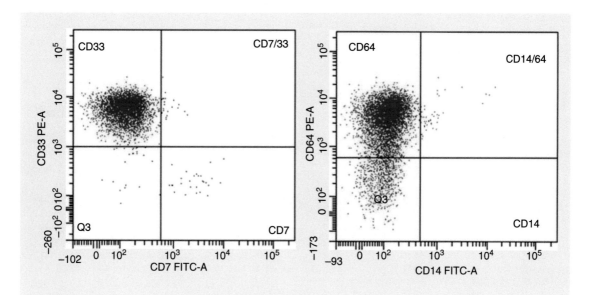

Note the CD34 and HLA-DR negativity, homogenous CD33+, heterogenous CD13+ and CD64 expression. This is a typical hypergranular acute promyelocytic leukaemia immunophenotype. Cytogenetic studies confirmed a t(15;17) (q22;q12) translocation.

WORKED EXAMPLE 5.5

A 50-year-old female presented with a similar short history and marked mucosal and skin haemorrhage. An FBC showed Hb 95 g/L, WBC 45×10⁹/L, (neutrophils 0.2) and platelets 55×10⁹/L. She also had a coagulopathy in keeping with DIC. Abnormal hypogranular promyelocytes were easily identified in peripheral blood. The absence of prominent granules should not detract from the diagnosis as the presence of bilobed, reniform nuclei is highly suggestive of the hypogranular variant of acute promyelocytic leukaemia.

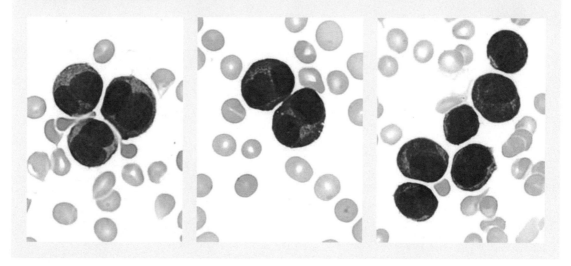

Immunophenotyping studies on bone marrow, using a CD34$^+$ gate, are shown below. Note a proportion of malignant promyelocytes are showing a degree of granularity and show increased side scatter in the lower portion of the gate.

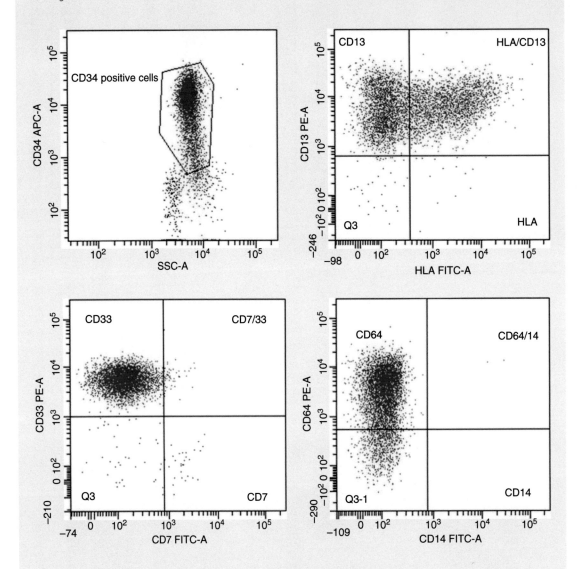

Note that although this case is expressing CD34 and HLA-DR, there are a number of similarities to the case above in terms of homogenous CD33$^+$, heterogenous CD13$^+$ and CD64 expression in the absence of CD14. Although CD34 and HLA DR are expressed this is also heterogenous, with cells showing a spectrum of positivity. Hypogranular APML has been misdiagnosed as acute monoblastic leukaemia so attention should be paid, not just to antigen positivity, but to the flow cytometric behaviour of the antigen positive cells. This case also was confirmed to have a t(15;17) (q22;q12) translocation.

WORKED EXAMPLE 5.6

A 49-year-old female presented with a short history of profound lethargy and pain from a deep dental infection that had failed to resolve with antibiotic therapy. An FBC showed Hb 70 g/L, WBC 350×10⁹/L, and platelets 27×10⁹/L. D dimers were markedly elevated but the PT, APTT and fibrinogen were normal. The peripheral blood smear was informative, showing predominantly undifferentiated partially granulated myeloid blasts, without typical features of APL, with prominent cup-like nuclear invaginations and pseudo Chediak granules (centre image).

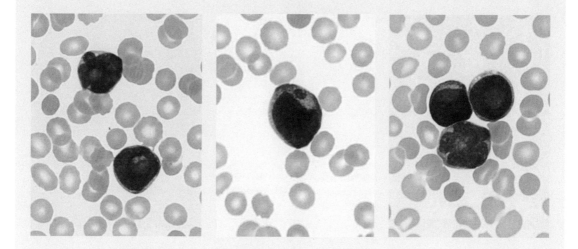

Flow cytometry analysis generated the following characteristics.

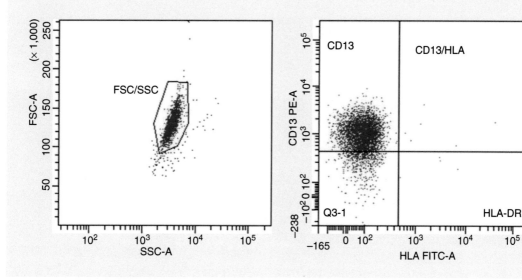

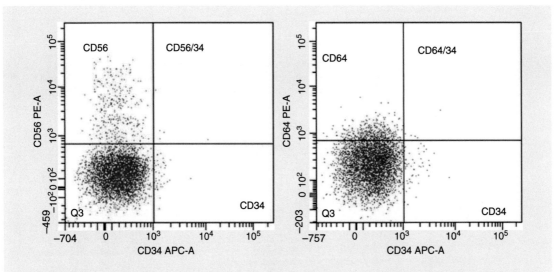

Note the CD34⁻, HLA-DR⁻, CD13⁺ homogenous, CD64⁻, CD56⁻ phenotype. Further studies showed normal standard cytogenetics: molecular studies identified a FLT3 ITD mutation alongside NPM1 positivity. Although there are some similarities with APL, a careful morphological and immunophenotypic study should differentiate the two prior to the cytogenetic/molecular workup.

WORKED EXAMPLE 5.7

A 63-year-old female presented with a short history of lethargy and bruising. FBC showed Hb 90 g/L, WBC 27×10⁹/L, and platelets 15×10⁹/L. The peripheral blood smear showed small granular myeloid blasts with prominent nuclear clefts and folds, but without cup-like forms, classic bilobed cells or faggots. Dysplastic neutrophils were evident. The coagulation profile was normal apart from elevated D dimers.

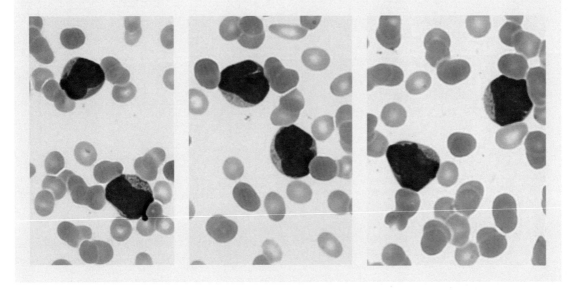

Flow cytometric analysis generated the following characteristics.

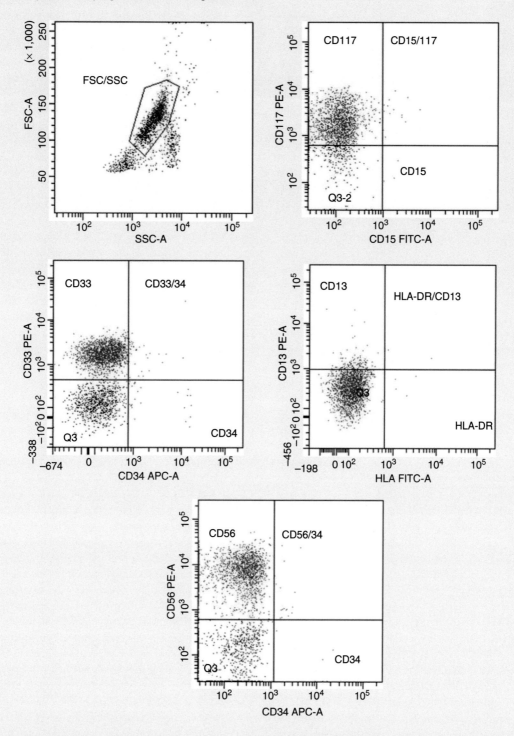

Note that in addition to the CD34⁻, HLA-DR⁻ phenotype these cells show relatively low FSC, loss of CD13, but with expression of CD33 and CD56. Cytogenetic and molecular studies revealed no abnormality. Further studies are needed to determine whether this leukaemia represents a distinct biological entity.

It can be seen that few patterns of antigen expression are specific for the subtype in question; however, some characteristic patterns are seen. Some of these have particular genetic and/or morphological associations and are important to recognize (e.g. to direct downstream genetic testing) and are discussed in greater detail below. Acute promyelocytic leukaemia has been discussed above.

1 Acute monocytic and monoblastic leukaemias: this subgroup of AML is characterized by a blast population (including promonocytes) of ≥ 20%, and typically ≥ 80% of leukaemic cells being of monocytic lineage. Identification and enumeration of neoplastic monoblasts, promonocytes and monocytes can be challenging for both the morphologist and cytometrist. Monoblastic leukaemias (M5a) often show very large blasts with prominent nucleoli with voluminous agranular cytoplasm. Monocytic leukaemia blasts (M5b) show more monocytic characteristics, with some preservation of nuclear convolution and folding, and pale blue vacuolated cytoplasm. These leukaemias have an affinity for extramedullary tissues and tend to cause gingival infiltration, leukaemia cutis and CNS involvement. Monocyte precursors may be difficult to differentiate morphologically from dysplastic, hypogranular myelocytes in AML and CMML, and CD34⁻ monoblasts may be difficult to differentiate by flow from more mature cells. Furthermore, neoplastic monocytes may occupy a similar position on SSC/CD45 plots to that of normal monocytes. Flow cytometry can resolve some of these difficulties. Bright CD14, CD15, CD33, CD64 and HLA-DR are useful to identify mature cells of monocytic lineage, although (with the exception of CD14) they are not specific. The expression of HLA-DR, CD14 and CD15 should distinguish them from hypogranular APL. Neoplastic monocytes may exhibit altered antigen intensity from normal; strong CD64 expression is particularly useful for distinguishing AML M5 from other CD64 dim AML [99]. Most cases of AML M5 are CD34 and CD117 negative (70%) [52], although in one study while CD117 was rarely detected in the more mature AML M5b it was seen frequently in AML M5a [88]. The more primitive monoblastic cases are often MPO negative as MPO is generally expressed from the promonocyte stage onwards. CD14, while specific for the monocytic lineage is, however, an insensitive marker for monocytic leukaemia (i.e. it is often negative) [52, 99]

although this can be epitope dependent (see Chapter 7). CD7 and/or CD56 are aberrantly expressed in up to 40% of cases [1]. For treatment purposes it is particularly important that AML of monocytic lineage be distinguished from CMML.

2 Acute erythroid leukaemia (AML M6): along with AML M7, AML M6 is a relatively rare form of AML (<5%) and case series are generally small, with variable use of antibody panels. Acute erythroid leukaemia comprises two entities: erythroleukaemia (comprising ≥50% erythroid precursors and ≥20% myeloblasts in the non-erythroid compartment) and the rare pure erythroid leukaemia (comprising ≥80% erythroblasts and lacking any significant myeloblast population) [1]. Morphological assessment is of central importance in the diagnosis of M6, as antibodies specific to early erythroblasts are lacking. The erythroid precursors generally exhibit marked dysplasia with vacuolation with frequent apoptotic cells, and an accurate differential count is required for proper classification (Figure 5.8). The erythroblast immunophenotype in both conditions is similar. In addition to absence of CD45 and CD34, the transferrin receptor CD71 is typically bright on erythroblasts, but is also expressed on precursor and activated cell types of other lineages and so lacks specificity. Likewise CD36, which is expressed on erythroid progenitors, appears also on monocytes and megakaryocytes. Glycophorin A and HLA-DR are variably expressed, and MPO is negative in erythroid cells, while the myeloblast population is usually CD13⁺, CD33⁺ and CD117⁺. CD41 and CD61 have variously been reported as positive on erythroblasts but this finding remains to be confirmed.

3 Acute megakaryoblastic leukaemia (AML M7): this condition is even less common than AML M6, and exhibits considerable biological and clinical heterogeneity. Megakaryoblasts are very variable in appearance, showing a spectrum of features: some blasts are small and retain some clues to identity such as fluffy, indistinct or blebbed cytoplasm amongst a background of megakaryocyte dysplasia. Other cases comprise large myeloid type blasts with few or no specific characteristics. This subtype of AML might be suspected according to clinical circumstances such as difficulty aspirating marrow, presentation in infants or as a late development in adults with a history of a myeloproliferative disorder. At least one of the commonly used megakaryocyte markers CD41a and CD61

WORKED EXAMPLE 5.8

A 56-year-old female presented with lethargy, bone pain, skin nodules and gingival swelling. An FBC showed Hb 60 g/L, WBC 56×109/L, and platelets 25×109/L. The peripheral blood smear showed a large population of monoblasts with a degree of attempted differentiation with nuclear folding, occasional vacuoles and pale blue cytoplasm.

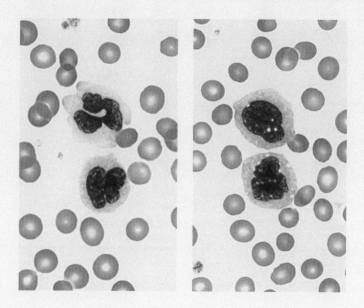

Immunophenotyping showed these cells to be CD34⁻, CD117⁻, CD13⁺, CD33⁺, HLA-DR⁺, CD38⁺ CD14/64⁺ in keeping with acute monoblastic leukaemia, M5b.

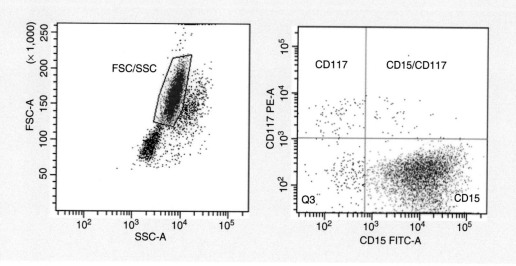

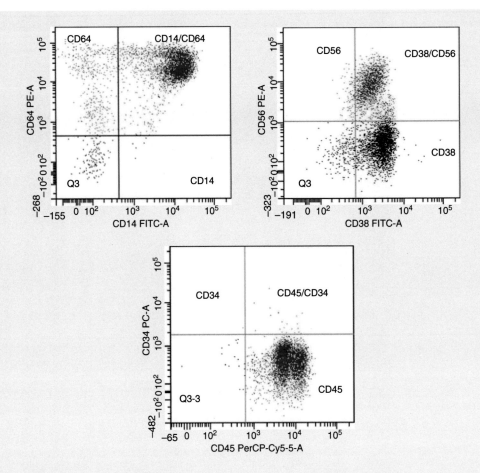

A second patient with a very similar presentation, but without cutaneous deposits, had a peripheral smear showing larger undifferentiated monoblasts with prominent nucleoli.

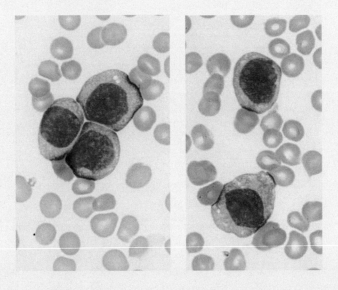

Immunophenotyping showed these cells to be CD34$^-$, CD117^{dim}, CD13$^+$, CD33$^+$, HLA-DR$^+$, CD14$^-$, CD64$^+$ in keeping with acute monoblastic leukaemia, M5a. Note that the lack of CD14 on the CD64$^+$ monoblast population defines a less mature immunophenotype. Cytogenetics and FISH identified an 11q23 (MLL) translocation.

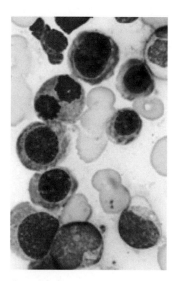 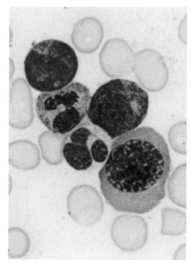 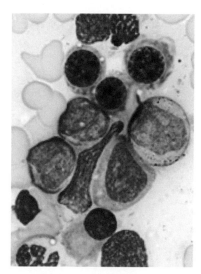

Figure 5.8 Bone marrow aspirate in erythroleukaemia showing pleomorphic dysplastic left shifted erythroid precursors alongside a myeloblast population.

were positive in 90% of a recent large series, with CD42b found less frequently [100]. Care must be taken to avoid false positivity with these antigens (as a result of adherent platelets to leucocytes) and cytoplasmic staining may be more specific [101]. CD13 and CD33 are commonly positive, as is CD36. CD34 may be detected (up to 75% in one study [100]) and aberrant CD7 is not uncommon. The diagnosis is often suspected morphologically (in the above series morphology was diagnostic or highly suspicious in almost 90% of cases), and can be used to select appropriate antibody panels. Many laboratories incorporate these antibodies routinely, but the authors' practice is to use them in morphologically suspicious cases or in cases with poorly differentiated blasts, including MPO negative cases.

4 Blastic plasmacytoid dendritic cell neoplasm: this rare and unusual tumour exhibits a typical clinical picture, presenting with ulcerating nodular skin lesions, followed later by bone marrow and blood involvement and sometimes lymphadenopathy. It is important to recognize for treatment purposes. Its typical immunophenotype is: CD4+ CD56+ CD123+ blast cells, occasionally with CD7, CD33 and/or TdT in some cases. CD34, CD117 and MPO are negative and rare cases are CD4 or CD56 negative. Given its clinical presentation and CD4/CD56 positivity there is a potential for it to be misinterpreted as a monoblastic leukaemia, but it is notably CD64 and CD14 negative. Acute myeloid leukemia, CMML, extranodal

NK/T lymphoma and mature T-cell lymphomas – all of which can involve the skin – should be excluded.

Precursor lymphoid neoplasms (acute lymphoblastic leukaemia/lymphoma)

There are two major categories of ALL, namely those of T or B-lineage. These are clearly distinguishable by flow cytometry. Flow may also be of use in further defining acute lymphoblastic *leukaemia* versus lymphoblastic *lymphoma* (using a cut-off of 25% marrow blasts, while keeping in mind the caveats on blast enumeration discussed previously). This is an important distinction to make as some treatment protocols alter therapy on that basis. The FAB classification of ALL (Table 5.1) is of little practical use (being based on cytomorphology of the blasts), while the WHO does not recognize a flow based subclassification of B or T-ALL and instead uses genetic and molecular findings. A very elegant flow based classification mirroring stages of normal lymphoid maturation is widely recognized in the literature and comes from the EGIL classification (Table 5.6 and Table 5.7). Several well-defined clinical-genotypic subtypes exist within these flow-defined subgroups and will be discussed further in this section.

As has already been discussed, the immunophenotype of ALL is generally much more homogeneous than for

WORKED EXAMPLE 5.9

A 74-year-old male with a ten-year history of primary polycythaemia, well controlled with hydroxycarbamide therapy, presented with a rapid onset of anaemia. Pleomorphic blasts, some primitive but some showing megakaryocyte differentiation, were evident in peripheral blood smears.

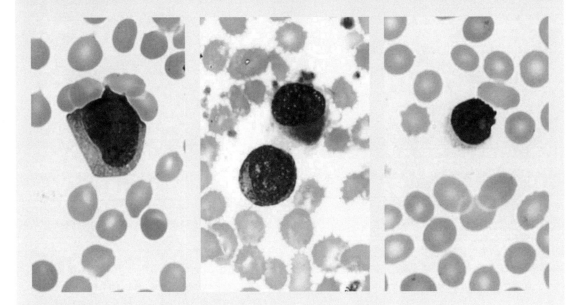

Bone marrow aspirate was dry, whilst the trephine showed almost maximal cellularity with a blastoid infiltrate. Immunophenotyping on peripheral blood, using a low SSC CD45^{dim} gating strategy gave the following data:

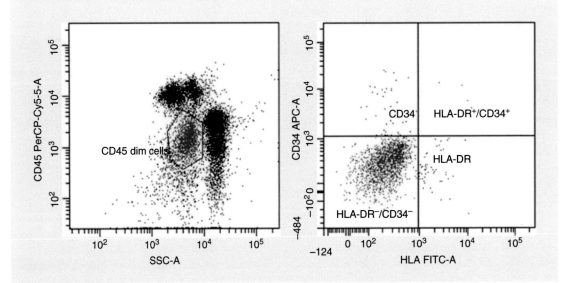

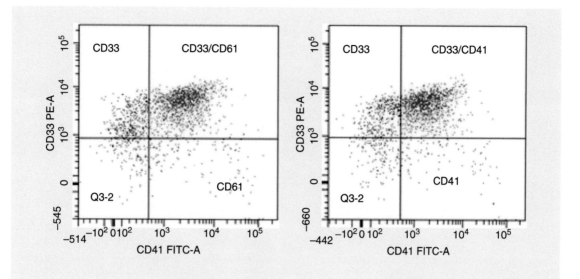

This CD34⁻, HLA-DR⁻, CD33⁺ (not shown) blast population was clearly expressing CD41 and CD61. These features are in keeping with acute megakaryoblastic leukaemia (AML M7). This was confirmed on immunohistochemical analysis of the trephine. Cytogenetics showed a near triploid karyotype.

WORKED EXAMPLE 5.10

A 58-year-old male presented with a three-month history of an enlarging ulcerating nodular lesion on the skin of his face. The first biopsy was inconclusive, showing largely necrotic material.

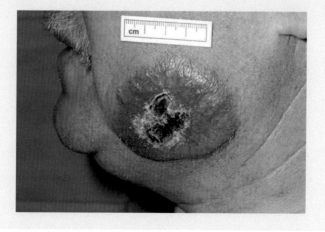

A pancytopenia developed and a bone marrow aspirate showed involvement by undifferentiated blast cells.

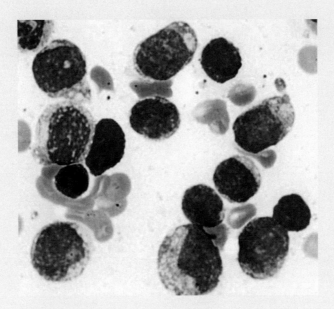

Flow cytometry studies were diagnostic by identifying a unique immunophenotype: the cells were CD45^{dim}, CD34$^-$, HLA-DR$^+$, CD117$^-$, MPO$^-$, CD33^{dim}, CD14/64$^-$, CD4$^+$, CD56$^+$, CD103$^+$.

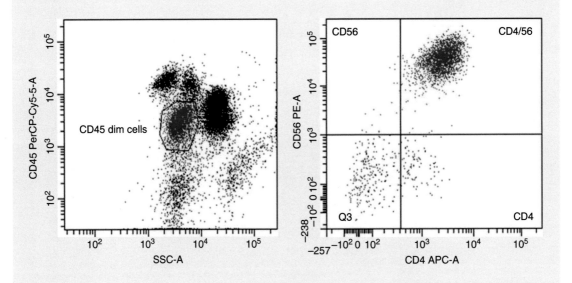

The clinical presentation and immunophenotyping studies were all in keeping with a blastic plasmacytoid dendritic cell neoplasm. In contrast to some reports using AML type therapy we treated this patient with CODOX M/IVAC (a Burkitt lymphoma regimen)

followed by autologous stem cell transplant in first remission. His skin lesion responded rapidly to the first cycle of therapy. The patient remained disease free at two years.

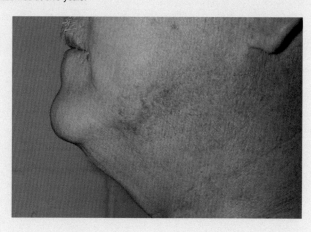

Table 5.6 Immunological subclassification of B-ALL. This table illustrates the widely accepted B-ALL subclassification based on the presence or absence of CD10 and immunoglobulin expression [1, 3]. Note that nearly all B-ALL is positive for CD19, CD22, CD79a and TdT. Mature ALL B-IV is of course now recognized as a variant of non-Hodgkin lymphoma, specifically Burkitt leukaemia variant with FAB L3 morphology. Other terminology in common use is early precursor B-ALL (cμ⁻) and precursor B-ALL (cμ⁺). The terminology is further confused by the historical use of the term B-ALL to indicate mature B-cell ALL, and readers should not be confused by the use of this term in older texts.

Immunological subtype (EGIL classification)	Discriminatory antigen pattern	Percentage of B-ALL adult cases (approx)	Percentage of B-ALL childhood cases (approx)
Pro-B-ALL (B-I)	CD10⁻, cμ⁻, sIg⁻	10–20	5
Common B-ALL (B-II)	CD10⁺, cμ⁻, sIg⁻	70	75
Pre-B-ALL (B-III)	CD10⁺, cμ⁺, sIg⁻	10–20	10–20
(mature B, B-IV, Burkitt lymphoma/leukaemia variant)	CD10⁺, sIg⁺(anti cμ⁻ and κ or λ)	5	2

AML, and in large part this lends itself to more straightforward diagnosis and reproducible immunological classification. Furthermore, because of the relative ease with which leukaemic lymphoblasts may be identified from within heterogeneous populations, MRD analysis is more straightforward (Chapter 9). This is not always possible for all cases (e.g. in acute lymphoblastic lymphoma with no detectable marrow disease).

B-cell acute lymphoblastic leukaemia/lymphoma

B-lineage ALL (B-ALL) was classified immunologically in 1995 based on the immunophenotype of the apparent maturation arrest stage as compared with normal lymphoid maturation [3]. These leukaemic populations are largely homogeneous and relatively easy to differentiate from the 'smear' of antigens expressed during sequential B-cell maturation (described in Chapter 4).

In broad terms, B-ALL is positive for CD19 (in nearly 100% of cases [22]), CD79a, cCD22, TdT, HLA-DR and is dim for CD45. CD19 and cCD22 are said to be the most sensitive markers for B-lineage. Note that CD45 can exhibit a range of staining intensity even within the same sample, and may even be negative in approximately 15–30% of cases [20, 85]. Relying solely on SSC/CD45^{dim} to identify blast cells may therefore not be well founded in all cases.

Table 5.7 Immunological subclassification of T-ALL.

Immunological subtype (EGIL Classification)	CD1a	CD2	cCD3	sCD3	CD4	CD5	CD7	CD8	CD34	TdT	Percentage of cases (adults and children, approx [117, 119])
Pro-T-ALL (T-I)	–	–	+	–	–	–	+	–	+/–	+	4–5
Pre-T-ALL (T-II)	–	+	+	–	–	+	+	–	+/–	+	25–47
Cortical-T- ALL (T-III)	+	+	+	–	+	+	+	+	–	+	40–60
Medullary-T-ALL (T-IV)	–	+	+	+	+/–	+	+	+/–	–	+/–	5–10

This table summarizes the widely recognized EGIL subclassification of T-ALL and LBL into four categories according to 'maturational' stage of thymic differentiation [3]. Note that cCD3, CD7 and TdT are the most frequently detected antigens (with cCD3 being the only T-lineage specific antigen). Cortical T-ALL is characterized by CD1a expression and double positivity for CD4 and CD8, whereas the medullary stage (sometimes referred to as mature) is restricted to either CD4 or CD8. T-LBL tends to be associated with a more mature maturational stage than T-ALL but there is significant overlap (e.g. T-IV T-ALL is generally associated with a T-LBL presentation). As with many other attempts at classification in haematological malignancy, cases exist which do not fit these well-defined 'maturational' stages.

The precursor nature of the cells is established by the presence of CD34 (in approximately 70% of cases [22, 102]), TdT (in >90% of cases [36]), and lack of cytoplasmic or surface *light-chain* expression. In a parody of normal B-cell maturation TdT and CD34 are more likely to be negative on later maturational stages [103], but overall only approximately 4% of cases lack both of these markers [19]. TdT expression in B-ALL is generally brighter than in T-ALL, which is in turn brighter than in AML [12]. While TdT negative B-ALL is rare (approximately 3% of cases), its absence does not preclude the diagnosis if an otherwise typical diagnostic profile is present.

B-ALL can be further subclassified based on the presence or absence of CD10 and cytoplasmic immunoglobulin *heavy chains* (cμ) (Table 5.6). In general terms surface immunoglobulin (s(Ig)) defines a mature B-cell malignancy; however, rare cases of B-ALL (discussed below) can occasionally cause confusion. Note that CD20 is not uncommonly positive on B-ALL (in approximately 20–40% [19, 22, 23]), an example of asynchronous antigen expression in conjunction with the markers of immaturity (i.e. CD34 and/or TdT). This pattern is not seen during normal maturation and CD20 expression has been shown to be a poor prognostic marker in adult B-ALL [104]. Recent studies suggest that the poor outcome for CD20+ paediatric cases [105] has been reversed with modern treatment protocols incorporating anti-CD20 [106]. CD20 expression may only be partial or weak. However, it may be increased in intensity following induction steroid therapy and this is one rationale for using anti-CD20 monoclonal antibodies in ALL clinical trials [23]. CD10

(formerly known as common ALL antigen, cALLa) is expressed on approximately 80–90% of adult and childhood B-ALL [19, 85]. It is brighter than when seen on haematogones, mature B-cell malignancies or on T-ALL [105]. It does of course lack any specificity for B-ALL as it is commonly found on mature B-cell malignancies including follicular, diffuse large B-cell and Burkitt lymphoma. Note the potential for misinterpretation here; on occasions these malignancies may lack surface immunoglobulin and CD10 should be interpreted in conjunction with the full immunophenotypic and genetic profile. There should also be full correlation with the clinical presentation, disease distribution and behaviour. The absence of CD10 in B-ALL is associated with MLL translocations and a poor outcome (i.e. pro-B-ALL, Table 5.6). Thus, analysis of CD10 is useful for full characterization of B-ALL but is neither specific nor required for the diagnosis.

It is worth noting that most B-ALL cases exhibit clonally rearranged *IGH* genes; however, TCR rearrangements may also be seen in up to 70% of cases. The reverse situation is also true; T-ALL exhibits TCR gene rearrangements but IGH genes are also rearranged in 20% of cases. Thus these genetic analyses are therefore not useful for lineage assignation [107, 108].

In keeping with a recurring theme in this book care must be taken when interpreting individual antigen expression, as morphology and immunophenotyping cannot be solely relied on in all cases to allow for correct classification. In particular, with regards B-ALL:

1 There are some notes of caution with regards specificity of B-cell markers in this setting. As has been

described above, CD19 may be expressed not uncommonly in AML and CD79a has been described on the surface of T-ALL blasts [10]. CD22 is also expressed on the surface of basophils, although confusion should not arise as they are universally CD19⁻ [91].

2 Rare but well-described cases exist demonstrating precursor B-cell immunophenotype (i.e. B-ALL), L3 morphology and MYC translocations (though not t(8;14) (q24;q32)). These are thought to be variants of Burkitt lymphoma/leukaemia and appear to have a good outcome with Burkitt type treatment regimens [29].

3 Other cases demonstrate both cytoplasmic and surface μ chain (but not associated light chains), lack L3 morphology and MYC translocations and have been termed transitional B-ALL [109]. These comprise approximately 3% of childhood B-ALL and have a good outcome with ALL treatment approaches.

4 A final, very rare group express cytoplasmic and surface monotypic light chains (sometimes in conjunction with intact IgM or IgD), lack L3 morphology and MYC translocations and often co-express markers of immaturity (TdT and CD34). Less than 2% of childhood ALL falls into this category and it appears to be particularly rare in adults [110, 111]. Many of these cases have B-ALL related genetic lesions and are best regarded as such.

Thus, expression of immunoglobulin, particularly monotypic light chains, must not be assumed to be indicative of a mature B-cell malignancy in all cases; genetic analysis and the full immunophenotyping profile must be taken into account.

Aberrant antigen expression in B-acute lymphoblastic leukaemia

Myeloid antigen expression in B-ALL is well described, although its frequency varies widely in published studies, likely for a number of technical reasons. In one large study of childhood cases one or more myeloid antigens (CD13, CD14, CD15, CD33 or CD65) was expressed in approximately a third of cases (31.9% of B-ALL and 28.8% of T-ALL) [112]. CD14 expression was the least frequently detected antigen (1% or so of cases), and 10% of cases expressed two or more. A particular association was noted with *MLL* gene rearrangements, where 82% expressed CD15, CD33 and CD65 either alone or in combination. Importantly, no independent prognostic significance was noted in relation to myeloid antigen expression. In a more recent study of both childhood

and adult cases of B-ALL, when CD11b, CD36 and CD64 were included in addition to the antigens above, over 80% of cases expressed one or more myeloid antigens with CD13 (54.5% of cases), CD33 (43%), CD15 (36%) and CD11b (20%) being seen most commonly [85]. Of note, little difference was seen between children and adults in terms of aberrant antigen patterns in B-ALL. Again CD15 expression was associated with *MLL* rearrangements (100% of cases), and over 90% of Ph + cases expressed myeloid antigens, as did those with t(12;21)(p13;q22). Clearly, the expression of myeloid antigens in ALL is a common phenomenon, with the latter study describing the highest proportion of myeloid positive ALL to date. Myeloid antigen expression, per se, does not necessarily indicate a poor prognosis but the presence of CD15, CD13 and CD33 should highlight the possibility that a recurring genetic lesion might be present; the nature of this may well influence response to treatment. For example, very good prognosis with t(12;21), but poor prognosis with t(4;11)(q21;q23). Confusion with AML should not arise, however. MPO expression is negative (and if positive indicates a mixed lineage AL), the myeloid antigen expression patterns are generally weak, and lymphoid antigens are clearly dominant in each case.

T-natural killer antigen expression in B-ALL is also reported in up to 9% of cases, most frequently CD4 or CD56, with the latter being seen more frequently in children [85]. The significance of CD25 expression in *BCR-ABL* positive ALL is discussed below.

Identifying B-acute lymphoblastic leukaemia subtypes by flow

The WHO genetically defined subtypes are illustrated in Figure 5.9, in accordance with their typical immunophenotype. While not absolute, some very strong correlations are noted. In particular, a CD10⁻ CD15⁺ Pro-B-ALL phenotype predicts strongly for the presence of abnormalities of the *MLL* gene, especially t(4:11); *MLL-AF4* [113, 114]. Indeed some investigators describe CD15 as 100% specific for the presence of an MLL rearrangement in infant B-ALL [114]. CD25 expression has been described in approximately 25% of *BCR-ABL* positive B-ALL but only 3% of *BCR-ABL* negative disease [94]. As up to 10% of *BCR-ABL* positive cases may be missed by conventional G-banding (i.e. Ph⁻) [115], detection of CD25 expression should prompt *BCR-ABL* PCR or FISH

Early or pro-
B-cell ALL

CD10⁻, CD19⁺, CD34⁺, TdT⁺, *CD15⁺*

WHO subtype: B-All with t[v;11q23]; *MLL* rearranged. Infants <1yr and adults with 11q23 (*MLL*) rearrangements most notably t(4;11); high WCC (>100), organomegaly and CNS disease common: poor outlook. Other myeloid antigens frequently expressed, such as CD33.

CD10⁺, CD19⁺, CD34⁺, TdT⁺, *CD25⁺, CD13⁺/CD33⁺*

WHO subtype: B-All with t(9;22); *BCR-ABL 1*. Variable immunophenotype but most commonly common B-ALL with high frequency of myeloid antigens (20–75% of CD13 and/or CD33 in different series). Found in15–30% of adults but only 2% of children and generally associated with a poor outcome.

CD10⁺, CD19⁺, CD34⁺, TdT⁺, *CD13⁺/CD33⁺*

WHO subtype: B-All with t(12;21); TEL-AML1 [ETV6-RUNX1]. Found in up to 30% of childwood ALL but <5% of adult cases. Myeloid antigens expressed in <50% of cases. Favourable outcome.

Common
B-cell ALL

CD10⁺, CD19⁺, CD34⁺, TdT⁺

WHO subtype: B-All with hyperdiploidy and B-ALL with hypodiploidy. The former is common in childhood (25%), rare in adults and is associated with a good prognosis. The latter is found in <5% of ALL and confers a poor outcome.

CD10⁺, CD19⁺, CD34⁺, TdT⁺

WHO subtype: B-All with t[5;14]; IL3-IGH. Rare (<1% of ALL), and associated with a marked polyclonal eosinophilia secondary to IL-3. Common ALL immunophemotype.

Pre-B-cell
ALL

CD10⁺, CD19⁺, *CD34⁻, cμ⁺*

WHO subtype: t(1:19); E2A-PBX1 (TCF3-PBX1). Generally more mature than cALL, (CD34⁻ and cμ⁻) typically termed pre-B All. CD45 often relatively strongly expressed as compared to other subtypes. Used to confer a poor prognosis; newer protocols seem to have reversed this. Seen in up to 6% of childhood ALL, less common in adults. Approximately 25% of all pre-B ALL exhibit this translocation.

Figure 5.9 Flow cytometric profiles of WHO defined ALL according to genotype. This schematic illustrates how the genetic subgroups of B-ALL relate to the widely accepted immunological classification. The typical antigen expression patterns are highlighted with the notable antigens (including aberrant antigen expression) highlighted in purple italics. Data is summarized from Swerdlow and Campo [1]; see text for further discussion and references.

in such cases. Finally, a strong correlation is noted between the presence of the t(1;19);*E2A-PBX1* translocation and a pre-B-ALL phenotype (namely CD34⁻, cμ⁺) in children.

T-cell acute lymphoblastic leukaemia/lymphoma

While only comprising approximately 15% of all childhood and 25% of all adult ALL, T-lineage disease is responsible for up to 90% of lymphoblastic lymphoma [1]. It is not formally subclassified by the WHO, but in an analogous way to B-lineage disease there exists a 'maturational' stage based immunophenotypic classification (Table 5.6). Historically it has had weak immunophenotypic/genetic correlations, although recent studies point to the immunological definition of a very poor risk subgroup (discussed further below).

The precursor origin of the tumour cells is indicated by the presence of TdT, CD1a and/or CD34 as well as a lack of sCD3. Aberrant co-expression of CD4 and CD8, or indeed expression of neither, is also suggestive of an immature phenotype. HLA-DR, while universally expressed in B-ALL is rarely expressed in T-ALL and is likely indicative of an early T-cell phenotype [10, 20, 116]: one small study documented its expression in 40–50% of pro- and pre-T-ALL but not in more mature cases [117]. Overall, TdT is the most commonly found precursor antigen (>90%) with CD34 expressed in only 30–40% [118, 119]. As with B-ALL, these antigens are more likely to be negative in the mature cases (i.e. medullary T-ALL), which may give, rise to some confusion with mature T-cell lymphomas. Furthermore, this is another situation where CD34⁻ HLA-DR⁻ blasts might be encountered. In general it would seem that the more

WORKED EXAMPLE 5.11

A 32-year-old female presented with anaemia, thrombocytopenia and high leucocytosis with a peripheral blood smear composed almost entirely of lymphoblasts.

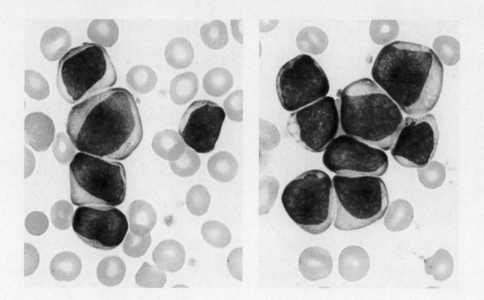

Immunophenotyping studies on peripheral blood were in keeping with a pro B-ALL. Note the absence of CD10 and strong CD15 expression on this precursor B-cell (cCD79a$^+$, CD19$^+$, TdT$^+$) neoplasm. No other myeloid markers were evident. A t(4;11) (MLL;AF4) translocation was identified. The patient received an allogeneic transplant in first remission because of the poor outcome predicted by this genetic lesion.

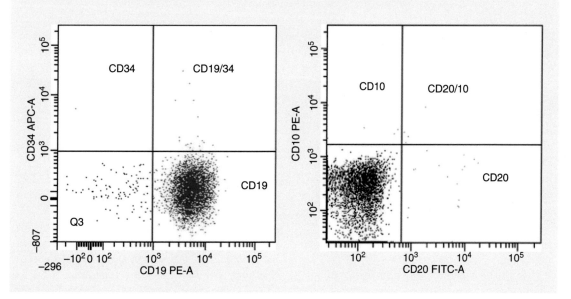

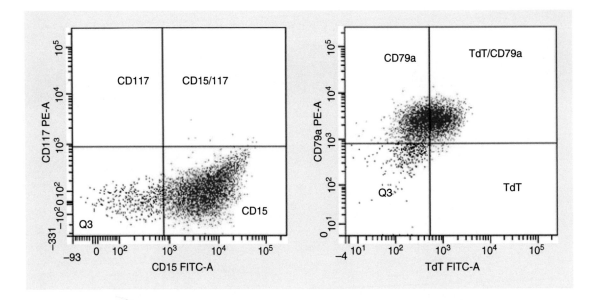

mature T-ALL subgroups have a better outlook than the pre-thymic ones [120, 121) with CD1a+(cortical) cases in particular having the best prognosis in most studies [119, 122, 123]. These observations extend to both adults and children.

CD10 appears transiently during normal T-cell maturation and is expressed in T-ALL (in approximately 30% of cases). It appears to have little or no prognostic impact in more recent studies using contemporary treatment protocols [119]).

A particularly immature T-ALL phenotype has recently been described in children with a very poor outcome using current treatment approaches [10]. This so-called early T-precursor phenotype (ETP) comprises 10–15% of all childhood T-ALL, and is characterized by a cCD3+, CD1a-, CD8-, CD5dim phenotype, with common co-expression of myeloid antigens (including CD117, CD13 and CD33) and markers of immaturity (i.e. CD34, HLA-DR, TdT and CD133). The risk of remission failure or relapse was 57% at two years in this group as compared to 14% for non-ETP T-ALL. The authors of this study now offer intensive therapy with allogeneic stem cell transplant upon identification of this immunophenotype. The incidence of this subgroup in adults remains unknown.

It is worth highlighting that in an analogous way to haematogones and B-ALL, normal thymocytes exhibit an immature T-cell phenotype and should not be confused with T-ALL. The latter exhibits a high degree of antigen aberrancy, and comparison of its abnormal maturation-arrest profile with the sequential maturation pattern of normal thymic T-cells should prevent confusion. It is always possible that biopsy of mediastinal lesions might contain otherwise normal thymic tissue, and particular care must be taken in this context.

Finally, as compared to AML and B-ALL, there are no strong relationships between immunophenotypic profiles and particular chromosomal abnormalities. Numerous genetic lesions are described in T-ALL but as yet they have little role in guiding treatment approach (see recent reviews [124, 125]).

Aberrant antigen expression in T-acute lymphoblastic leukaemia

Antigens aberrantly expressed by T-ALL include myeloid antigens, CD79a and CD56. CD56 has been discussed in some detail above where it is often co-expressed with myeloid antigens, CD34 and HLA-DR and predicts for reduced CR rates [83]. The presence of myeloid antigens (CD13 and CD33) may be indicative of an ETP phenotype in children. In adults these antigens are found in approximately 25% of cases [119] and may be associated

WORKED EXAMPLE 5.12

A nine-year-old boy presented with bone pain. The bone marrow aspirate showed a large pleomorphic lymphoblast population with prominent nucleoli and cytoplasmic projections known as 'hand mirror forms'.

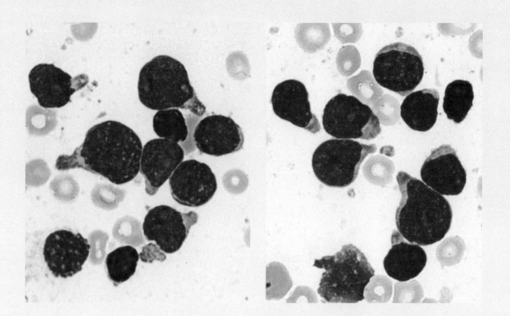

Immunophenotyping studies showed positivity for CD34, TdT, CD7, CD5, CD2, HLA-DR, CD38 and cCD3 in keeping with a pro-T-ALL. In addition, CD10 was positive but as discussed above was deemed not to carry independent prognostic significance.

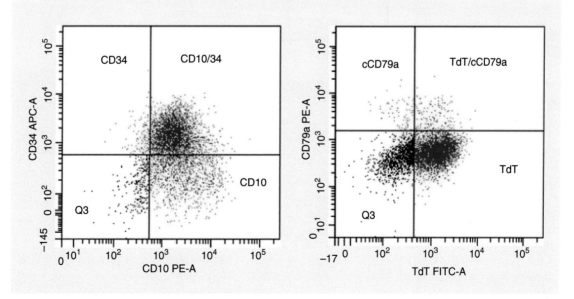

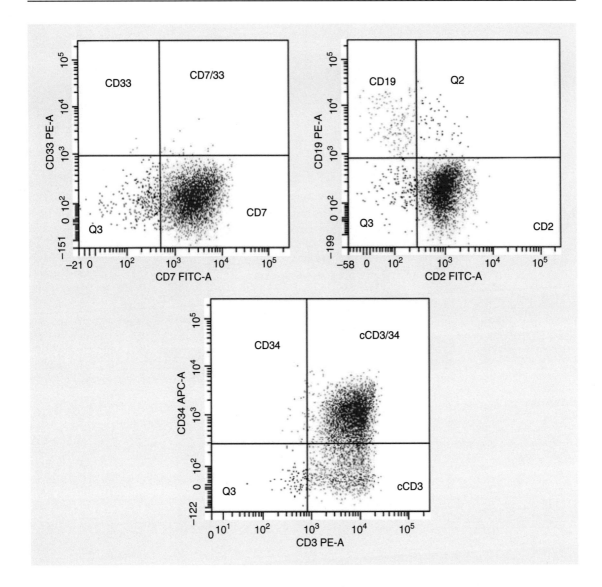

with lower CR rates (although in multivariate analysis only CD33, present in 10%, retained any significant prognostic impact). CD79a is described on a subset of predominantly cortical T-ALL; approximately 10% of T lymphoblastic lymphoma demonstrated significant staining by ICC in one study [126], although low level expression was described in up to 40–50% of cases in this and other studies [127]. When considered with other T-lineage markers (in particular cCD3), confusion with B-ALL should not arise.

Examination of cerebro-spinal fluid and serous effusions

Central Nervous System Disease in Acute Leukaemia

Prior to effective central nervous system (CNS) directed prophylaxis up to 50% of childhood ALL exhibited CNS relapse, usually in the form of leptomeningeal disease detectable by cytomorphology of the cerebro-spinal fluid (CSF) [128]. Central nervous system directed therapy is now a routine component of ALL treatment protocols for both adults and children and has dramatically reduced the incidence of CNS relapse (to approximately 5% [129]). However, some patients continue to present with evidence of CNS disease (approximately 2–3% of children with ALL [130]), which is not uncommonly detected on the initial lumbar puncture. Risk factors for CNS relapse in ALL include a T-ALL phenotype, high presenting WCC, blasts detectable in the CSF at diagnosis, traumatic lumber puncture and a pre-B-ALL phenotype with a t(1;19) translocation (129). The presence of a mediastinal mass may be an additional risk factor for adults [131].

Likewise, prior to the introduction of cytarabine chemotherapy, the incidence of CNS relapse for AML in children and adults was 20% and 16% respectively. Leptomeningeal disease at presentation is also recognized as a not infrequent complication of AML (being found in 11% of children at diagnosis in one large study [132]). Childhood AML protocols specify CNS prophylaxis as a routine, although this is not considered necessary for adults. Risk factors for CNS disease in AML include a monocytic component, relapsed APL, hyperleucocytosis, the presence of inv(16), age less than two years and CD56 expression [129].

The detection of CNS disease largely relies on sampling of CSF, with appropriate imaging often providing useful supportive information. In general several mL of CSF should be removed by lumbar puncture (LP) and sent promptly for analysis. Careful operator technique will avoid traumatic LP, in itself a risk factor for later CNS disease. Diagnostic CSF samples should be sent for a cell count and differential, protein and glucose measurement, Gram stain and culture (if infection is suspected), cytology (examination of appropriately stained cytospin slides) and flow cytometry and/or ICC (e.g. staining for TdT). If the initial sample is positive for blast cells, subsequent LPs should be studied to determine whether the blast cells are cleared with therapy.

Flow cytometry is an attractive technique in this situation given its ability to detect low numbers of tumour cells. Most published studies, however, have been performed in the lymphoma setting, where CNS disease may occur in up to 5% of patients with an aggressive histology [133]. Routine cytomorphology of AL CSF specimens is commonly practiced, but is relatively insensitive due to low cell numbers and difficulties in distinguishing malignant from reactive cells. In one study of patients with autopsy confirmed extensive leptomeningeal disease, only 66% of cases had demonstrated positive cytomorphology [134]. Reliable detection of neoplastic cells by cytomorphology requires that at least 5% of cells are neoplastic [135]. In contrast, flow can detect malignant cells when they comprise as few as 0.2% of all cells in the specimen, which often comprises significant numbers of reactive normal cells (e.g. T-cells, NK-cells and monocytes) [136]. Several studies have confirmed flow cytometry to be several-fold more sensitive than cytomorphology for the detection of tumour cells [137], and it is being increasingly viewed as a routine component of CSF analysis. It is now recommended in assessment of CSF samples in haematologic malignancy by the NCCN [138].

Issues remain, however, in terms of standardizing technical protocols and antibody panels, as well as determining what the criteria are for a sample being deemed positive [137]. There is a common consensus (that analysis should occur within a few hours) to prevent cell loss. Some centres advocate fixing samples to extend this timeframe (up to 24 hours [135]), which may allow shipping to a specialist flow laboratory. Antibody panels have yet to be standardized, but should be based upon the diagnostic immunophenotype as detected in marrow or blood. Analysis may, however, be limited because of low cell numbers. Other developments include the ability to accurately enumerate CSF blast cells using appropriate bead-calibration [139] and the use of flow-based detection of BCR-ABL (described below) to detect low levels of ALL cells in the CSF [140]. Indeed, if CSF samples contain adequate cell numbers confirmation of systemic disease genetic abnormalities (e.g. by FISH) can offer useful corroborative evidence of CNS disease.

Detection of acute leukaemia cells in serous effusions

Pleural, pericardial (and rarely peritoneal) effusions may be detected in patients at presentation, most typically in patients with lymphoblastic lymphoma. Analysis of fluid samples in these circumstances may be diagnostic as the bone marrow may be devoid of tumour cells and biopsy of any tumour masses technically difficult. Malignant involvement of serous cavities can be difficult to differentiate from reactive conditions using cytomorphology alone [141]. Serous effusions may comprise

WORKED EXAMPLE 5.13

A 51-year-old female with a history of common ALL treated with allogeneic transplant 18 months earlier presented with headache and papilloedema. The FBC was normal. A CSF specimen was hypercellular (cell count 0.05×10^9/L) with a protein level of 2.7 g/L and glucose 0.5 mM/L. A cytospin identified a population of blast cells with folded nuclei, nucleoli and blue cytoplasm, alongside a population of small mature lymphoid cells. Flow cytometry showed the large cells to have a CD45^{dim} CD19$^+$ CD10$^+$ CD20$^+$ phenotype with high FSC (red events) in keeping with meningeal relapse of common ALL. The smaller cells (blue events) with condensed chromatin, absent nucleoli and pale cytoplasm, were reactive T-cells with CD45^{bright}, low FSC, T-cell phenotype (data not shown).

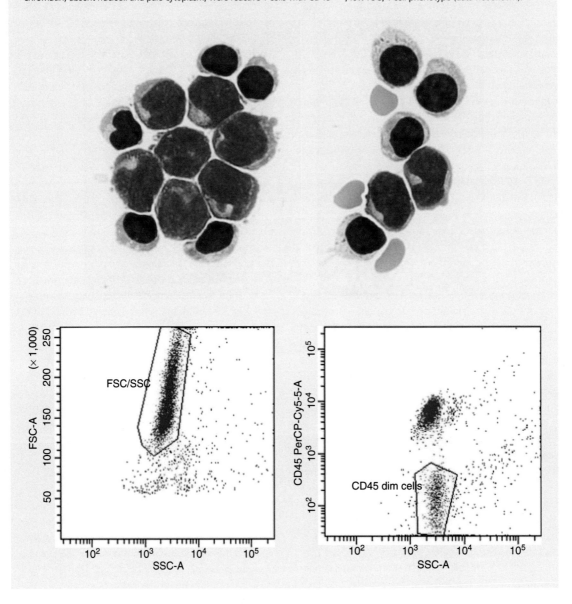

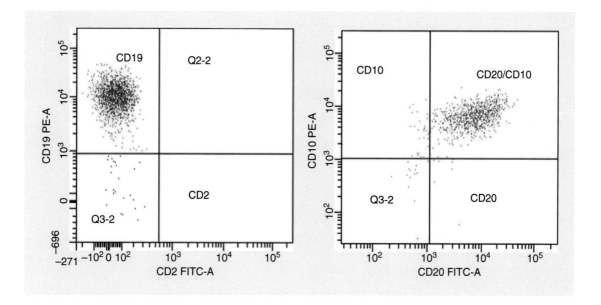

WORKED EXAMPLE 5.14

A 20-year-old female presented with cough, dyspnoea, hypotension and night sweats. The FBC was normal. A CXR showed a mediastinal mass and right pleural effusion.

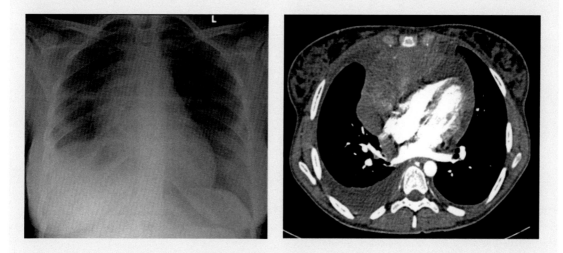

A cardiac echo identified a large pericardial effusion with ventricular compromise which was aspirated with symptomatic improvement. CT imaging confirmed a large anterior mediastinal mass with pleuropericardial involvement. A stained smear showed abnormal pleomorphic lymphoid cells. Immunophenotyping studies on the pericardial effusion cells confirmed a cortical type T lymphoblastic lymphoma. Note the absence of CD34 and TdT, expression of CD2, CD1a and CD4/CD8 together. The cells were also positive for surface CD7, CD5 and CD3 (not shown), This is a typical immunophenotype of a cortical T lymphoblastic lymphoma alongside a common presentation with antero-superior mediastinal mass of thymic origin.

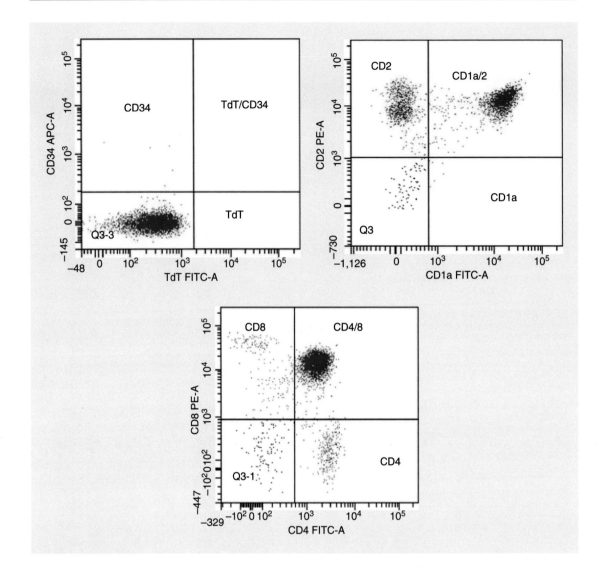

mesothelial cells, histiocytes and lymphocytes, and malignant cells may be infrequent. Flow lends itself to the detection of the latter. The few published studies on serous effusion flow cytometry incorporate lymphoma or even solid tumours, and little has been documented surrounding the detection of ALL cells. However, the general principles described thus far in this chapter seem likely to hold true. The authors' practice is to examine such samples promptly and assess cell viability prior to analysis with an appropriate antibody panel.

Identification of genetic abnormalities by flow

Currently, identification of the common fusion genes in AL relies on karyotyping, FISH or RT-PCR of fusion transcript mRNA. Taken together these techniques require a considerable body of expertise and as a consequence are generally carried out at larger centres only. One of the most exciting laboratory developments in recent years involves the detection of

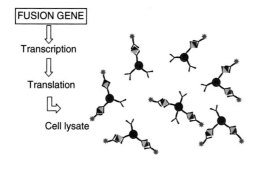

Transcription

Translation

Cell lysate

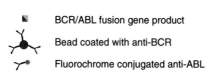

▶ BCR/ABL fusion gene product

Bead coated with anti-BCR

Fluorochrome conjugated anti-ABL

Figure 5.10 Detection of the BCR-ABL Fusion Gene by Flow Cytometry. Adapted from Dekking et al. [142], with permission from Elsevier.

chromosomal translocations by flow (comprehensively reviewed in [142]).

The first fusion protein to be reliably detected by such methodology was BCR-ABL, using a twin antibody technique (Figure 5.10) developed by the Euroflow Consortium [143]. It demonstrated 100% concordance with standard RT-PCR and sensitivity of this technique was measured at 1%. Further work by this group has led to the development of flow-based assays for PML-RARA, TEL- AML1, E2A-PBX1, MLL-AF4, AML1-ETO and CBFB-MYH11 fusion proteins. Flow cytometry has also been used successfully to demonstrate cytoplasmic (mutated) NPM1 in AML [44]. This protein is normally located in the nucleolus; however, the commonly reported AML mutations result in its aberrant cytoplasmic relocation, which is detectable using cell permeabilization techniques. It is hoped that once validated, commercially available antibodies may allow testing for these common genetic lesions in the flow cytometry laboratory.

Conclusion

Flow cytometry has gained a central role in the routine diagnosis and classification in AL. While the prognostic significance of single antigens remains controversial in most circumstances, many studies have demonstrated

immunophenotypic patterns of expression which correlate closely with underlying genetic abnormalities and in many cases, outcome. Ongoing development of techniques to allow flow-based detection of these genetic abnormalities is an exciting step and one that is likely to consolidate flow cytometry's central role in the diagnosis and management of these cases.

References

1 Swerdlow SH, Campo E, *et al. WHO Classification of Tumours of Haematopoietic and Lymphoid Tissues* (4th edn). 2008. IARC Press, Lyon, France.

2 Bennett JM, Catovsky D, Daniel MT, *et al.* Proposals for the classification of the acute leukaemias. French-American-British (FAB) co-operative group. *Br J Haematol* 1976, **33**(4): 451–8.

3 Bene MC, Castoldi G, Knapp W, *et al.* Proposals for the immunological classification of acute leukaemias. *Leukaemia* 1995, **9**: 1783–6.

4 Sekeres MA, Elson P, Kalaycio ME, *et al.* Time from diagnosis to treatment initiation predicts survival in younger, but not older, acute myeloid leukemia patients. *Blood* 2009, **113**(1): 28–36.

5 Erber WN. *Diagnostic techniques in hematological malignancies.* 2010. Cambridge University Press, Cambridge.

6 Wood BL. Myeloid malignancies: myelodysplastic syndromes, myeloproliferative disorders, and acute myeloid leukemia. *Clin Lab Med* 2007, **27**(3): 551–75, vii.

7 Bonnet D, Dick JE. Human acute myeloid leukemia is organized as a hierarchy that originates from a primitive hematopoietic cell. *Nat Med* 1997, **3**(7): 730–7.

8 Al-Mawali A, Gillis D, Hissaria P, Lewis I. Incidence, sensitivity, and specificity of leukemia-associated phenotypes in acute myeloid leukemia using specific five-color multiparameter flow cytometry. *American Journal of Clinical Pathology* 2008,**129**(6): 934–45.

9 Adriaansen H, te Boekhorst P, Hagemeijer A, van der Schoot C, Delwel H, van Dongen J. Acute myeloid leukemia M4 with bone marrow eosinophilia (M4Eo) and inv(16)(p13q22) exhibits a specific immunophenotype with CD2 expression. *Blood* 1993, **81**(11): 3043–51.

10 Coustan-Smith E, Mullighan CG, Onciu M, *et al.* Early T-cell precursor leukaemia: a subtype of very high-risk acute lymphoblastic leukaemia. *Lancet Oncol* 2009, **10**(2): 147–56.

11 Brooimans RA, Kraan J, van Putten W, Cornelissen JJ, Löwenberg B, Gratama JW. Flow cytometric differential of leukocyte populations in normal bone marrow: Influence of

peripheral blood contamination. *Cytometry Part B: Clinical Cytometry* 2009, **76B**(1): 18–26.

12 Farahat N, Lens D, Morilla R, Matutes E, Catovsky D. Differential TdT expression in acute leukemia by flow cytometry: a quantitative study. *Leukaemia* 1995, **9**: 583–7.

13 Bene MC, Bernier M, Casasnovas RO, *et al.* The reliability and specificity of c-kit for the diagnosis of acute myeloid leukemias and undifferentiated leukemias. *Blood* 1998, **92**(2): 596–9.

14 Thalhammer-Scherrer R, Mitterbauer G, Simonitsch I, *et al.* The immunophenotype of 325 adult acute leukemias. *American Journal of Clinical Pathology* 2002, **117**(3): 380–9.

15 Asnafi V, Beldjord K, Boulanger E, *et al.* Analysis of TCR, pT alpha, and RAG-1 in T-acute lymphoblastic leukemias improves understanding of early human T-lymphoid lineage commitment. *Blood* 2003, **101**(7): 2693–703.

16 Oelschlaegel U, Mohr B, Schaich M, *et al.* HLA-DRneg patients without acute promyelocytic leukemia show distinct immunophenotypic, genetic, molecular, and cytomorphologic characteristics compared to acute promyelocytic leukemia. *Cytometry B Clin Cytom* 2009, **76**(5): 321–7.

17 Ziegler-Heitbrock L. The CD14+ CD16+ blood monocytes: their role in infection and inflammation. *J Leukoc Biol* 2007, **81**(3): 584–92.

18 Craig FE, Foon KA. Flow cytometric immunophenotyping for hematologic neoplasms. *Blood* 2008, **111**(8): 3941–67.

19 Gorczyca W. *Flow Cytometry in Neoplastic Hematology: Morphologic-Immunophenotypic Correlation.* 2006. Taylor & Francis, London.

20 Bain BJ. *Leukaemia Diagnosis* (4th edn). 2012. Wiley-Blackwell, Oxford.

21 Pernick N. PathologyOutlines.com. 2011 (updated 18 November 2011; cited 2011); available from: http://www.pathologyoutlines.com/cdmarkers.html.

22 Hurwitz CA, Loken MR, Graham ML, *et al.* Asynchronous antigen expression in B-lineage acute lymphoblastic leukemia. *Blood* 1988, **72**(1): 299–307.

23 Dworzak MN, Schumich A, Printz D, *et al.* CD20 upregulation in pediatric B-cell precursor acute lymphoblastic leukemia during induction treatment: setting the stage for anti-CD20 directed immunotherapy. *Blood* 2008, **112**(10): 3982–8.

24 Bain BJ, Barnett D, Linch D, Matutes E, Reilly JT. Revised guideline on immunophenotyping in acute leukaemias and chronic lymphoproliferative disorders. *Clin Lab Haematol* 2002, **24**(1): 1–13.

25 Bene MC, Nebe T, Bettelheim P, *et al.* Immunophenotyping of acute leukemia and lymphoproliferative disorders: a consensus proposal of the European LeukemiaNet Work Package 10. *Leukemia* 2011, 1–8.

26 Voskova D, Schoch C, Schnittger S, Hiddemann W, Haferlach T, Kern W. Stability of leukemia-associated aberrant immunophenotypes in patients with acute myeloid leukemia between diagnosis and relapse: comparison with cytomorphologic, cytogenetic, and molecular genetic findings. *Cytometry B Clin Cytom* 2004, **62**(1): 25–38.

27 Khoury H, Dalal BI, Nevill TJ, *et al.* Acute myelogenous leukemia with t(8;21), identification of a specific immunophenotype. *Leukemia and Lymphoma* 2003, **44**(10): 1713–8.

28 Hans CP, Finn WG, Singleton TP, Schnitzer B, Ross CW. Usefulness of anti-CD117 in the flow cytometric analysis of acute leukemia. *Am J Clin Pathol* 2002, **117**(2): 301–5.

29 Navid F, Mosijczuk AD, Head DR, *et al.* Acute lymphoblastic leukemia with the (8;14)(q24;q32) translocation and FAB L3 morphology associated with a B-precursor immunophenotype: the Pediatric Oncology Group experience. *Leukemia* 1999, **13**: 135–42.

30 Li S, Eshleman JR, Borowitz MJ. Lack of surface immunoglobulin light chain expression by flow cytometric immunophenotyping can help diagnose peripheral B-cell lymphoma. *American Journal of Clinical Pathology* 2002, **118**(2): 229–34.

31 Majeti R. Monoclonal antibody therapy directed against human acute myeloid leukemia stem cells. *Oncogene* 2011, **30**(9): 1009–19.

32 Vardiman JW, Thiele J, Arber DA, *et al.* The 2008 revision of the World Health Organization (WHO) classification of myeloid neoplasms and acute leukemia: rationale and important changes. *Blood* 2009, **114**(5): 937–51.

33 Dohner H, Estey EH, Amadori S, *et al.* Diagnosis and management of acute myeloid leukemia in adults: recommendations from an international expert panel, on behalf of the European LeukemiaNet. *Blood* 2010, **115**(3): 453–74.

34 van Rhenen A, Feller N, Kelder A, *et al.* High stem cell frequency in acute myeloid leukemia at diagnosis predicts high minimal residual disease and poor survival. *Clin Cancer Res* 2005,**11**(18): 6520–7.

35 Casasnovas RO, Slimane FK, Garand R, *et al.* Immunological classification of acute myeloblastic leukemias: relevance to patient outcome. *Leukemia* 2003, **17**(3), 515–27.

36 Kaleem Z, Crawford E, Pathan MH, *et al.* Flow cytometric analysis of acute leukemias. *Archives of Pathology and Laboratory Medicine* 2003, **127**(1): 42–8.

37 Legrand O, Perrot JY, Baudard M, *et al.* The immunophenotype of 177 adults with acute myeloid leukemia: proposal of a prognostic score. *Blood* 2000, **96**(3): 870–7.

38 Baer MR, Stewart CC, Dodge RK, *et al.* High frequency of immunophenotype changes in acute myeloid leukemia at relapse: implications for residual disease detection (Cancer

and Leukemia Group B Study 8361). *Blood* 2001, **97**(11): 3574–80.

39 Peffault de Latour R, Legrand O, Moreau D, *et al.* Comparison of flow cytometry and enzyme cytochemistry for the detection of myeloperoxydase in acute myeloid leukaemia: interests of a new positivity threshold. *British Journal of Haematology* 2003,**122**(2): 211–6.

40 Bene MC, Castoldi G, Knapp W, *et al.* Proposals for the immunological classification of acute leukemias. European Group for the Immunological Characterization of Leukemias (EGIL). *Leukemia* 1995, **9**(10): 1783–6.

41 Jaffe E, Harris N, Stein H, Vardiman J. *World Health Organization Classification of Tumours. Pathology and Genetics of Tumours of Haematopoietic and Lymphoid Tissues.* 2001. IARC, Lyon, France.

42 van den Ancker W, Terwijn M, Westers TM, *et al.* Acute leukemias of ambiguous lineage: diagnostic consequences of the WHO2008 classification. *Leukemia* 2010, **24**(7): 1392–6.

43 Dong HY, Kung JX, Bhardwaj V, McGill J. Flow cytometry rapidly identifies all acute promyelocytic leukemias with high specificity independent of underlying cytogenetic abnormalities. *Am J Clin Pathol* 2011, **135**(1): 76–84.

44 Oelschlaegel U, Koch S, Mohr B, *et al.* Rapid flow cytometric detection of aberrant cytoplasmic localization of nucleophosmin (NPMc) indicating mutant NPM1 gene in acute myeloid leukemia. *Leukemia* 2010, **24**(10): 1813–6.

45 Cohen PL, Hoyer JD, Kurtin PJ, Dewald GW, Hanson CA. Acute myeloid leukemia with minimal differentiation. A multiple parameter study. *Am J Clin Pathol* 1998, **109**(1): 32–8.

46 Bain BJ. *Leukaemia Diagnosis* (3rd edn). 2003. Blackwell Pub., Malden, Mass, Oxford.

47 Reading C, Estey E, Huh Y, *et al.* Expression of unusual immunophenotype combinations in acute myelogenous leukemia. *Blood* 1993, **81**(11): 3083–90.

48 Cruse J, Lewis R, Wang H. *Immunology Guidebook.* 2004. Elsevier, San Diego.

49 Bradstock K, Matthews J, Benson E, Page F, Bishop J. Prognostic value of immunophenotyping in acute myeloid leukemia. Australian Leukaemia Study Group. *Blood* 1994, **84**(4): 1220–5.

50 Guglielmi C, Paola Martelli M, *et al.* Immunophenotype of adult and childhood acute promyelocytic leukaemia: correlation with morphology, type of PML gene breakpoint and clinical outcome. A cooperative Italian study on 196 cases. *British Journal of Haematology* 1998, **102**(4): 1035–41.

51 Lin P, Hao S, Medeiros LJ, *et al.* Expression of CD2 in acute promyelocytic leukemia correlates with short form of PML-RARA ± transcripts and poorer prognosis. *American Journal of Clinical Pathology* 2004, **121**(3): 402–7.

52 Dunphy CH, Orton SO, Mantell J. Relative contributions of enzyme cytochemistry and flow cytometric immunophenotyping to the evaluation of acute myeloid leukemias with a monocytic component and of flow cytometric immunophenotyping to the evaluation of absolute monocytoses. *Am J Clin Pathol* 2004, **122**(6): 865–74.

53 Dunphy CH. Comparative analysis of detecting monocytic cells and their aberrancy. *Appl Immunohistochem Mol Morphol* 2011, **19**(4): 336–40.

54 Villamor N, Zarco MA, Rozman M, Ribera JM, Feliu E, Montserrat E. Acute myeloblastic leukemia with minimal myeloid differentiation: phenotypical and ultrastructural characteristics. *Leukemia* 1998, **12**(7): 1071–5.

55 Teodosio C, García-Montero AC, Jara-Acevedo M, *et al.* Mast cells from different molecular and prognostic subtypes of systemic mastocytosis display distinct immunophenotypes. *The Journal of Allergy and Clinical Immunology* **125**(3): 719–26.e4.

56 Filion LG, Izaguirre CA, Garber GE, Huebsh L, Aye MT. Detection of surface and cytoplasmic CD4 on blood monocytes from normal and HIV-1 infected individuals. *J Immunol Methods* 1990, **135**(1–2): 59–69.

57 Lucey DR, Dorsky DI, Nicholson-Weller A, Weller PF. Human eosinophils express CD4 protein and bind human immunodeficiency virus 1 gp120. *J Exp Med* 1989, **169**(1): 327–32.

58 Louache F, Debili N, Marandin A, Coulombel L, Vainchenker W. Expression of CD4 by human hematopoietic progenitors. *Blood* 1994, **84**(10): 3344–55.

59 Larson RS, McCurley TL, 3rd. CD4 predicts nonlymphocytic lineage in acute leukemia. Insights from analysis of 125 cases using two-color flow cytometry. *Am J Clin Pathol* 1995, **104**(2): 204–11.

60 Barcena A, Muench M, Galy A, *et al.* Phenotypic and functional analysis of T-cell precursors in the human fetal liver and thymus: CD7 expression in the early stages of T- and myeloid-cell development. *Blood* 1993, **82**(11): 3401–14.

61 Al-Mawali A, Gillis D, Lewis I. The role of multiparameter flow cytometry for detection of minimal residual disease in acute myeloid leukemia. *Am J Clin Pathol* 2009, **31**(1): 16–26.

62 Mason KD, Juneja SK, Szer J. The immunophenotype of acute myeloid leukemia: is there a relationship with prognosis? *Blood Rev* 2006, **20**(2): 71–82.

63 Ogata K, Nakamura K, Yokose N, *et al.* Clinical significance of phenotypic features of blasts in patients with myelodysplastic syndrome. *Blood* 2002, **100**(12): 3887–96.

64 Suzuki R, Yamamoto K, Seto M, *et al.* CD7+ and CD56+ myeloid/natural killer cell precursor acute leukemia: a distinct hematolymphoid disease entity. *Blood* 1997, **90**(6): 2417–28.

65 Kita K, Nakase K, Miwa H, *et al.* Phenotypical characteristics of acute myelocytic leukemia associated with the t(8;21)(q22;q22) chromosomal abnormality: frequent expression of immature B-cell antigen CD19 together with stem cell antigen CD34. *Blood* 1992, **80**(2): 470–7.

66 Yin CC, Medeiros LJ, Glassman AB, Lin P. t(8;21)(q22;q22) in Blast Phase of Chronic Myelogenous Leukemia. *American Journal of Clinical Pathology* 2004, **121**(6): 836–42.

67 Coustan-Smith E, Behm FG, Hurwitz CA, Rivera GK, Campana D. N-CAM (CD56) expression by CD34+ malignant myeloblasts has implications for minimal residual disease detection in acute myeloid leukemia. *Leukemia* 1993, **7**(6): 853–8.

68 Walter K, Cockerill PN, Barlow R, *et al.* Aberrant expression of CD19 in AML with t(8;21) involves a poised chromatin structure and PAX5. *Oncogene* 2010, **29**(20): 2927–37.

69 Adriaansen HJ, van Dongen JJ, Kappers-Klunne MC, *et al.* Terminal deoxynucleotidyl transferase positive subpopulations occur in the majority of ANLL: implications for the detection of minimal disease. *Leukemia* 1990, **4**(6): 404–10.

70 Porwit-MacDonald A, Janossy G, Ivory K, *et al.* Leukemia-associated changes identified by quantitative flow cytometry. IV. CD34 overexpression in acute myelogenous leukemia M2 with t(8;21). *Blood* 1996, **87**(3): 1162–9.

71 Campana D, Hansen-Hagge TE, Matutes E, *et al.* Phenotypic, genotypic, cytochemical, and ultrastructural characterization of acute undifferentiated leukemia. *Leukemia* 1990, **4**(9): 620–4.

72 Robertson MJ, Ritz J. Biology and clinical relevance of human natural killer cells. *Blood* 1990, **76**(12): 2421–38.

73 Pittet MJ, Speiser DE, Valmori D, Cerottini JC, Romero P. Cutting edge: cytolytic effector function in human circulating CD8+ T-cells closely correlates with CD56 surface expression. *J Immunol* 2000, **164**(3): 1148–52.

74 Xu Y, McKenna RW, Karandikar NJ, Pildain AJ, Kroft SH. Flow cytometric analysis of monocytes as a tool for distinguishing chronic myelomonocytic leukemia from reactive monocytosis. *Am J Clin Pathol* 2005, **124**(5): 799–806.

75 Rothe G, Gabriel H, Kovacs E, *et al.* Peripheral blood mononuclear phagocyte subpopulations as cellular markers in hypercholesterolemia. *Arterioscler Thromb Vasc Biol* 1996, **16**(12): 1437–47.

76 Sconocchia G, Keyvanfar K, El Ouriaghli F, *et al.* Phenotype and function of a CD56+ peripheral blood monocyte. *Leukemia* 2005, **19**(1): 69–76.

77 Pileri SA, Ascani S, Cox MC, *et al.* Myeloid sarcoma: clinicopathologic, phenotypic and cytogenetic analysis of 92 adult patients. *Leukemia* 2007, **21**(2): 340–50.

78 Yang DH, Lee JJ, Mun YC, *et al.* Predictable prognostic factor of CD56 expression in patients with acute myeloid leukemia with t(8:21) after high dose cytarabine or allogeneic

79 hematopoietic stem cell transplantation. *Am J Hematol* 2007, **82**(1): 1–5.

79 Baer MR, Stewart CC, Lawrence D, *et al.* Expression of the neural cell adhesion molecule CD56 is associated with short remission duration and survival in acute myeloid leukemia with t(8;21)(q22;q22). *Blood* 1997, **90**(4): 1643–8.

80 Ferrara F, Morabito F, Martino B, *et al.* CD56 expression is an indicator of poor clinical outcome in patients with acute promyelocytic leukemia treated with simultaneous all-trans-retinoic acid and chemotherapy. *J Clin Oncol* 2000, **18**(6): 1295–300.

81 Montesinos P, Rayon C, Vellenga E, *et al.* Clinical significance of CD56 expression in patients with acute promyelocytic leukemia treated with all-trans retinoic acid and anthracycline-based regimens. *Blood* 2010, **117**(6): 1799–805.

82 Karandikar NJ, Aquino DB, McKenna RW, Kroft SH. Transient myeloproliferative disorder and acute myeloid leukemia in Down syndrome. An immunophenotypic analysis. *Am J Clin Pathol* 2001, **116**(2): 204–10.

83 Fischer L, Gokbuget N, Schwartz S, *et al.* CD56 expression in T-cell acute lymphoblastic leukemia is associated with non-thymic phenotype and resistance to induction therapy but no inferior survival after risk-adapted therapy. *Haematologica* 2009, **94**(2): 224–9.

84 Paietta E, Neuberg D, Richards S, *et al.* Rare adult acute lymphocytic leukemia with CD56 expression in the ECOG experience shows unexpected phenotypic and genotypic heterogeneity. *American Journal of Hematology* 2001, **66**(3): 189–96.

85 Seegmiller AC, Kroft SH, Karandikar NJ, McKenna RW. Characterization of immunophenotypic aberrancies in 200 cases of B acute lymphoblastic leukemia. *Am J Clin Pathol* 2009, **132**(6): 940–9.

86 Cornfield D, Liu Z, Gorczyca W, Weisberger J. The potential role of flow cytometry in the diagnosis of small cell carcinoma. *Arch Pathol Lab Med* 2003, **127**(4): 461–4.

87 Lewis RE, Cruse JM, Sanders CM, Webb RN, Suggs JL. Aberrant expression of T-cell markers in acute myeloid leukemia. *Experimental and Molecular Pathology* 2007, **83**(3): 462–3.

88 Khalidi HS, Medeiros LJ, Chang KL, Brynes RK, Slovak ML, Arber DA. The immunophenotype of adult acute myeloid leukemia: high frequency of lymphoid antigen expression and comparison of immunophenotype, French-American-British classification, and karyotypic abnormalities. *Am J Clin Pathol* 1998, **109**(2): 211–20.

89 Gazzola MV, Collins NH, Tafuri A, Keever CA. Recombinant interleukin 3 induces interleukin 2 receptor expression on early myeloid cells in normal human bone marrow. *Exp Hematol* 1992, **20**(2): 201–8.

90 Saito Y, Kitamura H, Hijikata A, *et al*. Identification of therapeutic targets for quiescent, chemotherapy-resistant human leukemia stem cells. *Science Translational Medicine* 2010, **2**(17): 17–9.

91 Han X, Jorgensen JL, Brahmandam A, *et al*. Immunophenotypic study of basophils by multiparameter flow cytometry. *Arch Pathol Lab Med* 2008, **132**(5): 813–9.

92 Lichtman MA, Segel GB. Uncommon phenotypes of acute myelogenous leukemia: basophilic, mast cell, eosinophilic, and myeloid dendritic cell subtypes: a review. *Blood Cells Mol Dis* 2005, **35**(3): 370–83.

93 Valent P, Sotlar K, Horny HP. Aberrant expression of CD30 in aggressive systemic mastocytosis and mast cell leukemia: a differential diagnosis to consider in aggressive hematopoietic CD30-positive neoplasms. *Leuk Lymphoma* 2011, **52**(5): 740–4.

94 Paietta E, Racevskis J, Neuberg D, Rowe JM, Goldstone AH, Wiernik PH. Expression of CD25 (interleukin-2 receptor alpha chain) in adult acute lymphoblastic leukemia predicts for the presence of BCR/ABL fusion transcripts: results of a preliminary laboratory analysis of ECOG/MRC Intergroup Study E2993. Eastern Cooperative Oncology Group/Medical Research Council. *Leukemia* 1997, **11**(11): 1887–90.

95 Imamura N. Sensitive detection technique of myeloperoxidase precursor protein by flow cytometry with monoclonal antibodies. *Am J Hematol* 1998, **58**(3): 241–3.

96 Zuo Z, Polski JM, Kasyan A, Medeiros LJ. Acute erythroid leukemia. *Arch Pathol Lab Med* 2010, **134**(9): 1261–70.

97 Duchayne E, Demur C, Rubie H, Robert A, Dastugue N. Diagnosis of acute basophilic leukemia. *Leuk Lymphoma* 1999, **32**(3–4): 269–78.

98 Shvidel L, Shaft D, Stark B, Shtalrid M, Berrebi A, Resnitzky P. Acute basophilic leukaemia: eight unsuspected new cases diagnosed by electron microscopy. *Br J Haematol* 2003, **120**(5): 774–81.

99 Dunphy CH, Tang W. The value of CD64 expression in distinguishing acute myeloid leukemia with monocytic differentiation from other subtypes of acute myeloid leukemia: a flow cytometric analysis of 64 cases. *Arch Pathol Lab Med* 2007, **131**(5): 748–54.

100 Duchayne E, Fenneteau O, Pages M-P, *et al*. Acute Megakaryoblastic Leukaemia: A National Clinical and Biological Study of 53 Adult and Childhood Cases by the Groupe Francais d'Hematologie Cellulaire (GFHC). *Leukemia and Lymphoma* 2003, **44**(1): 49–58.

101 Kafer G, Willer A, Ludwig W, Kramer A, Hehlmann R, Hastka J. Intracellular expression of CD61 precedes surface expression. *Ann Hematol* 1999, **78**(10): 472–4.

102 Borowitz MJ, Shuster JJ, Civin CI, *et al*. Prognostic significance of CD34 expression in childhood B-precursor acute lymphocytic leukemia: a Pediatric Oncology Group study. *J Clin Oncol* 1990, **8**(8): 1389–98.

103 Jennings CD, Foon KA. Recent advances in flow cytometry: application to the diagnosis of hematologic malignancy. *Blood* 1997, **90**(8): 2863–92.

104 Thomas DA, O'Brien S, Jorgensen JL, *et al*. Prognostic significance of CD20 expression in adults with de novo precursor B-lineage acute lymphoblastic leukemia. *Blood* 2009, **113**(25): 6330–7.

105 Borowitz MJ, Shuster J, Carroll AJ, *et al*. Prognostic significance of fluorescence intensity of surface marker expression in childhood B-precursor acute lymphoblastic leukemia. A Pediatric Oncology Group Study. *Blood* 1997, **89**(11): 3960–6.

106 Jeha S, Behm F, Pei D, *et al*. Prognostic significance of CD20 expression in childhood B-cell precursor acute lymphoblastic leukemia. *Blood* 2006, **108**(10): 3302–4.

107 van der Velden VH, Bruggemann M, Hoogeveen PG, *et al*. TCRB gene rearrangements in childhood and adult precursor-B-ALL: frequency, applicability as MRD-PCR target, and stability between diagnosis and relapse. *Leukemia* 2004, **18**(12): 1971–80.

108 Szczepanski T, Pongers-Willemse MJ, Langerak AW, *et al*. Ig heavy chain gene rearrangements in T-cell acute lymphoblastic leukemia exhibit predominant DH6-19 and DH7-27 gene usage, can result in complete V-D-J rearrangements, and are rare in T-cell receptor alpha beta lineage. *Blood* 1999, **93**(12): 4079–85.

109 Koehler M, Behm FG, Shuster J, *et al*. Transitional pre-B-cell acute lymphoblastic leukemia of childhood is associated with favorable prognostic clinical features and an excellent outcome: a Pediatric Oncology Group study. *Leukemia* 1993, **7**(12): 2064–8.

110 Vasef MA, Brynes RK, Murata-Collins JL, Arber DA, Medeiros LJ. Surface immunoglobulin light chain-positive acute lymphoblastic leukemia of FAB L1 or L2 type: a report of 6 cases in adults. *Am J Clin Pathol* 1998, **110**(2): 143–9.

111 Kansal R, Deeb G, Barcos M, *et al*. Precursor B lymphoblastic leukemia with surface light chain immunoglobulin restriction: a report of 15 patients. *Am J Clin Pathol* 2004, **121**(4): 512–25.

112 Pui CH, Rubnitz JE, Hancock ML, *et al*. Reappraisal of the clinical and biologic significance of myeloid-associated antigen expression in childhood acute lymphoblastic leukemia. *J Clin Oncol* 1998, **16**(12): 3768–73.

113 Burmeister T, Meyer C, Schwartz S, *et al*. The MLL recombinome of adult CD10-negative B-cell precursor acute lymphoblastic leukemia: results from the GMALL study group. *Blood* 2009, **113**(17): 4011–5.

114 Borkhardt A, Wuchter C, Viehmann S, *et al.* Infant acute lymphoblastic leukemia – combined cytogenetic, immunophenotypical and molecular analysis of 77 cases. *Leukemia* 2002, **16**(9): 1685–90.

115 Moorman AV, Harrison CJ, Buck GA, *et al.* Karyotype is an independent prognostic factor in adult acute lymphoblastic leukemia (ALL): analysis of cytogenetic data from patients treated on the Medical Research Council (MRC) UKALLXII/Eastern Cooperative Oncology Group (ECOG) 2993 trial. *Blood* 2007, **109**(8): 3189–97.

116 Digiuseppe JA. Acute lymphoblastic leukemia: diagnosis and detection of minimal residual disease following therapy. *Clin Lab Med* 2007, **27**(3): 533–49, vi.

117 Babusikova O, Stevulova L, Fajtova M. Immunophenotyping parameters as prognostic factors in T-acute leukemia patients. *Neoplasma* 2009, **56**(6): 508–13.

118 Porwit-MacDonald A, Bjorklund E, Lucio P, *et al.* BIOMED-1 concerted action report: flow cytometric characterization of CD7$^+$ cell subsets in normal bone marrow as a basis for the diagnosis and follow-up of T-cell acute lymphoblastic leukemia (T-ALL). *Leukemia* 2000, **14**(5): 816–25.

119 Vitale A, Guarini A, Ariola C, *et al.* Adult T-cell acute lymphoblastic leukemia: biologic profile at presentation and correlation with response to induction treatment in patients enrolled in the GIMEMA LAL 0496 protocol. *Blood* 2006, **107**(2): 473–9.

120 Uckun FM, Gaynon PS, Sensel MG, *et al.* Clinical features and treatment outcome of childhood T-lineage acute lymphoblastic leukemia according to the apparent maturational stage of T-lineage leukemic blasts: a Children's Cancer Group study. *J Clin Oncol* 1997, **15**(6): 2214–21.

121 Czuczman MS, Dodge RK, Stewart CC, *et al.* Value of immunophenotype in intensively treated adult acute lymphoblastic leukemia: Cancer and Leukemia Group B Study 8364. *Blood* 1999, **93**(11): 3931–9.

122 Schabath R, Ratei R, Ludwig WD. The prognostic significance of antigen expression in leukaemia. *Best Pract Res Clin Haematol* 2003, **16**(4): 613–28.

123 Marks DI, Paietta EM, Moorman AV, *et al.* T-cell acute lymphoblastic leukemia in adults: clinical features, immunophenotype, cytogenetics, and outcome from the large randomized prospective trial (UKALL XII/ECOG 2993). *Blood* 2009, **114**(25): 5136–45.

124 Onciu M. Acute lymphoblastic leukemia. *Hematol Oncol Clin North Am* 2009, **23**(4): 655–74.

125 Meijerink JP. Genetic rearrangements in relation to immunophenotype and outcome in T-cell acute lymphoblastic leukaemia. *Best Pract Res Clin Haematol* 2010, **23**(3): 307–18.

126 Pilozzi E, Pulford K, Jones M, *et al.* Co-expression of CD79a (JCB117) and CD3 by lymphoblastic lymphoma. *J Pathol* 1998, **186**(2): 140–3.

127 Asnafi V, Beldjord K, Garand R, Millien C, *et al.* IgH DJ rearrangements within T-ALL correlate with cCD79a expression, an immature//TCR[gamma][delta] phenotype and absence of IL7R[alpha]//CD127 expression. *Leukemia* 2004, **18**(12): 1997–2001.

128 Simone J. Acute lymphocytic leukemia in childhood. *Semin Hematol* 1974, **11**(1): 25–39.

129 Pui CH, Thiel E. Central nervous system disease in hematologic malignancies: historical perspective and practical applications. *Semin Oncol* 2009, **36**(4 Suppl 2): S2–S16.

130 Pui C-H, Howard SC. Current management and challenges of malignant disease in the CNS in paediatric leukaemia. *The Lancet Oncology* 2008, **9**(3): 257–68.

131 Lazarus HM, Richards SM, Chopra R, *et al.* Central nervous system involvement in adult acute lymphoblastic leukemia at diagnosis: results from the international ALL trial MRC UKALL XII/ECOG E2993. *Blood* 2006, **108**(2): 465–72.

132 Johnston DL, Alonzo TA, Gerbing RB, Lange BJ, Woods WG. The presence of central nervous system disease at diagnosis in pediatric acute myeloid leukemia does not affect survival: A Children's Oncology Group study. *Pediatric Blood and Cancer* 2010, **55**(3): 414–20.

133 Hill QA, Owen RG. CNS prophylaxis in lymphoma: who to target and what therapy to use. *Blood Rev* 2006, **20**(6): 319–32.

134 Glass JP, Melamed M, Chernik NL, Posner JB. Malignant cells in cerebrospinal fluid (CSF): the meaning of a positive CSF cytology. *Neurology* 1979, **29**(10): 1369–75.

135 Quijano S, Lopez A, Manuel Sancho J, *et al.* Identification of leptomeningeal disease in aggressive B-cell non-Hodgkin's lymphoma: improved sensitivity of flow cytometry. *J Clin Oncol* 2009, **27**(9): 1462–9.

136 Hegde U, Filie A, Little RF, *et al.* High incidence of occult leptomeningeal disease detected by flow cytometry in newly diagnosed aggressive B-cell lymphomas at risk for central nervous system involvement: the role of flow cytometry versus cytology. *Blood* 2005, **105**(2): 496–502.

137 Ahluwalia MS, Wallace PK, Peereboom DM. Flow cytometry as a diagnostic tool in lymphomatous or leukemic meningitis. *Cancer* 2012, **118**(7): 1747–53.

138 NCCN. Central Nervous System Cancers. 2011 (accessed 1 Feb 2012); v2.0.2011: Available from: http://www.nccn.org.

139 Kraan J, Gratama JW, Haioun C, *et al.* Flow cytometric immunophenotyping of cerebrospinal fluid. *Curr Protoc Cytom* 2008, Chapter 6: Unit 6, **25**.

140 D'Alessio F, Mirabelli P, Mariotti E, *et al.* Miniaturized flow cytometry-based BCR-ABL immunoassay in detecting leptomeningeal disease. *Leukemia Research* 2011, **35**(10): 1290–3.

141 Santos GC, Longatto-Filho A, de Carvalho LV, Neves JI, Alves AC. Immunocytochemical study of malignant lymphoma in serous effusions. *Acta Cytol* 2000, **44**(4): 539–42.

142 Dekking E, van der Velden VH, Bottcher S, *et al.* Detection of fusion genes at the protein level in leukemia patients via the flow cytometric immunobead assay. *Best Pract Res Clin Haematol* 2010, **23**(3): 333–45.

143 Weerkamp F, Dekking E, Ng YY, *et al.* Flow cytometric immunobead assay for the detection of BCR-ABL fusion proteins in leukemia patients. *Leukemia* 2009, **23**(6): 1106–17.

CHAPTER 6

Chronic Lymphoid Leukaemias and Exfoliating Lymphoma

The use of flow cytometry (FCM) in the study of chronic lymphoproliferative disorders (LPD) is particularly important. It is able to reliably discriminate between true clonal proliferations and the reactive lymphocytosis seen as a response to a variety of physiological stimuli. Before any potentially clonal disorder can be categorized it is important to have a basic understanding of T and B-cell lymphoid ontogeny. The pattern of surface cluster differentiation (CD) antigen expression indicates the degree of maturity, the possible relationship with the lymph node germinal centre and sometimes the function of the normal cell from which a malignant population is derived.

Normal peripheral blood lymphoid populations

It is clearly important to have an understanding of the characteristics of normal peripheral blood lymphocytes, which have an absolute level of 0.75 to 3.6×10^9/L [1]. T-cells normally account for 80–90% of lymphocytes in peripheral blood (absolute level 0.7 to 2.78×10^9/L) and are identified by the expression of surface(s) CD3. The presence of sCD3 indicates a cell that has matured beyond the precursor T-cell stage. Precursor T-cells are normally located in thymus and bone marrow and will express cytoplasmic (c)CD3 from a very early stage of T-cell differentiation. Furthermore, cCD3 is retained in mature T-cells as well as sCD3. Cytoplasmic CD3 expression, therefore, is the gold standard immunophenotypic marker of T-cell lineage. T-helper cells express surface CD4, whilst T-suppressor cells express surface CD8. The normal peripheral blood CD4/CD8 ratio is approximately 2:1 (range 1:1 to 3:1), whilst the normal bone marrow CD4/CD8 ratio is reversed at approximately 1:2.

Normal T-cells also express CD2, CD5 and CD7. T-cells which co-express both CD4 and CD8 are undergoing thymic maturation/migration and are encountered in normal peripheral blood at very low levels. It is important to remember that an apparent excess of CD4+ cells might be due to a congenital or acquired deficiency of CD8+ cells and vice versa. One should not, for example, report an apparent CD8 excess in patients with profound CD4 depletion due to human immunodeficiency virus infection. In these situations it is important to calculate absolute values – a normal CD4 count is $> 493 \times 10^6$/L and a normal CD8 count is $> 224 \times 10^6$/L [1]. A small population of natural killer (NK) cells (an important component of the innate immune system) are normally present in peripheral blood (up to 654×10^6/L). These cells express CD2 but not CD3 and this explains why peripheral blood lymphoid cell CD2+ population (T-cells and NK cells) are always slightly higher than the CD3+ population (T-cells only). With NK cells excepted, one should not normally encounter CD4 or CD8 negative cells in peripheral blood. Such a phenotype indicates T-cell immaturity, possibly a precursor T-cell neoplasm and often a clonal T-cell population.

Normal B-cells account for 10–20% of peripheral blood lymphocytes, with an absolute level of 0.07 to 0.52×10^9/L [1]. Mature B-cells express surface CD19, CD79a and usually CD20. Immature B-cells characteristically express cytoplasmic +/− surface CD19 and CD79a, but are usually CD20 negative. Cytoplasmic CD79a is our gold standard for identifying cells of B-cell lineage. CD19 is usually also a reliable B-cell marker but can be aberrantly expressed in some non-B-cell neoplastic diseases. Peripheral blood B-cells normally express CD22 and FMC7 with surface light chain expression, either kappa or lambda at a ratio of between 2:1 and 3:2. Normal

Practical Flow Cytometry in Haematology Diagnosis, First Edition. Mike Leach, Mark Drummond and Allyson Doig.
© 2013 John Wiley & Sons, Ltd. Published 2013 by John Wiley & Sons, Ltd.

B-cells express HLA-DR whereas normal non-activated T-cells do not.

It is important to recognize that normal T and B-cell antigens are expressed at a certain strength or brightness, this being quantified as mean fluorescence intensity (MFI). Each laboratory should have established a normal range of intensity of expression of important antigens ascertained on their flow cytometer using the antibodies and fluorochromes in daily use for a variety of normal cell populations. Such normal reference values are invaluable when interpreting clinical FCM studies.

Identification of clonal lymphoid populations

Having recognized the characteristics of normal peripheral blood lymphocytes we are now better placed to recognize abnormal populations. There are a number of factors which assist in this process and certain rules should be followed. On occasion, even with elaborate FCM studies, it can be difficult to determine whether an apparent abnormal population is clonal or not. This is particularly relevant to mature T-cell populations where definite ascertainment of clonality can sometimes be difficult. This is where careful correlation with other clinical and laboratory parameters is particularly important. We should always be careful not to cause unnecessary distress and anxiety to patients or precipitate additional needless investigations. We should therefore consider when it might be appropriate to perform FCM studies when considering a possible diagnosis of LPD. A list of potential indications is listed below:

- Significant lymphocytosis ($>6 \times 10^9$/L)
- Lymphadenopathy and lymphocytosis
- Abnormal lymphoid morphology
- Splenomegaly $^{+/-}$ cytopenias where an LPD is possible
- Unexplained cytopenias where an LPD is possible
- Persistent unexplained erythroderma
- Splenomegaly and lymphadenopathy where a node biopsy is not possible

The presence of a minor lymphocytosis (4 to 6×10^9/L) in isolation, is in our experience not a good indication for FCM studies; it often identifies normal or reactive populations and frequently identifies subclinical entities like monoclonal B lymphocytosis.

Identification of clonal B-cell disorders

Clonal B-cell disorders are usually easily recognized, as clonality is often indicated by grossly skewed kappa to lambda surface light chain ratios or dim light chain expression. In fact the light chain MFI on normal residual B-cells can act as an internal control which assists in the diagnostic process. However, a number of features are useful in making a diagnosis:

1 Skewing of kappa:lambda ratio greater than 10:1 or less than 1:10
2 Weak or absent surface light chain expression
3 Aberrant CD5 expression
4 CD10 expression
5 CD11c, CD103, CD123 and CD25 expression
6 CD23 expression.
7 Weak, dim or absent CD79a, CD19, CD22 or CD20 expression
8 Aberrant CD2, CD4, CD7 or CD8 expression

The absolute relevance of any of the above findings must always be interpreted with respect to the patient's clinical presentation, physical signs and peripheral blood cell morphology.

Diagnosis of B-cell disorders

Although B lymphocytes constitute a minority of normal peripheral blood lymphoid cells, B-cell lymphoproliferative disorders are significantly more common than their T-cell counterparts. Flow cytometry studies are often prompted by the recognition of a significant peripheral blood lymphocytosis. These cases are often analysed using a lymphoid gated CD2+ versus CD19+ plot (Figure 6.1).

An excess of CD19+ cells will generate further analysis using antibodies comprising a chronic B-cell panel as outlined below in Table 6.1.

Additional antibodies may be of value in patients presenting with splenomegaly, circulating hairy or villous lymphoid cells and cytopenias (summarized in Table 6.2). Positivity for each of the antigens is given a score of one point: this scoring system helps define classic hairy cell leukaemia (HCL) from disorders with a similar presentation (see below).

At the outset it is important always to distinguish the precursor T or B neoplasms from the mature LPD as the immunophenotypic analysis will differ significantly. Precursor neoplasms tend to present acutely with

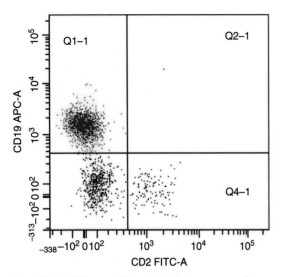

Figure 6.1 A CD19 versus CD2 analysis indicates an excess of B-cells, 77% of events (in red) compared to T-cells, 5% of events.

Table 6.1 A typical antibody panel selection for defining B-cell disorders.

Antigen	Cells on which normally expressed (surface)
CD19	Pro B to mature B-cells
CD20	Pre B to mature B-cells
CD79b	Pro B to mature B-cells
CD22	Pro B to mature B-cells
CD38	Activated B-cells, plasma cells, T and NK cells
CD23	Activated mature B-cells expressing IgM or IgD
CD5	Small subset of normal B-cells, T-cells
FMC7	Mature B-cells
CD10	Pre B lymphocytes and germinal centre B-cells
HLA-DR	Normal B-cells, activated T-cells
Kappa	Normal polyclonal mature B-cells
Lambda	Normal polyclonal mature B-cells

Table 6.2 A useful supplementary antibody panel for defining hairy cell leukaemia like disorders.

Antigen	Cells on which normally expressed (surface)
CD11c	Granulocytes, macrophages, NK cells, dendritic cells
CD103	Intraepithelial T lymphocytes
CD25	Activated B and T-cells, macrophages
CD123	Plasmacytoid monocytes

Table 6.3 Important immunophenotypic discriminator antigens in distinguishing precursor B-cell neoplasms from mature LPD.

Characteristic	Precursor B ALL	B LPD
Surface Ig	Negative	Positive
TdT	Often positive	Negative
FMC7	Negative	Positive (except CLL)
CD20	Sometimes positive	Positive
CD34	Often positive	Negative

CD5 positive B-cell lymphoproliferative disorders

The finding of aberrant CD5 expression on a B-cell LPD is very helpful in the diagnostic process as this narrows the differential very substantially. CD5 is a T-cell antigen, so aberrant expression on B-cells is strongly suggestive of a clonal B-cell disorder. Only a very small normal B-cell subset expresses CD5 [2]. Furthermore relatively few B-cell disorders express CD5, so it carries useful diagnostic potential; the relative frequency of expression varies between the conditions. Some, such as chronic lymphocytic leukaemia (CLL) and mantle cell lymphoma (MCL), express CD5 in the majority of cases, whereas others like lymphoplasmacytoid lymphoma (LPL) and splenic marginal zone lymphoma (SMZL) express it only in a minority. CD5 expression, however, is useful in starting to consider the differential diagnosis. The following entities should be considered.

Chronic lymphocytic leukaemia

This is the most commonly encountered LPD in clinical practice. CLL cells have a characteristic morphology and immunophenotype that should allow easy recognition.

B symptoms, bone marrow failure and often a high WBC, whereas the LPD are increasingly found incidentally and usually cause symptoms in more advanced stage disease. A careful assessment of the presentation, together with a detailed review of peripheral blood morphology will usually differentiate these disorders and allow the appropriate FCM antibody panel analysis to be performed. The main immunophenotypic differences of the precursor and mature B-cell disorders is summarized in Table 6.3.

CLL cells probably arise either from a naive pre-germinal centre B-cell (unmutated CLL) or a post-germinal centre memory B-cell (mutated CLL) [3]. Most patients are diagnosed following the finding of either an incidental lymphocytosis, after presenting with lymphadenopathy, following admission to hospital with infection or after developing an autoimmune haemolytic anaemia or thrombocytopenia. The disease is staged according to Rai or Binet (Table 6.4) and this is predictive of survival.

Table 6.4 The Binet staging system for CLL.

Stage	Feature	Median survival
A	Less than 3 nodal areas	10 years
B	More than 3 nodal areas	5 years
C	Hb <100 g/L, Platelets <100×10⁹/L	2 years

Reproduced from Binet et al. *Cancer* 1977; 40: 855–64, with permission from Wiley.

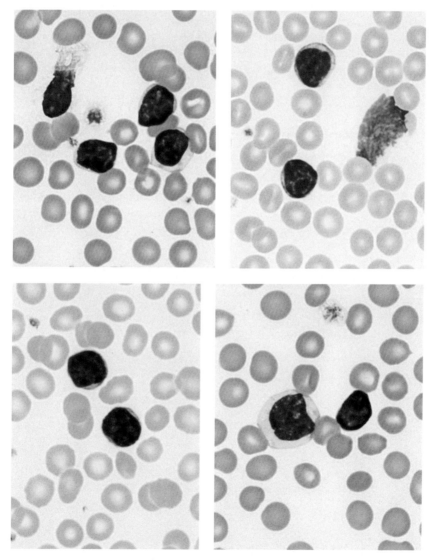

Figure 6.2 Typical morphology of lymphocytes in CLL. Note the condensed chromatin, sparse cytoplasm and absent nucleoli in addition to the smear cells (upper images) and the prolymphocyte (bottom right).

Morphology

CLL cells are typically small, with condensed nuclear chromatin, absent nucleoli, high nuclear to cytoplasmic ratio and round or ovoid nuclei. Nuclear clefts or folds are only seen in a minority of cells (Figure 6.2).

The morphology of some cases is atypical, with increased pleomorphism, occasional nucleoli and more abundant cytoplasm. Atypical morphology with an increased proportion of prolymphocytes is associated with cytogenetic abnormalities, most often trisomy 12 and del17p [4], progressive disease and refractoriness to therapy.

CLL and small lymphocytic lymphoma (SLL), is not infrequently associated with auto-immune haemolytic anaemia (AIHA). It is always worth considering the diagnosis in any new patient referred with a Coombs positive warm antibody mediated autoimmune haemolytic condition (Figure 6.3).

Immunophenotype

CLL cells show a number of characteristic features in addition to aberrant CD5 positivity which assists diagnosis. They show light chain restriction but MFI for kappa or lambda is usually dim. Similarly, CD20 expression is dim, CD79b and CD22 are often negative or dim and FMC7, which is an epitope of the CD20 molecule, is absent or dim. CD38 may be expressed in some cases and

this appears to correlate with CLL showing an unmutated IgVH gene or Zap 70 expression and therefore may carry prognostic significance [5], but it should be noted that the expression of CD38 may vary in any individual patient's cells over time. CLL scoring systems have been devised to take into account some of these features and indicate the likelihood of a diagnosis of CLL based on the immunophenotypic characteristics (Table 6.5) [4, 6].

True CLL will have a score of 3 or more in 96% of cases. The assessment through scoring can be further strengthened by paying attention to intensity of CD20 expression. A proportion of CLL, 7–20% [7], will not show CD5 expression, but because of the multiple parameters used in scoring the diagnosis should still not be difficult. Some CLL cases show absent surface light chains and others show oligoclonal or biclonal expression [8], for example one kappa and one lambda restricted clone. These cases should not be misinterpreted as polyclonal: the immunophenotype is otherwise that of CLL (CD5+ CD23+ CD79b−/dim CD20dim, FMC7−). Confirmation of clonality in those cases with absent surface light chains can be achieved by demonstrating cytoplasmic light chain restriction. More recently, the membrane glycoprotein CD200 has been shown to be useful in discriminating between CLL with immunophenotypic aberrancy and MCL; it is universally positive in the former but not the latter [9].

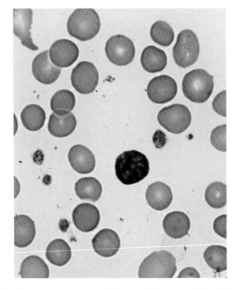 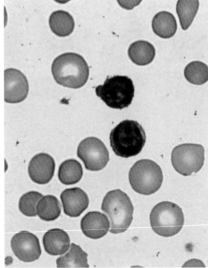

Figure 6.3 Prominent spherocytes in AIHA complicating early stage CLL.

Table 6.5 The CLL scoring system.

Antigen	Expression	Score
CD5	Positive	1
CD23	Positive	1
FMC7	Negative	1
Surface Ig	Weak/dim	1
CD79b	Negative or dim	1

Reproduced from Moreau et al. [6], with permission from American Society for Clinical Pathology.

Table 6.6 Cytogenetic aberrations and survival in CLL.

Cytogenetic finding	Median survival (months)
Normal	111
13q deletion	133
Trisomy 12	114
11q deletion	79
17p deletion	32

Cytogenetics

Standard cytogenetics using metaphase preparations are rarely useful in CLL as the cells are difficult to grow *in vitro*. Fluorescent *in situ* hybridization (FISH) studies (using fluorescent probes which align and hybridize with segments of the chromosome of interest), have identified a number of important abnormalities which assist in making a diagnosis in difficult cases but also carry prognostic significance (with del11q and del17p in particular, having an adverse outcome) (Table 6.6) [10]. The presence of such, together with IgVH gene mutation status, are important predictors of disease behaviour in early stage patients [11]. The presence of adverse cytogenetic findings is significantly more likely in unmutated IgVH gene patients. Detection of 17p del, reflecting loss of TP53 function, also indicates likely refractoriness to standard fludarabine based therapy.

Monoclonal B lymphocytosis

The term monoclonal B-cell lymphocytosis (MBL) was recently introduced to identify individuals with a small population of monoclonal B-cells, usually with an immunophenotype identical to CLL. There is absence of other features that are diagnostic of a B-cell lymphoproliferative disorder (such as cytopenias, lymphadenopathy and splenomegaly) and the absolute level of clonal cells is below that required for a diagnosis of CLL (5×10^9/L) [12, 13]. MBL is often identified through hospital investigation of a mild lymphocytosis. This entity is interesting and may provide insight into our understanding of the biology and evolution of CLL, familial CLL and other lymphoproliferative disorders [14]. Its recognition, however, can often generate unnecessary anxiety for patients. Only 1% of such individuals develop progressive disease requiring

treatment per year [15], analogous to the relationship between monoclonal gammopathy of uncertain significance (MGUS) and multiple myeloma.

Mantle cell lymphoma

This is another B-cell LPD derived from the mantle zone of the lymph node follicle, which often exfoliates into blood and frequently expresses CD5. This disease predominantly affects middle-aged to elderly males. Patients may present with incidental lymphocytosis, lymphadenopathy, splenomegaly, extra nodal periorbital disease or with diarrhoea, gastrointestinal bleeding, weight loss or abdominal bloating due to bowel involvement. Bone marrow involvement is common. A proportion of patients present with exfoliating disease and splenomegaly but with minimal nodal involvement.

Morphology

Mantle cells are often pleomorphic and demonstrate varied nuclear and cytoplasmic morphology in peripheral blood. The nuclei often show convolutions with clefts and may contain nucleoli, the cytoplasm is very variable in volume and the cells from a given case may vary considerably in size (Figure 6.4). Mantle cells can on occasion resemble monocytes. The blastoid and pleomorphic variants show large cells with prominent or multiple nucleoli and often show aggressive clinical behaviour with refractoriness or short-lived response to treatment (Figure 6.5).

Immunophenotype

CD5 is usually (but not always) expressed and MCL cells show pan B antigen expression with positivity for CD20, CD79a, CD22, FMC7 and HLA-DR. Light chain and CD20 expression is usually moderate in intensity; CD23 is usually negative and helps discriminate from CLL/SLL

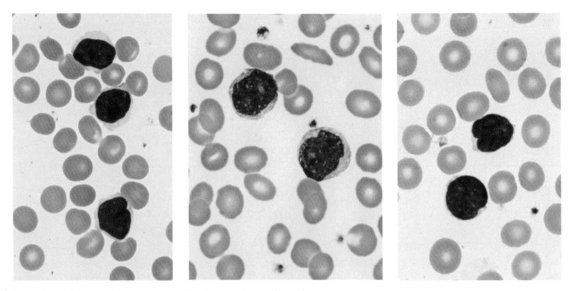

Figure 6.4 Typical morphology of mantle cell lymphoma cells in peripheral blood.

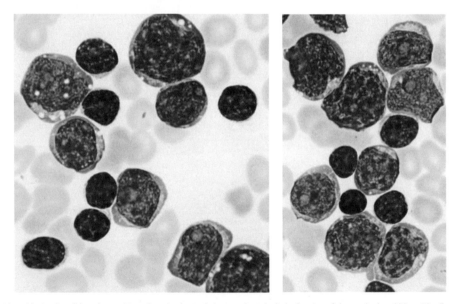

Figure 6.5 Blastoid mantle cell lymphoma. Note the mixed populations and particularly the size of the nucleolated blastoid cells.

but has been reported positive in up to 25% of patients in some series [16, 17]. Rare cases have been documented to also express CD10 and this sometimes correlates with blastoid morphology [18]. MCL can occasionally be confused with B prolymphocytic leukaemia (B-PLL) [19], particularly in cases presenting with blood and bone marrow disease with splenomegaly and without lym-phadenopathy. Such cases of MCL may show more indolent behaviour and longer survival [20]. The immunophenotype of MCL and B PLL, particularly if CD5 is not expressed, can appear very similar. Careful assessment of the clinical history and examination, morphology, immunohistochemistry (see below) and cytogenetics should differentiate the two.

Cytogenetics

MCL will typically show a t(11;14) (q13;q32) translocation, involving the Ig heavy chain gene and CCND1 gene leading to over expression of cyclin D1. This is considered to be the primary genetic event. The translocation can be identified using FISH and cyclin D1 over expression can be demonstrated using immunohistochemistry. Cyclin D1 positivity in MCL is not universal but such cases always show nuclear expression of a protein called SOX11 [21]. SOX11 expression is rare in other B-cell LPD. Furthermore, cases with a leukaemic, non-nodal presentation with splenomegaly are often cyclin D1 positive but SOX11 negative [22], so nuclear SOX11 status may indicate a better prognosis disease and might influence treatment decisions. Finally, MCL can show a large number of additional secondary cytogenetic abnormalities including rearrangements of the MYC gene at 8q24 and TP53 at 17p13; These findings are correlated with blastoid morphology and rapid disease progression [23].

Splenic marginal zone lymphoma

Splenic marginal zone lymphoma (SMZL) cells often appear in peripheral blood at low to medium levels and can, on occasion, express CD5 so the entity is considered here in the differential diagnosis. This condition most frequently affects patients over 50 years with equal male to female distribution and usually presents with a mild lymphocytosis, cytopenias and splenomegaly. It often pursues an indolent course, with around 70% of patients alive at ten years [24]. About one-third of patients have a small serum paraprotein and an association with hepatitis C virus infection has been noted. Some patients have coexistent lymphadenopathy, but this is usually a later feature. The degree of bone marrow involvement is variable but when seen is usually interstitial or nodular in pattern, with a notable affinity for the marrow sinusoids. This may relate to the SMZL cellular adhesion profile, which might also explain involvement of the splenic red pulp and liver sinusoidal vasculature. Peripheral blood cytopenias are most often due to hypersplenism but can also be due to autoimmune phenomena.

Morphology

Marginal zone lymphoma cells vary quite significantly in their morphological characteristics between patients. Most often these cells are small and compact, without nuclear pleomorphism or nucleoli. Some cells can be difficult to differentiate from normal lymphocytes but with careful searching the morphologist can usually find a number of cells with cytoplasmic convolutions, blebs or fronds, most typically in a bipolar distribution and often best found in the thicker part of the blood smear. This characteristic may be artefactual as it is often not apparent in cells examined in the thinner tail of the smear (Figure 6.6).

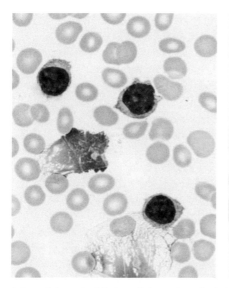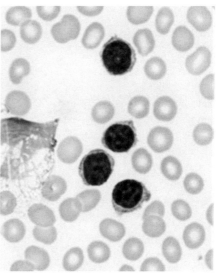

Figure 6.6 Typical morphology of exfoliating cells from a case of splenic marginal zone lymphoma.

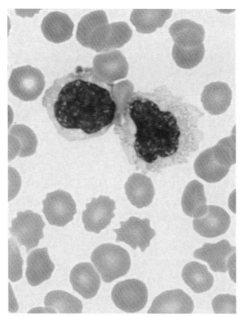
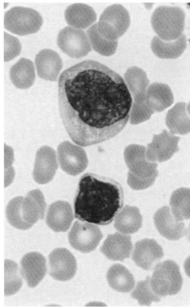

Figure 6.7 Pleomorphic nucleolated cells in TP53 mutated SMZL.

The absence of this feature, however, should not detract from the diagnosis if other investigations are suggestive. Some cases show larger cells with nucleoli and voluminous cytoplasm and these need differentiated from B prolymphocytic leukaemia (PLL) and HCL.

Such morphology has been associated with a more aggressive clinical behaviour and inferior outcome due to loss or mutation of the TP53 gene on chromosome 17p (Figure 6.7) [25].

Immunophenotype

Marginal zone lymphoma cells also show pan B antigen expression. Light chain and CD20 expression is usually moderate to strong in intensity, whilst CD23 and CD11c can be positive or negative. CD5 is expressed in a subset of cases (~20%) and may predispose to higher peripheral blood load and diffuse bone marrow involvement [26]. Marginal zone lymphoma is negative for CD103, CD25 and CD123, allowing discrimination from HCL, which can have a similar presentation and morphology.

Cytogenetics

The most frequent cytogenetic aberrations are del 7q and gain of 3q, but also reported are +3, +5, +9q, +12q, +18 and +20q [27]. As noted above, loss or mutation of TP53 does occur [28] and is often implicated in a more aggressive clinical course.

B Prolymphocytic leukaemia

This is a rare condition predominantly affecting middle-aged to elderly males with a median age at presentation of 70 years. It presents typically with a significant lymphocytosis, anaemia, thrombocytopenia and splenomegaly. Lymphadenopathy is very rare so if this is present the potential diagnosis should be questioned. Historically B PLL was thought to be a variant of CLL, or could evolve from it. Over the last decade it has become apparent that B PLL is a separate entity with important clinical and laboratory differences from CLL, though the mechanisms involved in its pathogenesis are still poorly understood.

Morphology

The cells of B PLL show a number of characteristic features. They are medium to large, with a round nucleus, fairly central nucleolus and moderate faint basophilic cytoplasm. Nuclear clefts are occasionally present but these are much more typical of MCL (Figure 6.8).

Advanced stage progressive CLL will often show marked pleomorphism of peripheral blood lymphoid cells with prominent atypical prolymphocytoid forms, particularly in cases which have acquired a TP53 mutation. However, if the clinical and laboratory characteristics are carefully considered, advanced CLL and B PLL should not be confused.

WORKED EXAMPLE 6.1 Splenic marginal zone lymphoma

A 74-year-old female presented with generalized lymphadenopathy, massive splenomegaly, lymphocytosis, anaemia and thrombocytopenia. The peripheral blood smear showed pleomorphic but mature lymphoid cells, some with cytoplasmic fronds. An excess of B-cells was noted in the CD2 versus CD19 plot and two populations were identified according to intensity of CD19 expression (CD19 versus SSC). Gating on each population, according to different CD19 fluorescence intensity, identified two clonal populations. The first and larger population (red) showed CD20^{strong}, CD5$^-$, FMC7$^+$, CD23$^-$, CD11c$^+$ and lambda^{strong}, and was in keeping with a splenic marginal zone lymphoma. The second population (blue) were CD20^{dim}, CD5$^+$, FMC7$^-$, CD23$^+$, CD11c$^-$ and lamda^{dim}, in keeping with a monoclonal B lymphocytosis, CLL or SLL according to further work-up.

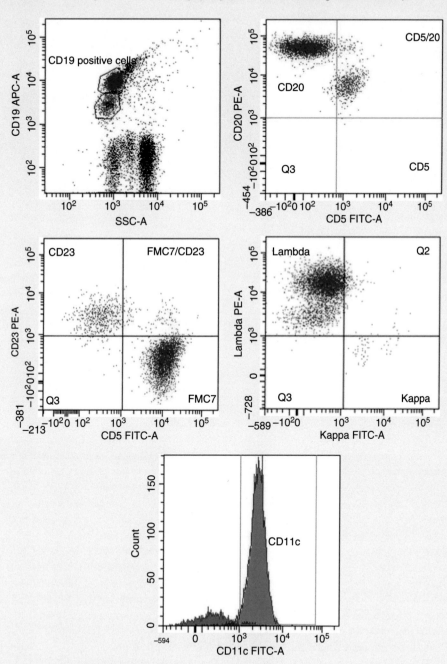

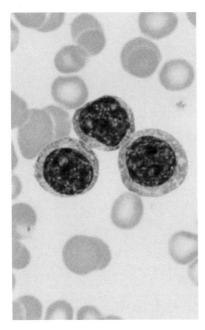
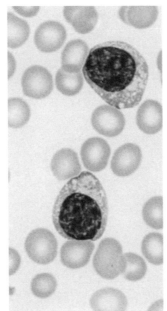
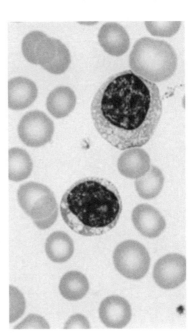

Figure 6.8 B prolymphocytic leukaemia.

Immunophenotype

CD5 is expressed in 20–30% of cases, whilst CD23 is positive in 10–20% [29]. The cells of B PLL show pan B antigen expression, moderate CD20, strong light chain MFI with FMC7 and CD11c positivity so it should not be confused with CLL, particularly if the presentation and morphology are carefully considered. In addition, most CLL patients with significant splenomegaly will also have widespread lymphadenopathy.

Cytogenetics

The cytogenetic findings are variable in B PLL, but perhaps the most frequent finding is of TP53 mutation, translocation or loss in 50% of cases. This at least partly explains the progressive course of this condition and its resistance to cytotoxic chemotherapy. In addition, aberrations of chromosome 1, 4 and 16 are encountered. Cases with t(11;14) invariably represent the leukaemic splenomegalic form of mantle cell lymphoma rather than B PLL [19].

Lymphoplasmacytoid lymphoma

Lymphoplasmacytoid lymphoma (LPL) is a neoplasm of mature B lymphocytes, plasmacytoid lymphocytes and plasma cells, which often involves bone marrow and occasionally peripheral blood. Lymph node and splenic involvement are variable. A paraprotein, IgG or IgM, is often present. It occurs at a median age of 60 years, with slight male predominance and shows an association with hepatitis C infection and type II cryoglobulinaemia. Some patients present with hyperviscosity symptoms due to high levels of IgM paraprotein or with neuropathies due to cryoglobulinaemia, incidental anti-myelin associated glycoprotein (anti-MAG) activity of the paraprotein or direct paraprotein deposition.

Morphology

Bone marrow involvement is frequent and shows a nodular diffuse or interstitial infiltrate of small lymphoid cells, plasmacytoid cells and plasma cells often accompanied by a striking mast cell infiltrate. Both CLL/SLL and MZL can show a degree of lymphoplasmacytoid differentiation in some cases and have to be considered in the differential diagnosis. The peripheral blood is occasionally involved, but the white cell count is rarely above 20×10^9/L (Figure 6.9). The cells of LPL are pleomorphic with variable degrees of plasmacytoid differentiation. Bone marrow involvement is much more frequent and more likely to generate a diagnosis (Figure 6.10).

Immunophenotype

The characteristic feature with this entity is the variable degree of surface and cytoplasmic light chain expression

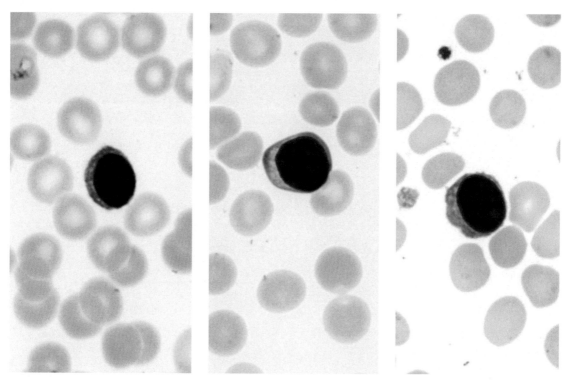

Figure 6.9 Lymphoplasmacytoid lymphoma cells in peripheral blood.

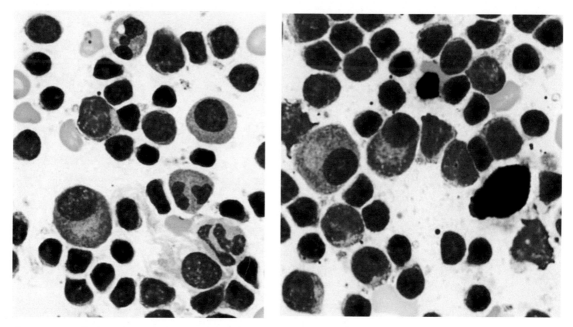

Figure 6.10 Lymphoplasmacytoid lymphoma in bone marrow aspirate. Note the variation in cell morphology, from small compact lymphoid cells to larger plasmacytoid cells. Mast cells are frequently seen (image right).

WORKED EXAMPLE 6.2

A 76-year-old male was referred with low volume lymphadenopathy, splenomegaly and a 30 g/L IgM paraprotein. A FBC showed a mild normocytic anaemia. A bone marrow aspirate was hypercellular with a prominent lymphoplasmacytoid lymphomatous (LPL) infiltrate. Flow cytometry studies on the bone marrow aspirate using a lymphoid gate on the FSC/SSC plot, are shown below. Note the surface kappa restricted CD19⁺ B-cell population, the subset of CD19⁺ CD38⁺ cells, the loss of FMC7 expression (a feature of LPL) and partial expression of CD23. The clinical presentation, morphology and immunophenotyping studies are all consistent with a diagnosis of lymphoplasmacytoid lymphoma.

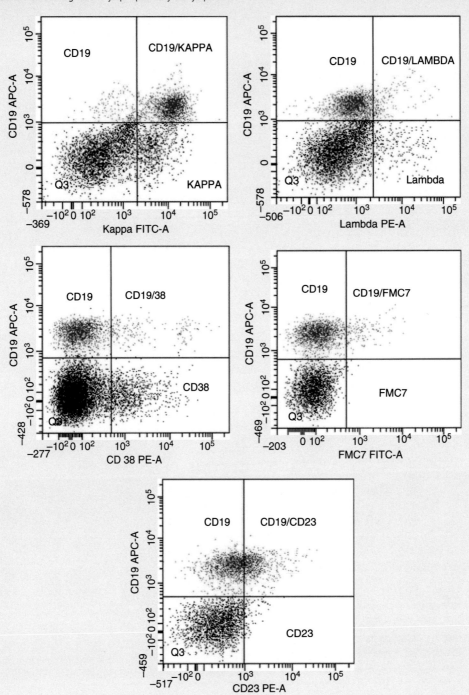

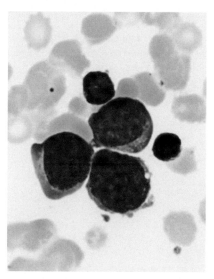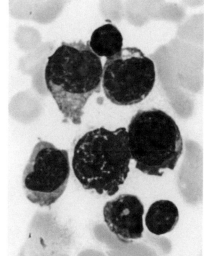

Figure 6.11 Richter type transformation of CLL in peripheral blood.

according to the degree of plasmacytoid differentiation. LPL cells normally show a mature pan B immunophenotype with expression of CD19, CD20, CD22 and CD79a. There are, however, some interesting characteristics of the immunophenotype. Although plasma cells are often a feature of LPL (admixed with lymphoid cells), these plasma cells (or perhaps plasmacytoid cells) do not show a malignant plasma cell immunophenotype as seen in myeloma. These cells have an immunophenotype similar to normal plasma cells, being CD45+, CD19+, CD20− and CD56− [30]. The lymphoid cells in LPL show restricted surface light chains and sometimes weak CD23 and CD5 expression and loss of FMC7 [31]. Furthermore, they often express CD38, CD11c and CD25 [31, 32], so if carefully considered, immunophenotyping can often be rewarding in LPL diagnosis.

Cytogenetics

There is no particular cytogenetic translocation associated with this lymphoma. Deletion 6q is seen in up to 50% of cases involving bone marrow but this finding is not specific.

Diffuse large B-cell lymphoma, Richter type

The exfoliation of diffuse large B-cell lymphoma (DLBC) cells into peripheral blood is not common but can be occasionally encountered, particularly in the setting of a transformation from CLL (Richter transformation) where the two entities may exist together. A Richter transforma-

tion may arise as a clonal evolution from CLL, often with an acquired TP53 mutation or as a *de novo* immunosuppression related DLBC following treatment with alemtuzumab or bone marrow transplant. The former may be CD5 positive whereas the latter are often CD5 negative. CD5 positivity is sometimes seen in DLBC NHL in the elderly and does not necessarily indicate an evolution from SLL/CLL but neoplastic cells are rarely seen in peripheral blood. Transformed DLBC NHL of Richter type presents with marked systemic upset, weight loss, sweats, bulky lymphadenopathy and a markedly raised serum lactate dehydrogenase (LDH). A Richter transformation is usually a nodal phenomenon, but can occur in virtually any extranodal site, bone marrow and blood.

Morphology

High grade lymphoma cells are often large and have blastoid morphology with frequent or multiple nucleoli and convoluted nucleus. The cytoplasm is plentiful and may show intense basophilic staining. There may be a background of smaller typical CLL cells in cases showing transformation (Figure 6.11).

Immunophenotype

High grade lymphoma cells will appear high in the blast gate on the FSC/SSC plot and may be missed in the analysis if a lymphoid gate is utilized. They will show pan B markers with strong CD20, FMC7, CD79a and CD22. Restricted light chain expression is usually dim to medium in intensity but in some cases is absent altogether. In transformed CLL, the morphology and immunophenotype of the high grade cells show clear contrasts with residual CLL cells in terms of intensity of antigen expression, but the basic immunophenotype (in terms of antigen positivity) is often similar to that of the pre-existing CLL [33].

Cytogenetics

These cases often show complex multiple abnormalities with hypo or even hyperdiploidy. Translocations and deletions of the TP53 gene are common in cases evolved from CLL. A summary of the immunophenotypic and clinical features of the CD5 positive LPDs is provided in Table 6.7.

Table 6.7 Summary of the CD5 positive lymphoproliferative disorders. % refers to percentage of cases that are positive for the antigen in question.

	CLL	MCL	SMZL	B PLL	LPL
CD20 (MFI)	Dim	Mod/bright	Mod/bright	Mod/bright	Mod
CD5 (%)	80	90	20	30	15
CD23 (%)	90	10	20	15	20
sIg (MFI)	Dim	Bright	Bright	Bright	Variable
FMC7	Neg	Pos	Pos	Pos	Variable
CD79b	Neg/dim	Pos	Pos	Pos	Pos
CD38 (%)	40	25	20	40	85
Lymph nodes	Yes	Yes	Yes/no	No	Yes/no
Splenomegaly	Yes/no	Yes/no	Yes	Yes	Yes/no
Paraprotein	Yes/no	No	Yes/no	No	Yes
AIHA/AITP	Yes	No	Yes	No	Yes/no

WORKED EXAMPLE 6.3 Peripheral blood Richter transformation of chronic lymphocytic leukaemia

A 72-year-old female with a long history of CLL presented with an acute clinical deterioration with weight loss and sweats. There was a marked leucocytosis with anaemia, rapid onset thrombocytopenia and significantly raised serum LDH. The peripheral blood showed two cell populations. The first was consistent with known CLL but a second population of large cells, with pleomorphic nuclei and nucleoli were evident

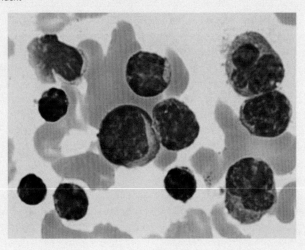

Flow cytometry studies confirmed two populations with the large cells (green) appearing high in the blast gate (FSC versus SSC), expressing CD20strong, CD5, CD79b, CD22 and kappastrong. These cells were high grade lymphoma cells evolving from CLL. The residual CLL population (red) remains in the lymphoid gate (FSC versus SSC) and has a typical phenotype; CD20dim, CD5+, CD79b−, CD22− and kappadim. There are therefore multiple characteristics that help not only to differentiate, but also to define the two populations.

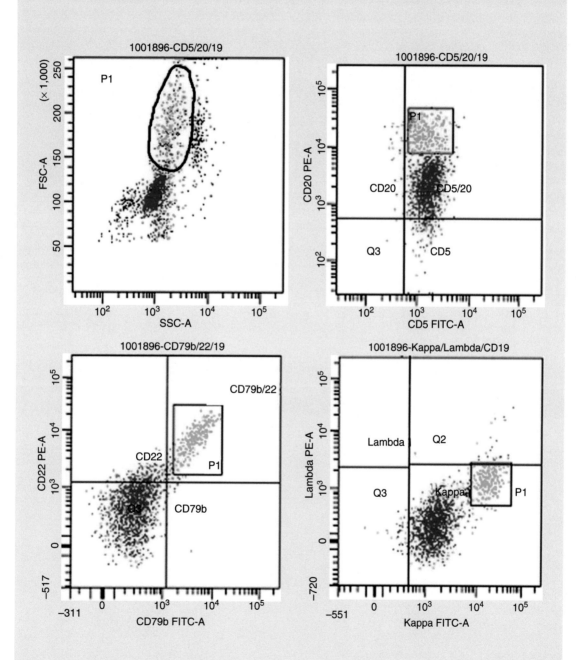

CD10 Positive B-cell lymphoproliferative disorders

Follicular lymphoma

Follicular lymphoma (FL) is a neoplasm derived from nodal germinal centre B-cells and accounts for 20% of all lymphomas registered. It typically presents with lymphadenopathy and paratrabecular bone marrow involvement, but peripheral blood exfoliation is not uncommon.

Morphology

Follicular lymphoma cells are often small with scant cytoplasm and a compact often cleaved nucleus without nucleoli. They are typically only a little larger than a red blood cell (7–10 μm) (Figure 6.12).

Occasional larger forms are sometimes apparent (Figure 6.13). The absolute PB leucocyte count is usually in the region of 10 to 30×10^9/L, but occasionally can be as high as 100×10^9/L. Of course, FL cells are more likely to be encountered in bone marrow specimens, but their tendency to generate paratrabecular infiltrates with associated fibrosis can mean that they are relatively underrepresented in aspirate material.

Immunophenotype

The derivation of FL from a germinal centre B-cell is indicated by CD10 positivity. This is a simple early means of discriminating from many other LPDs. FL demonstrates pan B-cell markers with expressing CD20, FMC7, CD79a and CD22. CD19 expression is often dim and this feature can help identify FL cells amongst a polyclonal B-cell background (see worked example below). Restricted light chain expression is usually dim to medium in intensity, but in some cases can be absent altogether. CD5 and CD23 are not normally expressed in FL cells from blood and bone marrow specimens but some discordance in CD23 expression has been reported in inguinal node samples [34].

Cytogenetics

The genetic hallmark of FL is the translocation t(14;18)(q32;q21) and BCL2 gene rearrangement which is present in a majority of cases. Additional cytogenetic abnormalities are frequent. It should be noted, however, that BCL2 over expression is encountered in a variety of other disorders so is not pathognomonic of this disorder. Acquisition of TP53 mutations is associated with high grade transformation and the presence of MYC

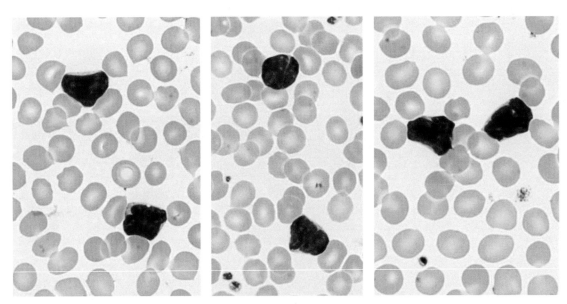

Figure 6.12 Follicular lymphoma cells in peripheral blood.

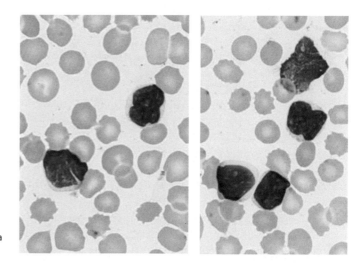

Figure 6.13 Larger pleomorphic follicular lymphoma cells in peripheral blood.

WORKED EXAMPLE 6.4 FOLLICULAR LYMPHOMA

A 70-year-old man presented with generalized lymphadenopathy and a peripheral blood lymphocytosis. A number of atypical small lymphoid cells with cleaved nuclei were noted in the peripheral blood smear. An excess of B-cells was noted in the CD2 versus CD19 plot and two populations were identified according to intensity of CD19 expression (CD19 versus SSC). The dim CD19+ cells (red) were CD10+, kappa restricted with dim CD20, in keeping with follicular lymphoma, which was later confirmed on lymph node biopsy. The polyclonal B-cells (blue) were non-light chain restricted, with normal CD19 and CD20 expression, but were CD10 negative.

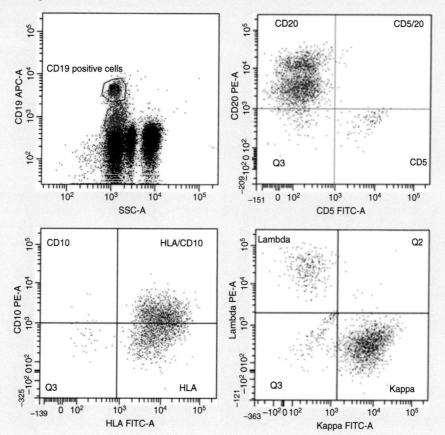

translocation is associated with aggressive clinical behaviour and resistance to therapy [35].

Diffuse large B-cell lymphoma

Diffuse large B-cell lymphoma (DLBCL) can be encountered in bone marrow, pleural and pericardial effusion specimens and occasionally in CSF. Very rarely it will appear in PB. It can occur *de novo*, evolve from FL or CLL (discussed above) or develop as a result of immunosuppressive therapy. The cell of origin is either a germinal centre centroblast (GC) or a germinal centre independent activated B-cell (ABC); these have contrasting immunophenotypes. This entity should be considered whenever abnormal clonal B-cells with blastoid morphology are encountered in diagnostic specimens.

Morphology

DLBCL cells are often large and have blastoid morphology with frequent or multiple nucleoli and convoluted nucleus. The cytoplasm is plentiful and may show intense basophilic staining (Figure 6.14).

Immunophenotype

DLBCL cells will appear in the blast gate on the FSC/SSC plot and may be missed in the analysis if a lymphoid gate is utilized. They show bright CD45 and pan B markers with strong CD20, FMC7, CD79a and CD22. Restricted light chain expression is usually dim to medium in intensity but in some cases is absent altogether. Some cases

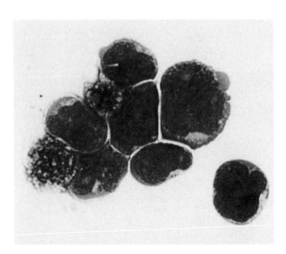

Figure 6.14 Diffuse large B-cell lymphoma cells in cerebrospinal fluid.

show dim CD19 and certain B-cell markers may be absent in selected cases; involved specimens often show apoptosis, cell trauma and free cell debris [36]. CD10 expression is seen in GC DLBCL, but not in the ABC subtype.

Cytogenetics

These cases often show complex multiple abnormalities with hypo or even hyperdiploidy. No particular cytogenetic aberration is characteristic in terms of assisting diagnosis. A hyperdiploid karyotype is well recognized and should not generate confusion with precursor B-cell neoplasms.

Burkitt lymphoma

Burkitt lymphoma (BL) is a highly aggressive neoplasm with a rapid proliferative rate which can present in blood, bone marrow or extranodal sites. It is derived from a pre-GC memory B-cell and can be encountered *de novo* or as a consequence of chronic immunosuppression and immune dysregulation (as seen in the context of EBV infection and endemic malaria, or as a result of HIV infection). The disease tends to be acute in onset with marked systemic upset. Patients show a rapid clinical deterioration so early accurate diagnosis is imperative; Circulating cells may be detectable in blood (particularly in cases with a leukaemia-like presentation) or on staging marrows. With appropriate intensive chemotherapy the outlook is often favourable in patients who are able to tolerate this approach.

Morphology

BL cells have highly characteristic morphology (Figure 6.15). They are medium sized, with an intense blue vacuolated cytoplasm and pleomorphic nucleus often showing nucleoli. Vacuoles may be seen within the nucleus. Mitotic figures are frequent; dead and dying cells are often seen.

Immunophenotype

BL cells have a mature precursor or early mature phenotype with expression of pan B markers (CD19, CD20, CD79a, CD22, FMC7) and early surface immunoglobulin which is often weak in intensity. In addition they express CD10 indicating their pre-GC origin. They are TdT negative, indicating their late precursor/early mature B-cell orientation. CD38 is frequently and brightly expressed [37] and can help differentiate true BL from MYC+ DLBCL.

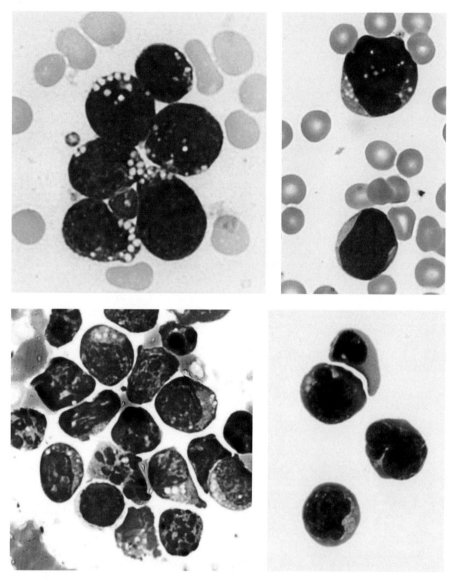

Figure 6.15 Burkitt lymphoma cells in blood (upper images), bone marrow (lower left) and CSF (lower right). Note the very prominent apoptosis and cell debris in the fresh bone marrow specimen.

Cytogenetics

The classic diagnostic hallmark of BL is t(8;14) (q24;q32), indicating rearrangement of the MYC gene against the IgH chain gene or less commonly MYC (8q24) in apposition to lambda (22q11) or kappa (2p12) light chain loci. It should be noted that MYC translocations are not themselves indicative of BL in isolation as they are not infrequently seen in other lymphomas (where they may nevertheless carry prognostic implications).

Precursor B acute lymphoblastic leukaemia

B acute lymphoblastic leukaemia (B-ALL) cells often demonstrate surface positivity for CD10. In fact CD10 is sometimes referred to as cALLa (common ALL antigen).

WORKED EXAMPLE 6.5

A 28-year-old female presented with a short history of abdominal bloating, weight loss and night sweats. An FBC showed a pancytopenia and the blood film showed atypical lymphoid cells with nucleoli, basophilic cytoplasm and vacuoles. CT imaging identified small bowel thickening and extensive intra-abdominal lymphadenopathy. Flow cytometry on a marrow aspirate generated the data presented below. Note the expression of CD22, CD79a, CD20 and CD10, together with strong CD38. Also note the FMC7 expression and weak restricted surface light chain expression which is often seen with Burkitt lymphoma/ leukaemia unlike the precursor B-cell neoplasms.

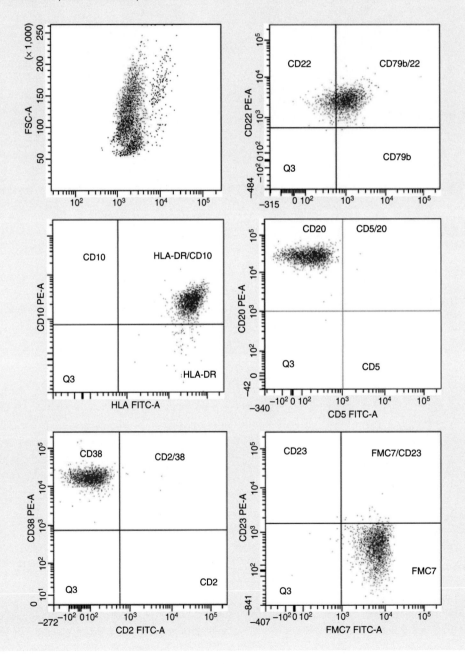

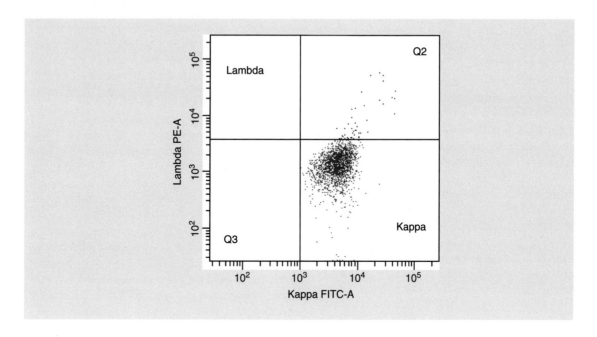

ALL is covered in detail in Chapter 5, but we should note that it should not be confused with the B lymphoproliferative disorders (Table 6.8).

Hairy cell leukaemia

Hairy cell leukaemia (HCL) is covered in detail in the next section. It should be noted, however, that CD10 positivity is not infrequent and hence it is listed here in the differential diagnosis of CD10 positive neoplasms. Put another way, if a B LPD has all the characteristics of HCL but also expresses CD10 then do not be dissuaded from this diagnosis.

B-cell disorders identified using an extended B-cell panel

When a B-cell LPD is encountered showing pan B antigen expression plus:
- Strong surface Ig
- Strong CD20
- Negative CD5
- Negative CD10

and particularly when the patient presents with cytopenias +/− splenomegaly, it is advisable to run an additional panel with antibodies to the following:
- CD11c
- CD103

Table 6.8 Summary of the CD10 positive LPD.

	FL	DLBCL	BL	B-ALL	HCL
CD20	Pos	Pos	Pos	Pos/neg	Pos
CD79b/CD19	Pos	Pos	Pos	Pos	Pos
FMC7	Pos	Pos	Pos	Neg	Pos
TdT	Neg	Neg	Neg	Pos	Neg
CD38	Neg	Pos/neg	Pos	Pos/neg	Neg
sIg	Pos	Pos/neg	Pos	Neg	Pos
Lymphadenopathy	Yes	Yes	Yes	Yes/no	No
Splenomegaly	Yes	Yes/no	Yes/no	No	Yes
High LDH	No	Yes/no	Yes	Yes/no	No
Marrow disease	Focal Frequent	Diffuse Infrequent	Diffuse Frequent	Diffuse Always	Yes
MYC expression	Rare	Infrequent	Always	No	No
t(14;18)	Frequent	Infrequent	No	No	No

- CD25
- CD123

This extended B-cell panel is useful in the identification of HCL and related disorders. Positivity for each of the above antigens is given a score of one point, generating a maximum score of 4 and minimum of 0. This approach is shown in Table 6.10.

Hairy Cell Leukaemia

Hairy cell leukaemia (HCL) is an indolent neoplasm of mature B-cells which characteristically infiltrates splenic red pulp and bone marrow with later peripheral blood involvement. The combination of diffuse bone marrow involvement with fibrosis and splenomegaly explains why patients commonly present with peripheral blood cytopenias. In addition, monocytopenia is a frequent finding. HCL can cause a severe pancytopenia in patients with a delayed diagnosis. Lymphadenopathy is uncommon but again can be seen in patients presenting late. Patients are predominantly middle aged to elderly males (male:female ratio is 5:1).

Morphology

It is important to consider this diagnosis in any patient presenting with cytopenias and splenomegaly. Hairy cells are often present at low levels in peripheral blood even in patients with long established disease so the morphologist needs to search the blood smear carefully, looking for the characteristic cells. Classic hairy cells are medium to large in size with an ovoid nucleus, without nucleoli and voluminous pale blue cytoplasm, often showing irregularity at the margin. This often resembles cytoplasmic hairs but can also appear as fronds, wisps or occasionally blebs. The cytoplasmic margin often appears indistinct (Figure 6.16).

Immunophenotype

Classic hairy cells are often infrequent in blood but have a unique immunophenotype which makes it the ideal entity for diagnosis using flow cytometry. Bone marrow aspirates are often dry so peripheral blood analysis is preferred in all cases. In addition to pan B markers, together with strong CD20 and surface Ig expression, classic HCL shows positivity for all the extended B-cell panel antigens in contrast to HCL variant (HCL-V) and splenic marginal zone lymphoma (SMZL). It is useful to apply a 'hairy cell score', analogous to that used in CLL, to discriminate between HCL, HCL-V, SMZL or other B-cell disorders with hairy or villous lymphocytes (see hairy cell leukaemia score in Table 6.10, p. 125) [38].

Cytogenetics

No cytogenetic abnormality is specific or prognostic for HCL so does not assist in diagnosis, which is normally straightforward. In addition, bone marrow aspirates are

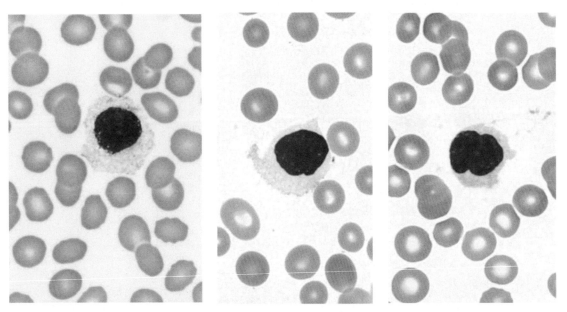

Figure 6.16 Classic hairy cell leukaemia cells showing typical morphology. Note the bilobed nucleus of the cell in the right image.

difficult to obtain and the hairy cells are often a minority population in peripheral blood.

Hairy Cell leukaemia variant

The term hairy cell leukaemia variant (HCL-V) variant refers to an entity that is probably not biologically related to classic HCL. This condition is described as variant for a variety of reasons; it differs in terms of presentation, morphology, immunophenotype and response to standard HCL treatment. This is a very rare condition, being some ten-fold less frequent than HCL, which in turn is ten-fold less frequent than CLL (Table 6.9).

Patients typically present with symptoms relating to either splenomegaly or cytopenias. The WBC is often high (typically 20 to 100×10^9/L) and without monocytopenia in contrast to HCL.

Table 6.9 Relative incidence of CLL, HCL and HCL-V in the Caucasian population.

Entity	Incidence, per 1,000,000 population per annum
CLL	30 cases
HCL	3 cases
HCL-V	0.3 cases

Morphology

Variant hairy cells are usually readily found in the peripheral blood smear. These cells are medium to large, with an ovoid and occasionally cleft nucleus, with frequent nucleoli and with moderate amounts of pale blue cytoplasm showing hairs, fronds or tufts. The morphology of HCL-V (Figure 6.17) is more variable between patients than the more consistent morphology of HCL (Figure 6.16). In contrast to HCL the bone marrow is often aspirable due to the absence of reticulin fibrosis.

Immunophenotype

HCL-V cells again show pan B antigen positivity but characteristically are often negative for CD25 and CD123. CD11c and CD103 may be positive so yielding a hairy cell score of 1 or 2 at most.

Cytogenetics

There is no specific cytogenetic aberration associated with this entity.

Splenic Marginal Zone Lymphoma

This condition, SMZL, has been discussed in relation to disorders exhibiting CD5 positivity above. However, it will more often be considered in the differential diagnosis of disorders presenting with cytopenias, splenomegaly and villous lymphoid cells and can be further analysed

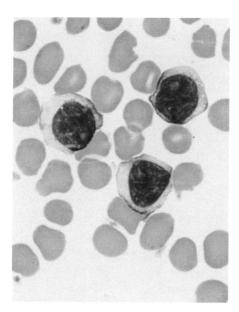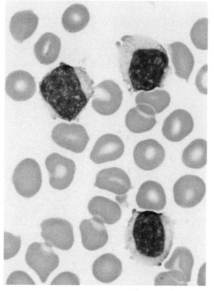

Figure 6.17 Hairy cell leukaemia variant. Note the cell size, nucleoli and more clearly defined cytoplasm compared to classic hairy cell leukaemia.

WORKED EXAMPLE 6.6 Hairy cell leukaemia

A 62-year-old patient presented with an incidental mild pancytopenia: Hb 105 g/L, WBC 2.1×10⁹/L, neutrophils 1.0×10⁹/L, monocytes 0.1×10⁹/L, platelets 104×10⁹/L. The peripheral film showed scarce medium to large lymphoid cells with irregular cytoplasm. The hairy cells (red) appear slightly larger, with more side scatter than the normal lymphoid cells (blue) (FSC versus SSC); this increased side scatter separates the hairy cells from the normal B-cells (CD19 versus SSC) and allows gating on the red events to confirm a classic hairy cell immunophenotype, with a score of 4 (CD11c⁺, CD25⁺, CD103⁺, CD123⁺).

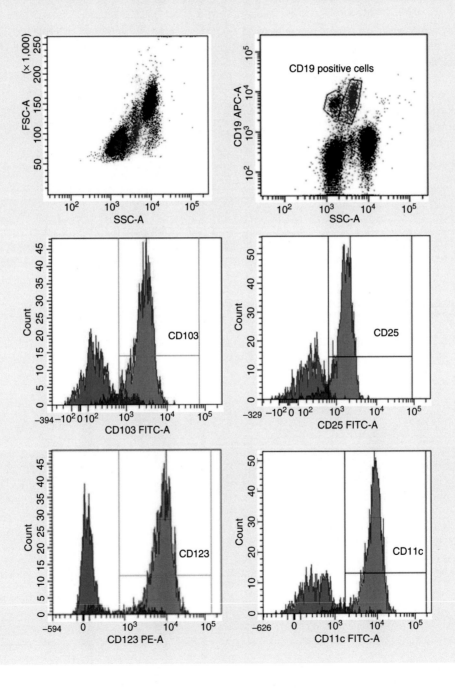

Table 6.10 Summary of the hairy cell leukaemia like conditions.

	HCL	HCL-V	SMZL
WBC count	Low	High	Variable
Cell size	Med/large cells	Medium/small	Medium/small
Cell cytoplasm	Hairy cytoplasm	Variable cytoplasm	Bipolar hairs
Cell nucleus	Absent nucleoli	Nucleoli	Rare nucleoli
Monocytopenia	Yes	No	No
Splenomegaly	Yes	Yes	Yes
Lymphadenopathy	No	No	Yes
Paraprotein	No	No	Yes (60%)
CD103	Pos	Pos/neg	Pos/neg
CD123	Pos	Neg	Neg
CD25	Pos	Neg	Pos/neg
CD11C	Pos	Pos	Pos/neg
SCORE	4	1 or 2	0, 1 or 2

using the extended hairy cell panel. The cells of SMZL may show expression of CD11C and/or CD25 but CD103 and CD123 are invariably negative, generating a hairy cell score of 0, 1 or 2. In addition to the above score, if CD5 or CD23 is co-expressed then a diagnosis of SMZL is highly likely and helps further to discriminate from other villous lymphoid disorders.

Identification of clonal T-cell disorders

Clonal T-cell disorders can be difficult to identify for certain as we do not have the benefit of skewed surface light chain expression that we so often utilize in mature B-cell disorders. There are, however, a number of features which can be used to identify clonal mature T-cell lymphoid proliferations, such as:

1 Skewing of the CD4:CD8 ratio to greater than 10:1 or less than 1:10
2 Loss of surface CD4 or CD8
3 Co-expression of CD4 and CD8
4 Loss of antigen expression, most often CD7 and CD5
5 Loss of intensity of antigen expression
6 Excess of $CD2^+$, $CD3^-$ negative cells

7 Additional antigen expression e.g. CD16, 56, 57, 25
8 Aberrant antigen expression

The absolute relevance of any of the above findings must be interpreted with respect to the patient's clinical presentation, physical signs and peripheral blood cell morphology. Antigen loss or aberrant expression is common in T and NK neoplasms. Assessment of the CD4:CD8 ratio in peripheral blood or bone marrow is a useful starting point, but minor deviances should be interpreted with caution and are often seen in reactive states. The expanded T-cell neoplastic clone will normally show a much more restricted antigen profile than that seen in reactive conditions. However, identification can still be difficult as reactive states often generate a restricted T-cell response. In infectious mononucleosis, for example, a reactive $CD8^+$ T-cell population with dim or absent CD7 is commonly seen. In contrast, many T-cell neoplasms can be partially obscured by the admixed polymorphous normal T-cell population. In such circumstances it often helps to consider potential diagnoses after considering the patient's presenting characteristics so allowing a better directed and focused analysis. Analysis of CD26 expression may be of value in discriminating between neoplastic and reactive T-cell populations as the former often show aberrant loss of this antigen. Its value has predominantly been reported in

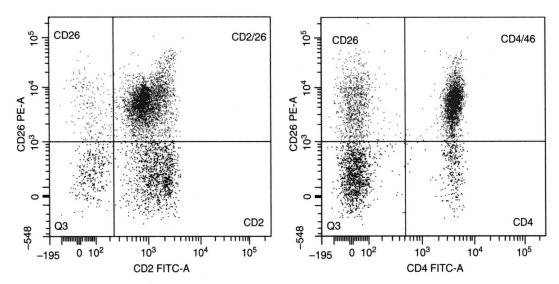

Figure 6.18 Normal range of CD26 expression encountered in peripheral blood T-cells. The majority of cells are positive but smaller numbers of CD26 negative T-cells are seen in both the CD4+ and CD2+ compartments (mean 7.2% and 26.8% negative, respectively, in our department) (unpublished observation).

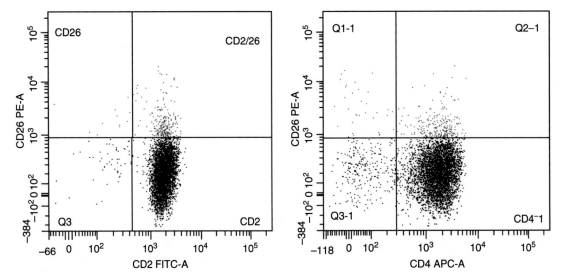

Figure 6.19 Loss of CD26 expression in Sezary Syndrome.

the identification of the neoplastic peripheral blood cells of Sezary syndrome/mycosis fungoides; both are CD26 negative [39, 40]. The interpretation of CD26 expression, however, is in itself difficult as normal T-cells show a heterogenous range of positivity for this antigen (Figure 6.18).

It is important, therefore, to assess the degree of antigen loss in comparison to control populations of known normal and reactive samples or to look at differential loss in say the CD8 subset compared to the CD4 subset in patients with CD8 proliferations and vice versa. The evaluation of the nature of CD26 expression as an aid to the identification of clonal versus reactive T-cell populations is ongoing. The plot in Figure 6.19 illustrates loss of CD26 expression in a case of CD2+, CD4+ Sezary syndrome.

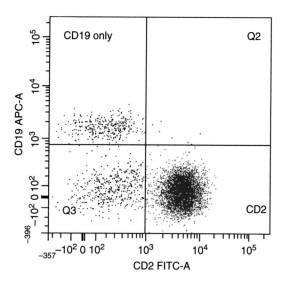

Figure 6.20 A CD19 versus CD2 analysis indicates an excess of T-cells, 86% of events (in red) compared to B-cells, 7% of events.

Table 6.11 A summary of CD antigens typically evaluated in the assessment of T-cell lymphoproliferative disorders.

Antigen	Cells on which normally expressed (surface)
CD2	T-cells and NK cells
CD3	Mature T-cells
CD5	Early to mature T-cells
CD7	Early to mature T-cells
CD4	T helper cells
CD8	T suppressor cells
HLA-DR	Activated T-cells, normal B-cells
CD16	NK cells, neutrophils
CD56	NK cells, large granular lymphocytes, activated T-cells
CD57	NK cell subset, cytotoxic T-cells
CD26	Mature T-cells (heterogenous)
CD25	Activated T- and B-cells, macrophages

Table 6.12 Antigens useful in discrimination of precursor from mature T-cell neoplasms.

Antigen	Precursor T ALL	T LPD
TdT	Often positive	Negative
CD4 or CD8	Only mature T ALL	Frequent
Loss of CD7	Rare	Frequent
Surface CD3	Only mature T ALL	Frequent
HLA-DR	Occasionally positive	Negative

Conversely, uniform positive expression of CD26 can also be indicative of a clonal T-cell disorder (see worked example of T-cell prolymphocytic leukaemia below). On occasion the degree of T-cell antigen loss in T-cell LPDs is so profound as to make lineage establishment difficult. In these cases assessment of cytoplasmic antigen expression can be helpful as well as surface expression of antigens like CD56 and CD30 and possibly the myeloid antigens CD13, CD33 and CD15. This will be discussed in more detail in the appropriate sections below.

It is of course essential that flow results from blood, bone marrow or body fluid specimens is closely compared to the histopathological assessment of any nodal, organ parenchymal or bone marrow material available. Furthermore, any information from cytogenetic or molecular studies should be assimilated before a final diagnosis is issued. These assessments should complement each other and be integrated into a multidisciplinary report after the free sharing of ideas between the specialists in each discipline. This is particularly important in T-cell disorders where diagnosis and classification remains a challenge.

Diagnosis of specific T-cell disorders

An excess of CD2+ cells should lead to a T-cell and a limited B-cell panel analysis, as in Figure 6.20.

A typical T-cell panel to evaluate potential T-cell LPD will incorporate the following antibodies to antigens as summarized in Table 6.11.

As noted above for the B-cell disorders, it is important always to distinguish the precursor T-cell neoplasms from the mature T LPD in terms of assessment of the clinical presentation and peripheral blood morphology before the appropriate analysis is performed. In addition, the classification of T and NK-cell neoplasms is less well established than that of the B-cell disorders so it is important that all available information is assimilated. The main immunophenotypic differences of the T-cell disorders is summarized in Table 6.12.

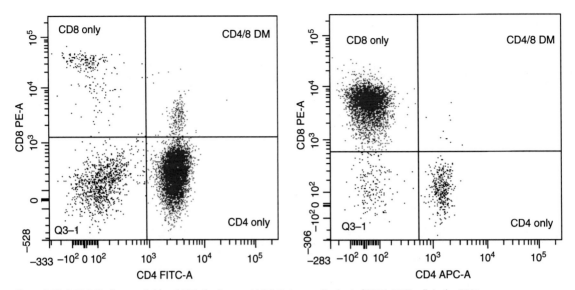

Figure 6.21 A CD4+ T-cell excess (left) and CD8+ T-cell excess (right). Note a small subset of CD4+, CD8+ cells in the CD4+ case.

The presence of an excess of CD4+ or CD8+ cells often serves as an initial indicator of the type of disorder which might be present, as in Figure 6.21.

CD4 Positive T-cell disorders

Sezary syndrome/cutaneous T-cell lymphoma

Sezary syndrome/cutaneous T-cell lymphoma (SS/CTCL) constitutes a triad of generalized erythroderma, lymphadenopathy and the presence of neoplastic T-cells in blood, lymph nodes and skin. Furthermore, one or more of the following criteria must also be met:

1 Absolute Sezary cell count $>1 \times 10^9$/L
2 Expanded CD4+ T-cell population with CD4:CD8 ratio > 10:1
3 Neoplastic CD4+ clone with loss of one or more antigens

This is a rare condition, accounting for only a small proportion of CTCL, which predominantly affects those over 60 years of age. It can be a devastating illness through the generation of intractable itch, alopecia (including loss of eyebrows and eyelashes), hyperkeratosis and onychodystrophy. It is an aggressive disease with a five-year survival rate of only 20%. There is a substantial overlap between SS and the diffuse non-plaque, non-tumour form of mycosis fungoides, but this apparent separation may be artificial. Indeed a leukaemic phase of CTCL may evolve in patients with longstanding disease. The diagnosis can be delayed as skin biopsies are often indeterminate or reported as a non-specific dermatitis and the peripheral blood lymphocytosis can be minor and not readily apparent if admixed with normal T-cells. If this diagnosis is being considered it is important that blood films are carefully scrutinized and that FCM studies are performed with this entity in mind.

Morphology

Sezary cells have very characteristic morphology. They are generally small cells with a high nuclear to cytoplasmic ratio and complex folded nuclei. This nuclear folding is often superimposed on the nucleus and may not be immediately apparent as a cleft, so they are often overlooked (Figure 6.22).

The bone marrow is often infiltrated by Sezary cells in a diffuse interstitial pattern but lymph nodes tend to show a complete effacement of architecture.

Immunophenotype

Sezary cells are typically CD4+, CD3+, CD5+, with loss of, or dim CD7 and loss of CD26. Some cases, however, retain CD7 positivity and the level of expression can vary in individual patients over time [39]. Dim expression of

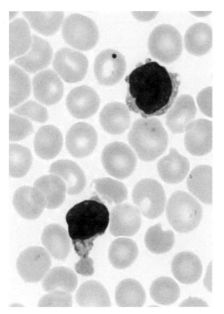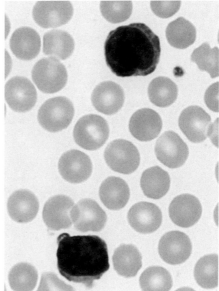

Figure 6.22 Sezary cells in peripheral blood. Note the nuclear clefts.

CD2 and CD3 is also described and may assist in making a diagnosis [40, 41]. CD25 is normally not expressed but has been reported in a subset of cases.

Cytogenetics

These are often complex in structure and number; recurrent abnormalities have not been identified. T-cell receptor genes are often rearranged.

T-cell prolymphocytic leukaemia

T-cell prolymphocytic leukaemia (T PLL) is a rare aggressive disorder which typically affects adults with a median age of onset of 65 years. It usually presents with lymphadenopathy, splenomegaly, high leucocytosis, anaemia, thrombocytopenia and skin lesions. Skin lesions are present to some degree in the majority of patients and can vary from a localized or diffuse erythema to plaques and nodules. The WBC count varies from 20 to 1000×10^9/L and late presentations can show gross organomegaly, effusions and oedema. It is rarely seen in childhood, but when it does occur, the clinician should consider the disorder ataxia telangiectasia which is an immunodeficiency syndrome with a much increased incidence of T-cell lymphomas, and is the result of a mutation in the AT gene located at 11q22-23. Mutations at this locus are well documented in sporadic

T PLL. Some patients have a more indolent presentation with an incidental leucocytosis, but are in danger of rapid disease progression with clinical deterioration, so most patients need consideration for treatment at the outset.

Morphology

The cells have a characteristic morphology. They are often medium to small with a high nuclear:cytoplasmic ratio, often have nucleoli and cytoplasmic blebs and projections, with occasional nuclear clefting and folds. The morphological appearance of these cells, with a typical presentation, is often highly suggestive of this disorder prior to confirmation with immunophenotyping (Figure 6.23).

Immunophenotype

T PLL cells have a post-thymic T-cell phenotype, demonstrating positivity for CD4, CD8 or both, absence of CD1a and TdT, together with pan T marker antigen positivity for CD2, CD3, CD5 and CD7. T PLL is most frequently CD4 positive but can also co-express CD4 and CD8 together and least often CD8 alone [41]. Cells strongly express CD52, which is relevant to the clinical application of the monoclonal anti-CD52 antibody alemtuzumab. Expression of NK and cytotoxic T-cell

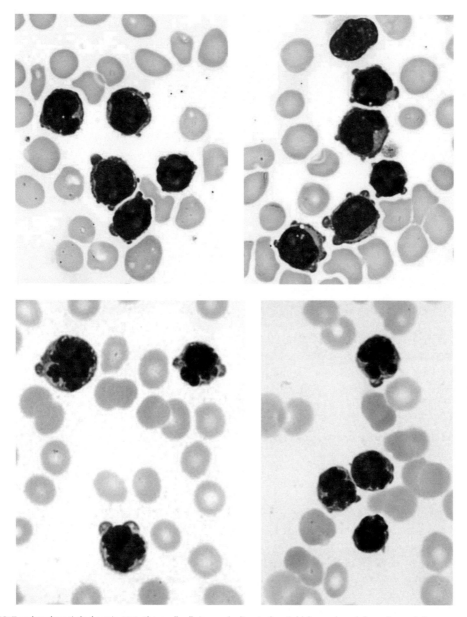

Figure 6.23 T prolymphocytic leukaemia. Note the small cell size, nucleoli, cytoplasmic blebs, nuclear clefts and convolutions.

antigens CD16, CD56 and CD57 is not commonly seen. CD26 is often uniformly positive in T PLL (and some peripheral T-cell lymphomas, notably anaplastic large cell lymphoma) [42], unlike normal T-cells. This feature can assist in the diagnosis of this entity which is known for showing a pan T phenotype, without the antigen loss which is so characteristic of many clonal T-cell disorders.

Cytogenetics

Chromosomal abnormalities are common in T PLL and most frequently involve chromosomes 8, 11 and 14. The most characteristic finding is inv(14) (q11;q32) which is present in two-thirds of cases and juxtaposes the TCRα gene to the oncogene TCL1 at 14q32. Most cases over express TCL1, which can be identified by

WORKED EXAMPLE 6.7 T-cell prolymphocytic leukaemia

A 72-year-old female presented with a patchy erythematous itchy rash. An FBC showed Hb 72 g/L, WBC 117×10⁹/L, platelets 15×10⁹/L. The blood film showed small lymphoid cells with multiply cleaved nuclei and cytoplasmic blebs. Immunophenotyping confirmed a CD4⁺ T-cell disorder with pan T antigen expression. Note the uniform strong expression of CD26 and subset of cells which are CD4⁺ CD8⁺.

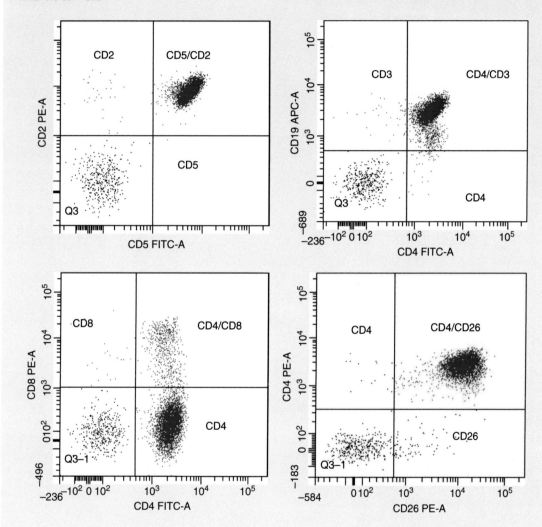

immunohistochemistry, suggesting that this gene is inherent to the pathogenesis of this disease. Interestingly, disruptions at 11q22-23 are not often seen in standard cytogenetic preparations but molecular analysis frequently detects mutations at the ATM locus. Additional chromosome aberrations are common, including 17p deletions, but these probably arise during disease evolu-tion and are not necessarily involved in the initial dis-ease pathogenesis.

Acute T-cell leukaemia/lymphoma

Acute T-cell leukaemia/lymphoma (ATLL) is another rare CD4⁺ T-cell disorder that often affects peripheral blood, the aetiology of which is strongly correlated with

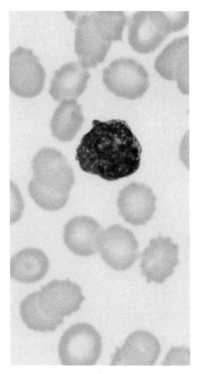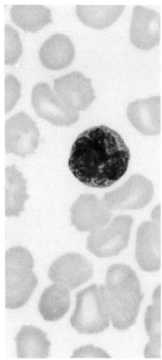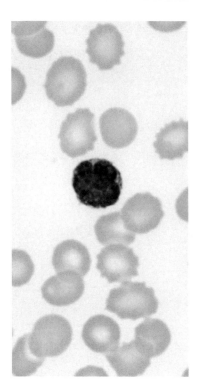

Figure 6.24 Adult T-cell leukaemia/lymphoma.

human T-cell leukaemia virus (HTLV) virus infection. This virus shows blood borne transmission and is endemic in some parts of Japan, the Caribbean, Africa and South America. The disease can have a long latency; however, less than 5% of the infected population develop the disease, suggesting that a secondary oncogenic mutation is necessary in infected cells [43].

Most patients present with the acute form, typified by peripheral blood involvement, lymphadenopathy, skin infiltrates (erythema, papules or nodules), bone lesions, hypercalcaemia and B symptoms. A pure lymphomatous, smouldering presentation is also well recognized, where neoplastic cells are not necessarily present in peripheral blood. In all cases, a peripheral blood eosinophilia is common. These patients exhibit a profound acquired immunodeficiency as a result of the HTLV infection on the CD4+ T-cell compartment. Deaths due to infection with atypical T-cell dependent organisms, like pneumocystis, cryptococcus and fungi are not uncommon.

Morphology
ATLL cells are medium to large, typically with a complex folded, etiolated or flower head like nuclear morphology

(Figure 6.24). Nuclear chromatin is often clumped, whilst presence of nucleoli is variable between cases.

Immunophenotype
ATLL cells normally have a pan T-cell phenotype but are typically lacking in CD7 [41]. The majority of cases are CD4+, but similarly to T PLL, a minority are CD8+ or CD4/CD8+. The typical finding is of strong expression of CD25 (the IL-2 receptor). CD26 is often absent [44]. Occasional cases will express CD30 but ALK protein is not expressed.

Cytogenetics
No common or pathognomonic aberration has been identified.

Anaplastic large cell lymphoma
Anaplastic large cell lymphoma (ALCL) is another uncommon CD4+ entity typified by an advanced stage lymphomatous presentation with a predilection for extranodal sites, such as skin, bone, lung and liver. The small cell variant, however, can appear in peripheral blood and all forms can be encountered in bone marrow specimens. Anaplastic large cell lymphoma expressing

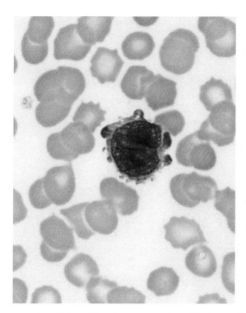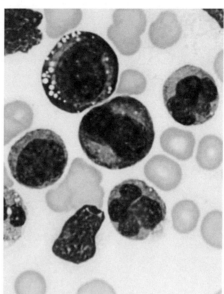

Figure 6.25 Anaplastic large cell lymphoma in peripheral blood, ALK⁻ (left) and ALK⁺ (right).

anaplastic lymphoma kinase (ALK) typically affects children and young adults and has a good prognosis, whilst ALK negative ALCL is predominantly a disease of middle-aged to elderly adults and has a much less favourable outcome.

Morphology

The cytological characteristics of ALCL in blood or bone marrow are highly variable and often without typical features, giving hints as to the diagnosis. The cells vary in size and often show nuclear/cytoplasmic complexity; cytoplasmic vacuoles are not uncommon (Figure 6.25). The morphology can vary quite markedly between cases and there are no particular features associated with ALK status.

Immunophenotype

ALCL normally retains some T antigen expression, most commonly CD2 and CD4. CD3, CD5 and CD7 are often absent and some cases have an apparent null immunophenotype. Strong surface CD30 expression is characteristic of this condition but is not diagnostic in isolation (see CD30 expressing neoplasms, Table 6.13). Interestingly, ALCL may show weak myeloid antigen expression, particularly CD13, CD15 and CD33 so this may cause confusion with AML on the basis of immunophenotyping. However, if the clinical presenta-

tion is carefully considered and the presence of strong CD30 and absence of cytoplasmic MPO, together with potential ALK expression, is taken into account then this dilemma should not arise in the diagnostic laboratory.

Cytogenetics

In ALK⁺ ALCL the most frequent translocation generating ALK overexpression is t(2;5) (p23;q35), juxtaposing the ALK gene and nucleophosmin genes on chromosomes 2 and 5, respectively. However, variant translocations involving ALK and numerous other partner genes have been described. There is no cytogenetic or molecular marker of ALK⁻ ALCL. A number of non-specific secondary chromosome losses and gains have been described, including loss of 17p.

Angio-immunoblastic T-cell Lymphoma

Angio-immunoblastic T-cell lymphoma (AITL) is a subtype of peripheral T-cell lymphoma, which predominantly affects middle-aged to elderly adults. It presents with a variety of constitutional symptoms, including sweats, fever and weight loss, which can mimic infection. Presentations with skin rash, effusions and arthralgias can mimic a connective tissue disorder. However, small volume lymphadenopathy and variable degrees of hepatosplenomegaly are invariably present. Patients show a

WORKED EXAMPLE 6.8 Anaplastic large cell lymphoma

A 60-year-old male presented with a recent development of large fleshy nodules in the skin. The FBC was normal. Computed tomography imaging showed no other sites of disease. Skin biopsy showed an undifferentiated, likely T-cell neoplasm, expressing CD30. A provisional diagnosis of a CD30 positive cutaneous T-cell lymphoma was made. Within one week the patient became unwell with fever, sweats and prostration; the peripheral blood suddenly showed large numbers of pleomorphic blast cells. Immunophenotyping studies indicated that the cells had a null phenotype but HLA-DR and weak CD10 was expressed, together with strong CD30, confirming a diagnosis of systemic anaplastic large cell lymphoma.

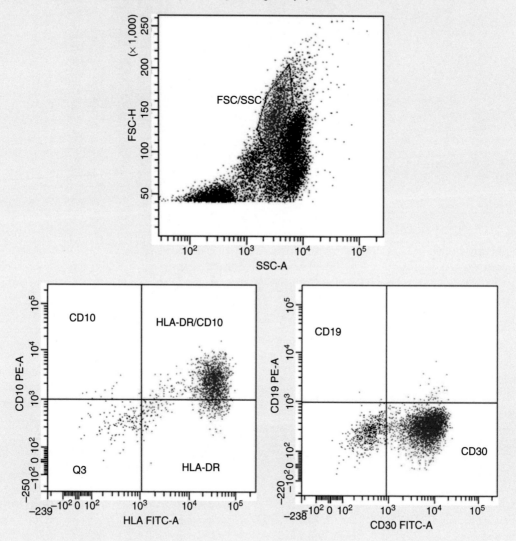

polyclonal rise in immunoglobulins, raised ESR and sometimes a positive direct Coombs test. The bone marrow is often involved but significant peripheral blood involvement is rare. Low level blood involvement is often present if carefully sought [45].

Morphology

The morphology of AITL is pleomorphic, with no particular defining features. There is often an admixed population of eosinophils and plasma cells in cases showing bone marrow involvement (Figure 6.26).

Table 6.13 Summary of the immunophenotype and clinical features of CD4 positive T-cell LPD.

Antigen	Sezary	T PLL	ATLL	ALCL	AITL
CD2	Pos	Pos	Pos	Pos	Pos
CD3	Pos	Pos	Pos	Pos/neg	Pos
CD5	Pos	Pos	Pos	Pos/neg	Pos
CD7	Often neg	Pos	Neg	Pos/neg	Neg/dim
CD25	Rare pos	Neg	Pos	Neg	Neg
CD30	Neg	Neg	Neg	Pos	Neg
CD10	Neg	Neg	Neg	Neg	Pos
Myeloid	Neg	Neg	Neg	Wk pos	Neg
Skin	Erythema	Variable	Variable	Variable	Rashes
Nodes	Yes	Yes	Yes	Yes/no	Yes
Blood	Yes	Yes	Often	Rare	Rare
Extranodal	No	No	Yes	Yes	Yes
BM disease	Yes	Yes	Yes	Variable	Yes
Other	Pruritis Nails Alopecia	Effusions Organomegaly	High Ca+ HTLV+	High LDH Stage IV	Fever Organomegaly Arthralgias

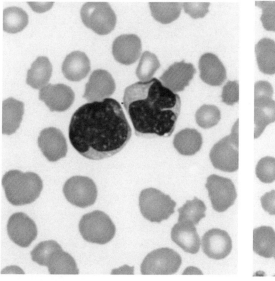
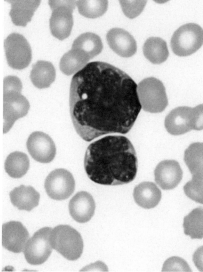

Figure 6.26 Angioimmunoblastic T-cell lymphoma.

Immunophenotype

Angio-immunoblastic T-cell lymphoma commonly expresses CD4, together with pan T antigens CD2, CD3 and CD5. CD7 expression is commonly lost. Characteristically the tumour cells show aberrant CD10 expression which helps to differentiate this entity from reactive phenomena and from other peripheral T-cell lymphomas. This also aids the detection of AITL cells in peripheral blood; these can be detected in up to 50% of cases using careful screening [46].

Cytogenetics

The most frequent abnormalities are trisomy 3, trisomy 5 and gain of X chromosome but none of these are diagnostic in isolation.

CD8 Positive T-cell disorders

T-cell large granular lymphocyte leukaemia

This is the most frequent CD8 positive neoplasm encountered in FCM studies. T-cell large granular lymphocyte leukaemia (T-LGL) is thought to be of cytotoxic T-cell derivation. As normal cytotoxic T-cell numbers can increase in response to a variety of stimuli, from infection to neoplasia, it is important that T-LGL is not overdiagnosed and mistaken for these reactive proliferations. Many cases are idiopathic, but there is a clear association between LGL proliferations and underlying diseases with inherent or acquired immune deficiency or immune dysregulation. There also appears to be an association with clonal LGL proliferations and haematological abnormalities in patients without evidence of underlying inflammatory or auto-immune disease [47]. The majority of patients with a clonal proliferation present with an absolute count of more than 2×10^9/L in distinction to those with non-clonal reactive states. Most patients with T-LGL are asymptomatic and the diagnosis is made incidentally. However, there is a definite association with neutropenia as 80% of patients will encounter this during their disease course, with 45% of patients developing severe neutropenia (absolute neutropenia $<0.5 \times 10^9$/L) [48]. A number of mechanisms underlying the neutropenia have been proposed, including auto-immune neutropenia, myeloid maturation arrest and the neutropenia of Felty syndrome. Infection is not necessarily encountered in all patients.

Anaemia, thrombocytopenia and splenomegaly may also be seen, whilst lymphadenopathy is uncommon. Anaemia, encountered in half of patients, may be due to red cell aplasia, auto-immune mechanisms, bone marrow infiltration or hypersplenism. The anaemia may also be due to a chronic inflammatory disease such as rheumatoid arthritis, Sjögren disease or systemic lupus erythematosis, with which conditions the leukaemia is associated. Rheumatoid arthritis shows the strongest association with T-LGL and both appear predisposed by the HLA-DR4 haplotype, suggesting a common immunogenic mechanism. Finally, T-LGL may be seen as a result of iatrogenic immune suppression in patients undergoing organ transplantation, so should be considered in the differential diagnosis in the spectrum of post-transplant related lymphoproliferative disorders [49]. For example, we have encountered a case of refractory red cell aplasia, developing post-renal transplantation, due to an immunosuppression related LGL leukaemia. The aplasia resolved after effective treatment with cyclophosphamide and steroids.

Morphology

Large granular lymphocytes have characteristic morphology. They are medium to large cells, with non-nucleolated nuclei, plentiful cytoplasm and coarse azurophilic granules (Figure 6.27). They cannot be reliably differentiated on morphological grounds from natural killer (NK) cells, whether reactive or clonal. Large granular lymphocytes are often prominent in peripheral blood smears from patients with other haemopoietic neoplasms, solid tumours, infective and inflammatory disorders. Their presence can detract attention from the true underlying disorder, so the clinical circumstances in which these cells appear will always need careful consideration.

Immunophenotyping

The vast majority of LGL leukaemias are CD8 positive (though rare CD4+ cases have been described [50]) and they typically co-express CD2, CD3, CD16 and CD57. CD5 and CD7 loss or dim expression is most frequently encountered and is helpful in identifying likely clonal proliferations [51], but antigen loss is not universal. The presence of CD16 is important as it is not expressed by normal T-cells: a CD16 positive population comprising more than 30% of total T-cells is suggestive of a clonal disorder [52]. CD56 is expressed in a proportion of cases to a variable degree; this antigen is most often associated

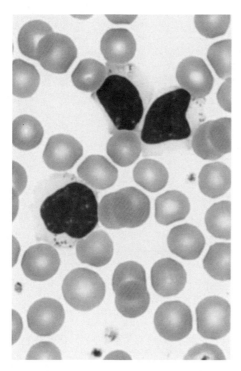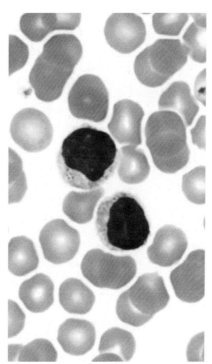

Figure 6.27 Large granular lymphocytic leukaemia.

with NK proliferations. An alpha/beta T-cell receptor (TCR) gene rearrangement is most frequently encountered in contrast to the gamma/delta TCR configuration. Demonstration of a TCR gene rearrangement, either by flow cytometry or PCR based methods is strongly supportive of a clonal LGL proliferation and should be pursued in any likely case showing co-existent cytopenias that need therapy. A potential FCM diagnosis can be made using peripheral blood analysis but bone marrow assessment is essential in patients with significant cytopenias. Serological studies for rheumatoid factor, antinuclear antibody, anti-Ro and La can be useful in selected patients presenting with associated symptoms.

Cytogenetics
Cytogenetic studies rarely generate useful diagnostic or prognostic information in suspected LGL leukaemia.

Natural killer cell chronic lymphoproliferations
Chronic proliferations of NK cells are rare. They are characterized by an NK cell population, usually $>2 \times 10^9$/L,

persisting for over six months without an apparent cause. Distinguishing reactive from clonal populations is difficult as NK cells often lack aberrant immunophenotypic characteristics and do not show TCR gene rearrangement. Chronic proliferations are usually seen in patients older than 60 years. The majority of patients are asymptomatic and there is only a weak association with anaemia, neutropenia or infection. Systemic upset, fever, lymphadenopathy, hepatomegaly and splenomegaly are very rare: the presence of such is more in keeping with aggressive NK neoplasms (these are discussed later in this chapter).

Morphology
Peripheral blood NK cells have morphology indeterminate from large granular lymphocytes (Figure 6.28). Only FCM studies can reliably differentiate the two conditions.

Immunophenotyping
As NK cells and cytotoxic T-cells are closely related in their ontogeny and function as part of the innate immune

WORKED EXAMPLE 6.9 Large granular lymphocytic leukaemia

A 60-year-old female with a known history of rheumatoid arthritis was referred on account of a persisting neutropenia, neutrophils 1.2×10^9/L. The remainder of the FBC was unremarkable, though the total lymphocyte count was marginally high at 5×10^9/L. The blood film showed prominent large granular lymphocytes. The FCM studies identified a CD8$^+$ CD26$^-$ CD16$^+$ CD57$^+$ CD7$^-$ population. The TCR gene rearrangement studies showed a clonal peak in a polyclonal background. Note the CD8 to CD4 excess (81% to 12%), CD57 positivity and loss of CD26 in this case.

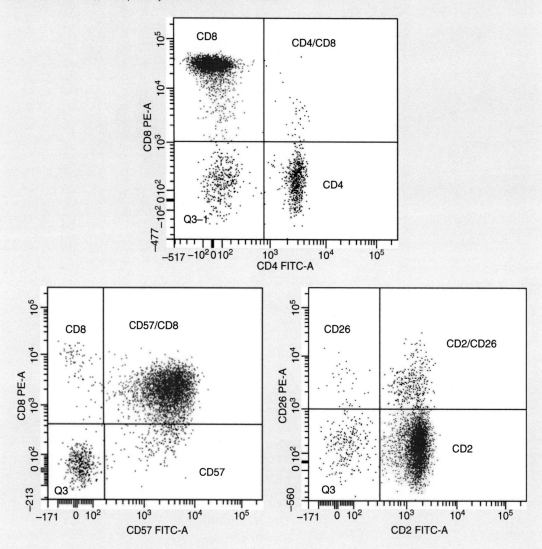

system it is not surprising that they share some immunophenotypic attributes. For example, CD16, CD56 and CD57 are expressed on both. One major difference is that NK cells lack a fully assembled CD3 surface complex so most cases are negative using anti-CD3 by flow cytometry. They do, however, express surface subunits of CD3, such as CD3ε, which may be detected by some immunohistochemical antibodies used in paraffin sections.

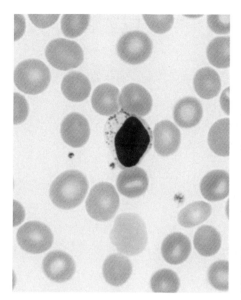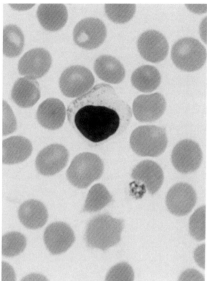

Figure 6.28 Chronic natural killer leukaemia.

Natural killer cells typically express CD2, weak CD8 and CD7, together with CD16, CD56 and sometimes CD57. A typical case is shown in Figure 6.29. Note the CD2$^+$, CD3$^-$, CD4$^-$, CD5$^-$, CD7dim, CD16$^+$ phenotype (red events) as compared to the normal T-cells (blue events). CD8 was not expressed (not shown) unlike most LGL proliferations.

Clonal NK proliferations may show subtle immunophenotypic variances which can assist in identifying non-reactive populations (see Table 6.14) [53]. In addition it is possible to evaluate surface expression of killer cell immunoglobulin receptors (KIRs). A number of KIRs are expressed in populations of normal NK cells: each is reactive to particular clusters of major histocompatibilty antigens as a means of recognizing non-self cells. Killer cell immunoglobulin receptor directed antibodies such as anti-CD158a, CD158b and CD158e can be useful as restricted expression is seen in two-thirds of cases with clonal proliferations [54, 55]. Other antibodies to epitopes, such as CD161 and CD94, are directed at other surface NK molecules which are part of the extended NK receptor (NKR) complex, of which KIRs form a part. The flow cytometric characteristics which are suggestive of clonal NK populations are summarized in Table 6.14.

Cytogenetics
Cytogenetic studies rarely generate useful diagnostic or prognostic information in suspected clonal NK proliferations.

Hepatosplenic T-cell lymphomas
When considering disorders of cytotoxic T-cells, the most common being T LGL, it is important to consider hepatosplenic T-cell lymphomas (HSTCL) in the differential diagnosis, although the clinical presentation of the two diseases is likely to be very different. Hepatosplenic T-cell lymphoma usually affects young adults, often males, who present with B symptoms, fever, hepatosplenomegaly, cytopenias and circulating granular large pleomorphic T-cells. Bone marrow infiltration with a particular affinity for the sinusoids is common [56] and haemophagocytosis is often evident. It is derived from a subset of cytotoxic $\gamma\delta$ T-cells though rare cases show an $\alpha\beta$ T-cell receptor derivation. Up to 20% of patients have a history of current or prior immunosuppression associated with organ transplantation, chemotherapy for solid tumours, relapsing malaria or treatment of inflammatory bowel disease [57]. This disease is extremely aggressive in its clinical behaviour and the prognosis is poor with current anthracycline based therapies.

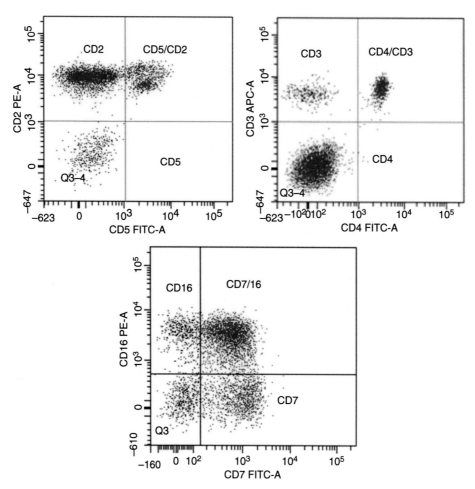

Figure 6.29 Natural killer cell proliferation.

Table 6.14 Immunophenotypic characteristics which can help define clonal from reactive NK proliferations.

Character	Normal NK cells	Clonal NK cells
CD16	Positive	Positive bright
CD56	Positive	Positive dim
CD8	Dim	Positive bright
CD7	Positive	Positive dim
CD5	Negative	Positive dim
CD2	Positive	Positive dim
CD158a,b,c	Polyclonal	Restricted
CD161	Positive	Negative or dim
CD94	Positive	Positive bright

Morphology

Hepatosplenic T-cell lymphoma cells are usually present in peripheral blood if carefully sought. They are very large cells, often with pleomorphic nuclei. Nucleoli may be seen and the cytoplasm may show azurophilic granules – the latter being the clue to their cytotoxic T-cell derivation (Figure 6.30).

Immunophenotype

Most cases express CD2, CD3, CD7 and CD56; CD8 may on occasion be expressed (hence its inclusion in this section), but most cases are CD4 and CD8 negative. CD16 is occasionally expressed, but CD57 is not usually a feature.

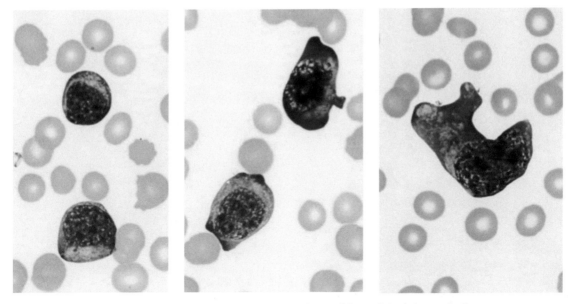

Figure 6.30 Hepatosplenic T-cell lymphoma cells in peripheral blood. Note the size of these cells in relation to red cells.

Cytogenetics

There is a strong association with isochromosome 7q [58], with or without trisomy 8.

T-prolymphocytic leukaemia

Please note that a subset of cases, 10–20%, are CD8 positive. Pan T-cell antigen expression is seen as per the more typical CD4 positive cases and clinical outcome is similar.

CD4/CD8 positive T-cell disorders

T PLL, ATLL and cortical T ALL can all express dual CD4/CD8 positivity. The former two are discussed in the section on CD4 positive T-cell disorders above and the latter in the section on precursor acute lymphoblastic leukaemia.

CD4/8 Negative disorders

Aggressive natural killer/T-cell neoplasms

Aggressive NK cell leukaemia and extranodal NK/T-cell lymphoma nasal type have many pathological and immunophenotypic features in common. Both are CD3-, CD56+ neoplasms which appear EBV driven with a high

serum LDH. Their clinical presentation, however, differs in that the latter is normally tissue based with an affinity for nasopharyngeal structures, whilst the former generates hepatosplenomegaly, haemophagocytosis and cytopenias. As the name implies NK cell leukaemia can often be detected in peripheral blood and it frequently infiltrates bone marrow. These are relatively rare lymphomas in the Western world, being most frequently encountered in Asia. Both are serious disorders and can affect young patients; they often express multi-drug resistant proteins and have a poor outcome despite intensive chemotherapy or even following transplantation procedures in those achieving remission.

Morphology

Natural killer/T-cell lymphoma is rarely encountered in blood or bone marrow specimens, other than in advanced relapsed or refractory disease, so the description here relates largely to NK leukaemia/lymphoma; the morphology and immunophenotypes of each have much in common. Natural killer leukaemia/lymphoma cells have a morphology which is predictable from their aggressive behaviour and NK cell origin. They are large pleomorphic cells with folded nuclei, nucleoli and a cytoplasm with prominent granules (Figure 6.31). They can usually be identified in peripheral blood if sought but rarely cause a peripheral leucocytosis. Bone marrow

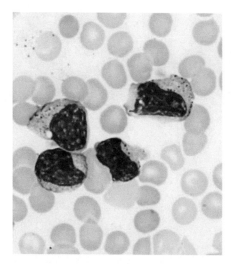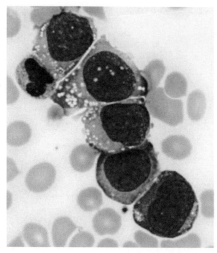

Figure 6.31 Two examples of aggressive NK leukaemia/lymphoma involving peripheral blood. Note the retention of 'NK-like' features with some nuclear chromatin condensation (despite nucleoli) in the image left, but more primitive blastoid morphology, absence of granules and vacuolation in the image right. Both showed aggressive clinical behaviour and were refractory to treatment.

involvement is frequent; the disease often triggers a profound haemophagocytic macrophage reaction and disseminated intravascular coagulation.

Immunophenotype

It is important that this condition is considered in patients presenting with B symptoms, hepatosplenomegaly and cytopenias as the condition can easily be missed if not considered and if appropriate gating strategies on blood and marrow samples are not generated. Neoplastic cells often constitute a minor population in the above specimens. They are typically CD2+, CD3−, CD56+, HLA-DR+ and CD57− and are likely to appear in the high blast gate, often with some increase in side scatter as a reflection of their morphological complexity and granularity. Cytoplasmic CD3ε is present but surface CD16 is often expressed in contrast to extranodal NK/T lymphoma nasal type [34]. Some cases express CD7 but other T-lineage antigens are present infrequently [35]. This condition needs to be considered in the differential diagnosis of acute leukaemias expressing CD56 with few other lineage specific antigens (see Chapter 5).

Cytogenetics

The most commonly encountered abnormalities involve chromosome 6 at 6q21–25 and loss of TP53 function at 17p13 due to 17p del or i17q [36].

CD56 expression is seen in a number of cytotoxic T-cell and NK-cell derived neoplasms as summarized in Table 6.15.

Enteropathy associated T-cell lymphoma

This is a small bowel lymphoma derived from a malignant transformation of the inflammatory intra-epithelial T lymphocytes associated with the gluten allergy of coeliac disease. Most cases arise in patients with subclinical or undiagnosed coeliac disease, though some arise in patients who are non-compliant with a gluten free diet. This lymphoma is very rare in patients with gluten free diet compliance. The disease is aggressive in presentation, causing anorexia, abdominal pain and weight loss. Small bowel perforation presenting as an acute abdomen often leads to a histological diagnosis. The condition is normally localized to small bowel and adjacent nodes but it can appear in peripheral blood and/or bone marrow so is included here for completeness.

Morphology

The cells are large and pleomorphic, with voluminous cytoplasm, often with azurophilic granules and a complex folded nucleus (Figure 6.32). The cell morphology is unlikely to prompt a diagnosis but, again, correlation with the known clinical circumstances and clinical history is of utmost importance.

WORKED EXAMPLE 6.10 Natural killer/T-cell lymphoma

A 35-year-old man was referred to our centre for assessment on account of an unexplained clinical deterioration with weight loss, night sweats, fever and progressive pancytopenia. An infective aetiology had been suspected. A bone marrow aspirate demonstrated an abnormal infiltrate of pleomorphic granular lymphoid cells. There was active haemophagocytosis; activated macrophages were consuming bone marrow cells of all lineages. Flow cytometry identified the cells to be of NK-lineage; the clinical presentation was in keeping with a diagnosis of an aggressive NK/T lymphoma.

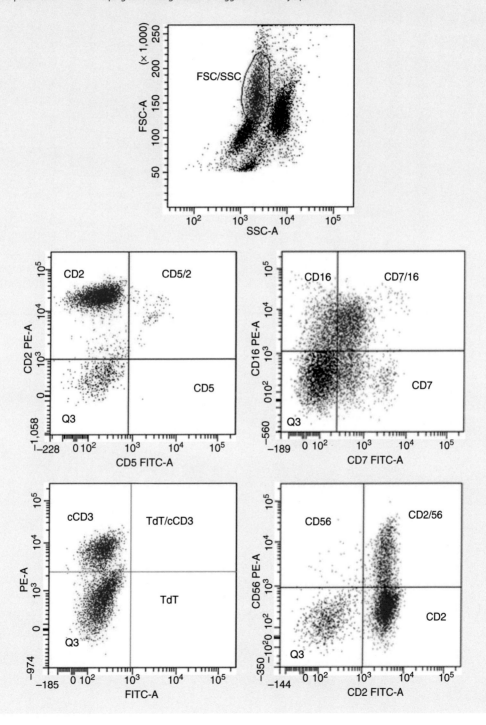

Table 6.15 Summary of cytotoxic T-cell and NK-cell neoplasms (CD56 positive).

Feature	LGL leukaemia	Chronic NK	HSTCL	EATL	Aggressive NK
Incidental diagnosis	Often	Often	No	No	No
Anaemia	Yes/no	Rare	Yes	Yes	Yes
Neutropenia	Yes/no	Rare	Yes/no	No	Yes/no
Thrombocytopenia	Yes/no	Rare	Yes	No	Yes
Autoimmune disease	Yes	Rare	No	Coeliac	No
Immune suppression	Yes	Yes/no	Yes	No	Yes/no
B symptoms	No	No	Yes	Yes	Yes
Organomegaly	No	No	Yes	No	Yes
CD3	Pos	Neg	Pos	Pos	Neg
CD8	Pos	Weak	Pos/neg	Neg	Neg
CD5	Pos/neg	Neg	Neg	Neg	Neg
CD7	Pos/neg	Pos	Pos/neg	Pos	Pos/neg
CD16	Pos	Pos	Pos/neg	Neg	Pos
CD56	Pos/neg	Pos	Pos	Pos	Pos
CD57	Pos	Pos/neg	Neg	Neg	Neg
Other Ag	–	CD158	TCR γδ	CD103$^+$(CD30$^+$)	EBV$^+$

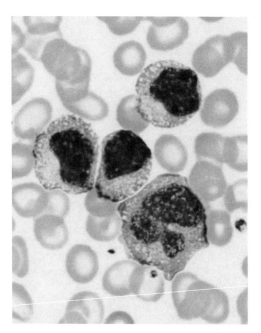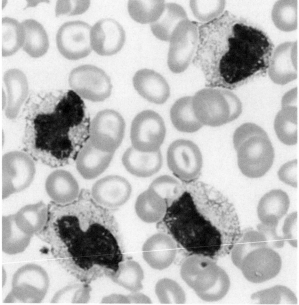

Figure 6.32 EATL cells circulating in peripheral blood, a rare phenomenon.

	ALCL	PTCL	EATL	ATLL	DLBC	HL
Nodes	Yes	Yes	Yes/no	Yes	Yes/no	Yes
Mediastinum	Yes/no	Yes/no	Rare	Yes/no	Yes	Yes
Extranodal	Yes	Yes	Yes	Yes	Rare	Yes/no
Blood	Rare	Rare	Rare	Yes	Rare	No
Bone marrow	Yes/no	Yes/no	Rare	Yes	Rare	Yes/no
Skin	Yes	Yes	Rare	Yes	Rare	No
CD20	Neg	Neg	Neg	Neg	Pos	Neg
CD15	Neg	Neg	Neg	Neg	Neg	Pos/neg
CD3	Pos	Pos/neg	Pos	Pos	Neg	Neg
CD4	Pos/neg	Pos/neg	Neg	Pos	Neg	Neg
CD45	Pos	Pos	Pos	Pos	Pos	Neg

Table 6.16 Neoplasms expressing CD30 which might be encountered in blood and bone marrow specimens (HL, Hodgkin lymphoma).

Immunophenotype

Enteropathy associated T-cell lymphoma (EATL) has a characteristic immunophenotype, being CD4 and CD8 negative, with absence of CD5. The inflammatory small bowel intraepithelial cells of advanced refractory coeliac disease (ulcerative jejunitis) are also CD4 and CD8 negative; it is likely that these cells are precursors of this high grade T-cell lymphoma. Most cases express CD3 and CD7; CD103, an antigen expressed by intraepithelial T lymphocytes, is often positive. EATL will often express CD56 and also CD30 in a proportion of cases.

Cytogenetics

Gains or rearrangements of chromosome 9q33-34 have recently been identified as a characteristic of this disorder. Studies using FISH might assist in making a diagnosis in atypical cases.

Hepatosplenic T-cell lymphomas

This is covered in detail under CD8 positive disorders above but please note that some cases are CD8⁻.

Peripheral T-cell lymphoma, not otherwise specified

The term peripheral T-cell lymphoma (PTCL) includes a whole spectrum of conditions with a nodal or extranodal tissue presentation. They can occasionally appear in peripheral blood or bone marrow and show a CD4 and CD8 negative phenotype, with very variable expression of other T-cell antigens. The presence of CD30 may lead the diagnostician to consider these disorders in a differential diagnosis of an exfoliating T-cell disorder. They, as might be expected, have a very variable morphology and immunophenotype as this entity in the WHO classification represents a spectrum of T-cell lymphomas with aggressive presentation and largely similar treatment approach.

CD30 positive tumours

A number of lymphoproliferative disorders may be difficult to categorize in terms of their clinicopathologic presentation. Many show a scarcity of lineage specific antigen expression, but the presence of CD30 can be of value in the differential diagnosis. Many of these diseases show significant clinicopathologic overlap, so all available clinical, morphological, immunophenotypic and cytogenetic/molecular information should be considered in making a diagnosis. Table 6.16 summarizes the conditions in which CD30 may be expressed; this finding can be a substantial aid to diagnosis. In cases where the immunophenotype appears bare or null, assessment of CD30 expression can be ultimately informative.

Flow cytometric assessment of serous effusions

The diagnostic laboratory will frequently encounter specimens of pleural, pericardial and peritoneal fluid for assessment in patients with a suspected lymphoproliferative disorder. In contrast to CSF examination, the presence of a pleural or peritoneal effusion indicates an established disease process; CSF has a fixed volume so sampling by nature is anticipatory at best.

A number of neoplasms, notably ALL, BL, DLBCL, FL and MZL commonly induce effusions. Such fluid collections can be a result of direct lymphomatous involvement of the pleura/peritoneum or as a secondary phenomenon due to mediastinal/abdominal lymph node involvement and impairment of lymphatic drainage from the associated viscera. As a rule chylous effusions due to impairment of thoracic duct drainage are due to mediastinal lymph node diseases and the neoplastic cells are rarely evident in the effusion fluid. In keeping with the physiological nature of lymphatic fluid, it is rich in normal lymphocytes, protein and lipid, the latter being responsible for its turbid macroscopic appearance.

The cytometrist has to be made aware, not only of the clinical circumstances, but also of the diseases which might be encountered. The majority of lymphoid neoplasms responsible for direct inducement of pleural effusions are B-cell disorders. It is important to focus, therefore, on the nature of the B-cells encountered in the specimen. As always, reactive and activated T-cells are often prominent, whilst neoplastic B-cells can form relatively minor populations. In some samples the neoplastic cells form the predominant population so that their recognition and characterization should not cause problems. The cytometric application has to be focused in accordance with the clinical history; if there is no prior diagnosis the usual diagnostic algorithm as outlined above, needs to be followed.

Primary effusion lymphoma

Primary effusion lymphoma (PEL) is a rare HIV-associated B-cell lymphoma which accounts for approximately 4% of lymphomas in this patient group [59]. It has been described in other immunocompromised T-cell depleted patients following organ transplant and during immunosuppression. It is a curious entity in that it has an affinity for the body cavities such as pleura, pericardium and peritoneum, often in the absence of nodal

involvement. It therefore presents with dyspnoea (pleuropericardial disease) and abdominal distension from malignant ascites. By definition, cases of PEL must show evidence of infection by HHV-8, a herpes virus which has also been implicated in the aetiology of Kaposi sarcoma [60]. Many of these patients also show evidence of EBV infection but its role in the pathogenesis of this lymphoma remain unclear. The cell of origin appears to be a post-GC activated B-cell. Morphologically, the neoplastic cells are large with pleomorphic nuclei, nucleoli and variable sometimes vacuolated cytoplasm; some cases have plasmacytoid/plasmablastic morphology.

Immunophenotypically, the cells often express CD45, but with limited evidence of lymphoid derivation; standard B-cell and T-cell markers are often absent, whereas markers of activation including CD30, CD38, HLA-DR and CD71 are usually present [61]. Some cases with plasmacytoid differentiation express CD138. Cytogenetic analysis normally reveals complex karyotypes but without a common recurring abnormality.

In terms of diagnosis, as applied to serous effusions generally, we utilize the same approach as discussed in relation to blood and bone marrow analysis. The cytometrist is looking for features of B or T-cell clonality and characteristics indicating a degree of maturity of the neoplasm. The same rules apply, but we need to be aware of the 'noise' in such specimens generated by debris, natural cell death, mesothelial cells and neoplastic cell apoptosis.

Flow cytometric assessment of cerebrospinal fluid

Lymphoid neoplasms also have a propensity to escape and survive within the tissues of the central nervous system (CNS). Furthermore, many treatment protocols designed to optimize systemic disease control have poor penetrance beyond the normal blood-brain barrier. The current optimal first-line chemotherapy for DLBCL, R CHOP, gives excellent outcome for the majority of patients able to tolerate this regimen [62], but has poor CNS penetrance and is not able to rescue the small proportion of patients who are destined for a CNS relapse. Flow cytometry on cerebrospinal fluid has two main applications with respect to the mature lymphoproliferative neoplasms, namely the identification of both overt and of subclinical disease.

Identification of overt central nervous system disease

Patients can present with meningeal lymphoma at diagnosis or at the time of localized or systemic relapse. They are often symptomatic, with headache, confusion and cranial nerve palsies. A CSF examination often shows a high cell count and elevated protein level [63]. Often the neoplastic cells are obvious on cytometry of a cytospin, though cell morphology is often distorted by this preparation process and the effects of the hypotonic CSF milieu. Cells often show distortion of nuclear and cytoplasmic architecture, but reliable morphological features of maturity and lineage, such as cell size, nucleoli and granulation, are often preserved.

Flow cytometry on CSF specimens is a reliable means of identifying meningeal involvement by lymphoma [64]. The same principles in diagnosis apply but the choice of antibodies needs tailoring to the disorders likely to be encountered. The CSF specimens are small volume and contain relatively few cells. Furthermore, reactive T-cells are often prominent and should not divert attention from the sometimes minor malignant cell population. The diseases most likely to be encountered are DLBCL, BL

and MCL [65]. ALL also has an affinity for CNS involvement; this is covered in Chapter 5. A concise panel of antibodies directed at CD45, CD2, CD19, CD5, CD10 and sIg, for example, is therefore appropriate for an initial assessment of possible involvement by lymphoma [66]. Attempts have been made in standardizing flow protocols for the analysis of CSF [67]. Flow cytometry is important, not just in making a diagnosis but repeated analyses are also important in assessing response to intrathecal and systemic chemotherapy treatment.

Parenchymal CNS relapse of B-cell lymphoma is also encountered. In these cases the meninges and CSF are often free of disease cells so flow cytometry often fails to isolate clonal B-cells. A diagnosis in these circumstances can be achieved with brain biopsy, but intracerebral relapse, where MRI shows focal enhancing lesions with marked oedematous response, is often presumed in appropriate clinical circumstances.

Identification of subclinical disease

A small proportion of patients presenting with DLBCL are ultimately destined to develop a CNS relapse, despite achieving a systemic complete response to

WORKED EXAMPLE 6.11 Central nervous system involvement by peripheral t-cell lymphoma

A 75-year-old man presented with an acute onset of fatigue, night sweats and weight loss, together with a two-day history of diplopia and headache. He was found to be systemically unwell and confused, with generalized lymphadenopathy and a sixth cranial nerve palsy. An MRI scan of his brain showed diffuse meningeal enhancement, particularly involving the brain stem. A CSF specimen was obtained; the cell count was 500×10^6/L, protein 3 g/dL and glucose 2 mM/L. A cytospin, shown below, was grossly abnormal with an undifferentiated lymphoid infiltrate accompanied by neutrophils and a brisk reactive eosinophilic response.

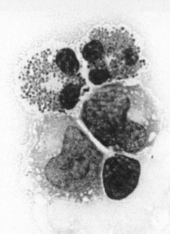
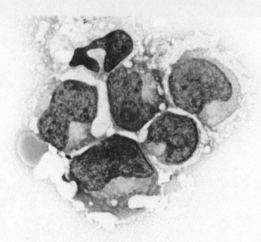

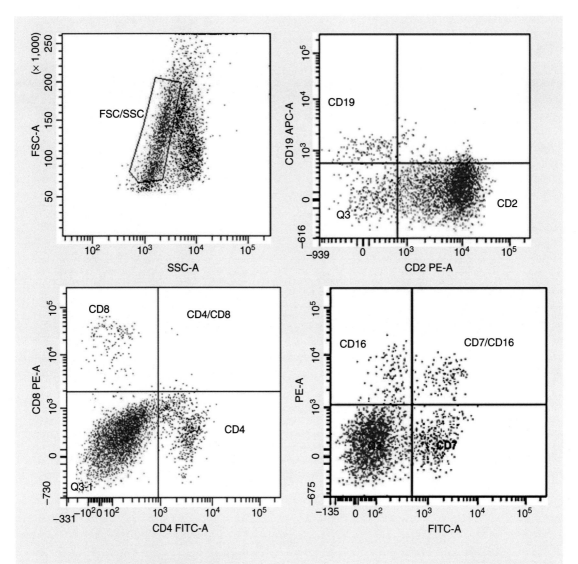

Flow cytometry studies indicated that the neoplastic population was likely to represent a peripheral T-cell lymphoma with a presumed IL-5 induced reactive eosinophilia. Note the pleomorphic lymphoid infiltrate on the FSC/SSC plot, with a CD2+ (CD5+ CD3+, not shown) phenotype but absence of CD7, CD4 and CD8. Most precursor T ALLs will express CD7 as this is one of the earliest antigens to be acquired. This aberrant phenotype was confirmed as a PTCL on lymph node biopsy.

chemotherapy. Less than 5% of patients with advanced stage DLBCL will relapse in the CNS when treated with R CHOP chemotherapy [68, 69], but when it occurs this complication is incurable and carries devastating consequences for the patient and their family. Attempts at treatment also carry significant toxicity and the clinical and radiological responses are often disappointing.

This problem has concerned haemato-oncologists for many years.

Although prophylactic treatment may reduce the incidence of CNS relapse it increases the toxicity of systemic therapy, may cause treatment delays and is unnecessary in the majority of patients. A number of clinical risk algorithms have therefore been developed; it appears that involved site, advanced stage, multiple foci of extranodal disease, together with a high serum LDH are particular features most often associated with a tendency toward this complication [70, 71]. However, the predictive value of these algorithms unfortunately remains low. It seems likely that CNS relapse occurs because of the survival of low levels of lymphoma cells which were present at the outset, but which have escaped the effects of systemic therapy which has poor penetration beyond the blood brain barrier.

There has been much interest, therefore, in the use of flow cytometry as a means of identifying patients with sub-clinical lymphomatous CSF involvement at diagnosis, who might have an increased risk of CNS relapse. Furthermore, it seems logical that if these patients were given additional CNS directed therapy then a potential relapse may be prevented.

A number of studies have addressed this issue. There is little doubt that flow cytometry is a far more sensitive than morphological cytometry in the diagnosis of occult CSF involvement, even in specimens without an increased cell count or protein level, but a positive result does not necessarily predict CNS relapse [72]. Other studies have identified very low level involvement which was predictive, but unfortunately despite additional CNS targeted therapy, a significant proportion still relapsed. In the study by Hegde et al. 22% of patients had occult CSF involvement but despite targeted therapy 45% of these developed a CNS relapse. Furthermore, 8% of those patients without detectable disease developed the same complication [73]. This indicates not only the difficulty in identifying patients at risk but also the limited and relatively ineffective prophylactic treatment options currently available for these patients. This is an interesting area for the application of flow cytometry, but still remains an area for significant development and refinement.

Summary

Many lymphoproliferative disorders and exfoliating lymphoid lymphomas can be encountered in clinical practice. These disorders are extremely different in their biological basis, presentation, morphology and immunophenotype. An accurate diagnosis can only be made when all these characteristics are carefully considered together and not assessed in isolation.

References

1 Barnett D, et al. Absolute CD4+ T-lymphocyte and CD34+ stem cell counts by single-platform flow cytometry: the way forward. Br J Haematol 1999, 106(4): 1059–62.

2 Durrieu F, et al. Normal levels of peripheral CD19(+) CD5(+) CLL-like cells: toward a defined threshold for CLL follow-up - a GEIL-GOELAMS study. Cytometry B Clin Cytom 2011, 80(6): 346–53.

3 Hamblin TJ, et al. Unmutated Ig V(H) genes are associated with a more aggressive form of chronic lymphocytic leukemia. Blood 1999, 94(6): 1848–54.

4 Matutes E, et al. The immunological profile of B-cell disorders and proposal of a scoring system for the diagnosis of CLL. Leukemia 1994, 8(10): 1640–5.

5 Damle RN, et al. Ig V gene mutation status and CD38 expression as novel prognostic indicators in chronic lymphocytic leukemia. Blood 1999, 94(6): 1840–7.

6 Moreau EJ, et al. Improvement of the chronic lymphocytic leukemia scoring system with the monoclonal antibody SN8 (CD79b). Am J Clin Pathol 1997, 108(4): 378–82.

7 Cartron G, et al. CD5 negative B-cell chronic lymphocytic leukemia: clinical and biological features of 42 cases. Leuk Lymphoma 1998, 31(1–2): 209–16.

8 Hsi ED, Hoeltge G, Tubbs RR. Biclonal chronic lymphocytic leukemia. Am J Clin Pathol 2000, 113(6): 798–804.

9 Alapat D, et al. Diagnostic usefulness and prognostic impact of CD200 expression in lymphoid malignancies and plasma cell myeloma. Am J Clin Pathol 2012, 137(1): 93–100.

10 Dohner H, et al. Genomic aberrations and survival in chronic lymphocytic leukemia. N Engl J Med 2000, 343(26): 1910–6.

11 Stilgenbauer S, et al. Genetics of chronic lymphocytic leukemia: genomic aberrations and V(H) gene mutation status in pathogenesis and clinical course. Leukemia 2002, 16(6): 993–1007.

12 Rawstron AC, et al. Monoclonal B-cell lymphocytosis and chronic lymphocytic leukemia. N Engl J Med 2008, 359(6): 575–83.

13 Rawstron AC, et al. Monoclonal B lymphocytes with the characteristics of 'indolent' chronic lymphocytic leukemia are present in 3.5% of adults with normal blood counts. Blood 2002, 100(2): 635–9.

14 Aurran-Schleinitz T, et al. Identification of a new monoclonal B-cell subset in unaffected first-degree relatives in familial chronic lymphocytic leukemia. Leukemia 2005, 19(12): 2339–41.

15 Rawstron AC, Monoclonal B-cell lymphocytosis. Hematology Am Soc Hematol Educ Program, 2009: 430–9.

16 Kelemen K, et al. CD23+ mantle cell lymphoma: a clinical pathologic entity associated with superior outcome

compared with CD23- disease. *Am J Clin Pathol* 2008, **130**(2): 166–77.

17 Gao J, *et al.* Immunophenotypic variations in mantle cell lymphoma. *Am J Clin Pathol* 2009. **132**(5): 699–706.

18 Morice, WG, *et al.* An unusual case of leukemic mantle cell lymphoma with a blastoid component showing loss of CD5 and aberrant expression of CD10. *Am J Clin Pathol* 2004, **122**(1): 122–7.

19 Ruchlemer R, *et al.* B-prolymphocytic leukaemia with t(11;14) revisited: a splenomegalic form of mantle cell lymphoma evolving with leukaemia. *Br J Haematol* 2004, **125**(3): 330–6.

20 Orchard J, *et al.* A subset of t(11;14) lymphoma with mantle cell features displays mutated IgVH genes and includes patients with good prognosis, nonnodal disease. *Blood* 2003, **101**(12): 4975–81.

21 Mozos A, *et al.* SOX11 expression is highly specific for mantle cell lymphoma and identifies the cyclin D1-negative subtype. *Haematologica* 2009, **94**(11): 1555–62.

22 Fernandez V, *et al.* Genomic and gene expression profiling defines indolent forms of mantle cell lymphoma. *Cancer Res* 2010, **70**(4): 1408–18.

23 Vaishampayan UN, *et al.* Blastic mantle cell lymphoma associated with Burkitt-type translocation and hypodiploidy. *Br J Haematol* 2001, **115**(1): 66–8.

24 Arcaini L, *et al.* Splenic marginal zone lymphoma: a prognostic model for clinical use. *Blood* 2006, **107**(12): 4643–9.

25 Baldini L, *et al.* Poor prognosis in non-villous splenic marginal zone cell lymphoma is associated with p53 mutations. *Br J Haematol* 1997, **99**(2): 375–8.

26 Baseggio L, *et al.* CD5 expression identifies a subset of splenic marginal zone lymphomas with higher lymphocytosis: a clinico-pathological, cytogenetic and molecular study of 24 cases. *Haematologica* 2010, **95**(4): 604–12.

27 Matutes E, *et al.* Splenic marginal zone lymphoma: proposals for a revision of diagnostic, staging and therapeutic criteria. *Leukemia* 2008, **22**(3): 487–95.

28 Gruszka-Westwood AM, *et al.* p53 abnormalities in splenic lymphoma with villous lymphocytes. *Blood* 2001, **97**(11): 3552–8.

29 Del Giudice I, *et al.* IgVH genes mutation and usage, ZAP-70 and CD38 expression provide new insights on B-cell prolymphocytic leukemia (B-PLL). *Leukemia* 2006, **20**(7): 1231–7.

30 Seegmiller AC, *et al.* Immunophenotypic differentiation between neoplastic plasma cells in mature B-cell lymphoma vs plasma cell myeloma. *Am J Clin Pathol* 2007, **127**(2): 176–81.

31 Konoplev S, *et al.* Immunophenotypic profile of lymphoplasmacytic lymphoma/Waldenstrom macroglobulinemia. *Am J Clin Pathol* 2005, **124**(3): 414–20.

32 Morice WG, *et al.* Novel immunophenotypic features of marrow lymphoplasmacytic lymphoma and correlation with Waldenstrom's macroglobulinemia. *Mod Pathol* 2009, **22**(6): 807–16.

33 Kroft SH, Dawson DB, McKenna RW. Large cell lymphoma transformation of chronic lymphocytic leukemia/small lymphocytic lymphoma. A flow cytometric analysis of seven cases. *Am J Clin Pathol* 2001, **115**(3): 385–95.

34 Olteanu H, *et al.* CD23 expression in follicular lymphoma: clinicopathologic correlations. *Am J Clin Pathol* 2011, **135**(1): 46–53.

35 Ouansafi I, *et al.* Transformation of follicular lymphoma to plasmablastic lymphoma with c-myc gene rearrangement. *Am J Clin Pathol* 2010, **134**(6): 972–81.

36 Bertram HC, Check IJ, Milano MA. Immunophenotyping large B-cell lymphomas. Flow cytometric pitfalls and pathologic correlation. *Am J Clin Pathol* 2001, **116**(2): 191–203.

37 Rodig SJ, *et al.* Characteristic expression patterns of TCL1, CD38, and CD44 identify aggressive lymphomas harboring a MYC translocation. *Am J Surg Pathol* 2008, **32**(1): 113–22.

38 Matutes E, *et al.* The immunophenotype of hairy cell leukemia (HCL). Proposal for a scoring system to distinguish HCL from B-cell disorders with hairy or villous lymphocytes. *Leuk Lymphoma* 1994, **14**(Suppl 1): 57–61.

39 Jones D, *et al.* Absence of CD26 expression is a useful marker for diagnosis of T-cell lymphoma in peripheral blood. *Am J Clin Pathol* 2001, **115**(6): 885–92.

40 Kelemen K, *et al.* The usefulness of CD26 in flow cytometric analysis of peripheral blood in Sezary syndrome. *Am J Clin Pathol* 2008, **129**(1): 146–56.

41 Foucar K. Mature T-cell leukemias including T-prolymphocytic leukemia, adult T-cell leukemia/lymphoma, and Sezary syndrome. *Am J Clin Pathol* 2007, **127**(4): 496–510.

42 Verstovsek S, Cabanillas F, Dang NH. CD26 in T-cell lymphomas: a potential clinical role? *Oncology (Williston Park)* 2000, **14**(6 Suppl 2): 17–23.

43 Nicot C. Current views in HTLV-I-associated adult T-cell leukemia/lymphoma. *Am J Hematol* 2005, **78**(3): 232–9.

44 Kondo S. *et al.* Expression of CD26/dipeptidyl peptidase IV in adult T cell leukemia/lymphoma (ATLL). *Leuk Res* 1996, **20**(4): 357–63.

45 Diaz-Alderete A, *et al.* Lymphocyte immunophenotype of circulating angioimmunoblastic T-cell lymphoma cells. *Br J Haematol* 2006, **134**(3): 347–8.

46 Baseggio L, *et al.* Identification of circulating CD10 positive T cells in angioimmunoblastic T-cell lymphoma. *Leukemia* 2006, **20**(2): 296–303.

47 Sabnani I, Tsang P. Are clonal T-cell large granular lymphocytes to blame for unexplained haematological abnormalities? *Br J Haematol* 2007, **136**(1): 30–7.

48 Lamy T, Loughran TP Jr. Clinical features of large granular lymphocyte leukemia. *Semin Hematol* 2003, **40**(3): 185–95.

49 Swerdlow SH. T-cell and NK-cell posttransplantation lymphoproliferative disorders. *Am J Clin Pathol* 2007, **127**(6): 887–95.

50 Dadu T, Rangan A, Bhargava M. CD4+/NKa+/CD8(dim+) T-cell large granular lymphocytic leukemia: a rare entity. *Journal of Postgraduate Medicine* 2010, **56**(3): 223–4.

51 Lundell R, et al. T-cell large granular lymphocyte leukemias have multiple phenotypic abnormalities involving pan-T-cell antigens and receptors for MHC molecules. *Am J Clin Pathol* 2005, **124**(6): 937–46.

52 Cady FM, Morice WG. Flow cytometric assessment of T-cell chronic lymphoproliferative disorders. *Clin Lab Med* 2007, **27**(3): 513–32, vi.

53 Morice WG, et al. Demonstration of aberrant T-cell and natural killer-cell antigen expression in all cases of granular lymphocytic leukaemia. *Br J Haematol* 2003, **120**(6): 1026–36.

54 Morice WG. The immunophenotypic attributes of NK cells and NK-cell lineage lymphoproliferative disorders. *Am J Clin Pathol* 2007, **127**(6): 881–6.

55 Hoffmann T, et al. Natural killer-type receptors for HLA class I antigens are clonally expressed in lymphoproliferative disorders of natural killer and T-cell type. *Br J Haematol* 2000, **110**(3): 525–36.

56 Belhadj K, et al. Hepatosplenic gammadelta T-cell lymphoma is a rare clinicopathologic entity with poor outcome: report on a series of 21 patients. *Blood* 2003, **102**(13): 4261–9.

57 Falchook, GS, et al. Hepatosplenic gamma-delta T-cell lymphoma: clinicopathological features and treatment. *Ann Oncol* 2009, **20**(6): 1080–5.

58 Wang CC, et al. Consistent presence of isochromosome 7q in hepatosplenic T gamma/delta lymphoma: a new cytogenetic-clinicopathologic entity. *Genes Chromosomes Cancer* 1995, **12**(3): 161–4.

59 Simonelli C, et al. Clinical features and outcome of primary effusion lymphoma in HIV-infected patients: a single-institution study. *J Clin Oncol* 2003, **21**(21): 3948–54.

60 Cesarman E, et al. Kaposi's sarcoma-associated herpesvirus-like DNA sequences in AIDS-related body-cavity-based lymphomas. *N Engl J Med* 1995, **332**(18): 1186–91.

61 Gaidano G, Carbone A. Primary effusion lymphoma: a liquid phase lymphoma of fluid-filled body cavities. *Adv Cancer Res* 2001, **80**: 115–46.

62 Coiffier B, et al. CHOP chemotherapy plus rituximab compared with CHOP alone in elderly patients with diffuse large-B-cell lymphoma. *N Engl J Med* 2002, **346**(4): 235–42.

63 Bromberg JE, et al. CSF flow cytometry greatly improves diagnostic accuracy in CNS hematologic malignancies. *Neurology* 2007, **68**(20): 1674–9.

64 Quijano S, et al. Identification of leptomeningeal disease in aggressive B-cell non-Hodgkin's lymphoma: improved sensitivity of flow cytometry. *J Clin Oncol* 2009, **27**(9): 1462–9.

65 Valdez R, et al. Cerebrospinal fluid involvement in mantle cell lymphoma. *Mod Pathol* 2002, **15**(10): 1073–9.

66 Roma AA, et al. Lymphoid and myeloid neoplasms involving cerebrospinal fluid: comparison of morphologic examination and immunophenotyping by flow cytometry. *Diagn Cytopathol* 2002, **27**(5): 271–5.

67 Kraan J, et al. Flow cytometric immunophenotyping of cerebrospinal fluid. *Curr Protoc Cytom* 2008. Chapter 6: Unit 6, 25.

68 Boehme V, et al. Incidence and risk factors of central nervous system recurrence in aggressive lymphoma–a survey of 1693 patients treated in protocols of the German High-Grade Non-Hodgkin's Lymphoma Study Group (DSHNHL). *Ann Oncol* 2007, **18**(1): 149–57.

69 Kridel R, Dietrich PY. Prevention of CNS relapse in diffuse large B-cell lymphoma. *Lancet Oncol* 2011, **12**(13): 1258–66.

70 Haioun C, et al. Incidence and risk factors of central nervous system relapse in histologically aggressive non-Hodgkin's lymphoma uniformly treated and receiving intrathecal central nervous system prophylaxis: a GELA study on 974 patients. Groupe d'Etudes des Lymphomes de l'Adulte. *Ann Oncol* 2000, **11**(6): 685–90.

71 Feugier P, et al. Incidence and risk factors for central nervous system occurrence in elderly patients with diffuse large-B-cell lymphoma: influence of rituximab. *Ann Oncol* 2004, **15**(1): 129–33.

72 Alvarez R, et al. Clinical relevance of flow cytometric immunophenotyping of the cerebrospinal fluid in patients with diffuse large B-cell lymphoma. *Ann Oncol* 2012, **23**(5): 1274–9.

73 Hegde U, et al. High incidence of occult leptomeningeal disease detected by flow cytometry in newly diagnosed aggressive B-cell lymphomas at risk for central nervous system involvement: the role of flow cytometry versus cytology. *Blood* 2005, **105**(2): 496–502.

CHAPTER 7

Myelodysplastic Syndromes and Myeloproliferative Neoplasms

Introduction

Within current disease classification systems, diagnosis of the myelodysplastic syndromes (MDS) and myeloproliferative neoplasms (MPN) rely on a combination of clinical and peripheral blood findings, bone marrow pathology, cytogenetic and molecular techniques. The role of flow cytometry for routine diagnostic purposes has hitherto been seen to be of less importance than in many other areas of haematology. For example, while flow has been used to characterize (and enumerate) myeloblasts in MDS and determine blast cell lineage in advanced phase chronic myeloid leukaemia (CML), the diagnosis of such conditions has been made largely by morphological and, in the case of CML, genetic criteria (i.e. the presence of the *BCR-ABL* translocation).

Aside from its obvious role in characterizing populations of blast cells, there is a groundswell of interest in placing flow cytometry at the centre of the diagnostic process, in particular in MDS. The ability of flow to detect aberrant and asynchronous antigen expression is useful in this group of conditions characterized by abnormal cell maturation and function, and significant efforts are under way to develop consensus antibody panels for detection of the numerous flow cytometric abnormalities described on MDS cells. For both CML and the *BCR-ABL* negative MPNs its role is less clear, although several publications have identified abnormalities of antigen expression in these disorders. Finally, it may be of considerable clinical utility in the diagnosis of rare myeloid neoplasms such as mastocytosis and also the detection of associated abnormalities that may support a marrow disorder (e.g. small PNH clones or reduced B-cell progenitors in MDS).

Its role in determining prognosis in this group of conditions is under ongoing investigation.

Myelodysplastic syndromes

These are a heterogeneous group of clonal haematopoietic stem cell (HSC) disorders characterized by abnormal maturation and differentiation of haematopoietic cells. They occur most commonly in older adults, and manifest principally as peripheral blood cytopenias in one or more lineages (as a result of disordered and ineffective haematopoiesis), frequently exhibit disease progression and may terminate in acute myeloid leukaemia (AML) or rarely granulocytic sarcoma [1]. Note that transformation into an acute lymphoblastic leukaemia (ALL) does not occur, and although it has been very rarely observed such cases may represent coincidental ALL [2]. The thresholds for definition of cytopenias have been set at a haemoglobin of <100 g/L, neutrophils $<1.5\times10^9$/L and platelets $<100\times10^9$/L, although blood counts outwith these ranges may not necessarily exclude a diagnosis of MDS [3]. By definition MDS exhibits marrow blast counts <20%, as above this threshold the diagnosis is AML.

Approximately 50% of MDS will demonstrate a cytogenetic abnormality, but the remainder have a normal karyotype. For many cases the demonstration of objective abnormalities will make diagnosis easy (e.g. presence of increased marrow blasts, gross morphological dysplasia and a karyotypic abnormality), but other cases may demonstrate much more subtle morphological changes and lack the other objective criteria. Furthermore, other insults to the marrow may cause similar appearances,

Practical Flow Cytometry in Haematology Diagnosis, First Edition. Mike Leach, Mark Drummond and Allyson Doig.
© 2013 John Wiley & Sons, Ltd. Published 2013 by John Wiley & Sons, Ltd.

such as B12 or folate deficiency, alcohol excess, infection, copper deficiency and lead toxicity. It is important to exclude these problems during the initial assessment and investigation of the patient. It is hoped that the routine use of flow cytometry to aid the diagnosis will reduce the reliance on these subjective criteria.

The morphological assessment of cells in peripheral blood and bone marrow has been one of the cornerstones of MDS diagnosis. Firm data with regard to cytogenetic aberrancy is not available in many cases so the diagnosis remains presumptive, in the presence of otherwise unexplained cytopenias, together with abnormalities of cellular nuclear and cytoplasmic anatomy in standard stained smears. The range of morphological abnormalities encountered in MDS is extensive and a full review is beyond the scope of this text, but a few are highlighted which are relevant to how these cells behave in standard FSC versus SSC plots which may influence gating strategy when myeloid cells are assessed by flow. A bone marrow aspirate is the prime tissue for the assessment of morphological aberrancy in MDS, and of course it allows the detection of excessive blast populations. Peripheral blood is also fruitful in providing useful information on nuclear and cytoplasmic configuration. Figures 7.1a, 7.1b and 7.1c illustrate the diversity of morphological features in peripheral blood myeloid cells in MDS.

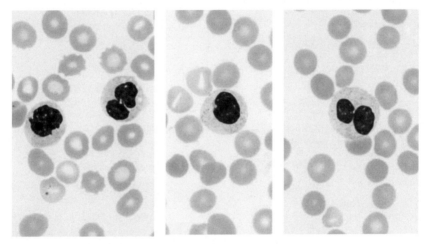

Figure 7.1a Abnormal nuclear hypo-segmentation and reduced cytoplasmic granulation in peripheral blood neutrophils in myelodysplastic syndromes.

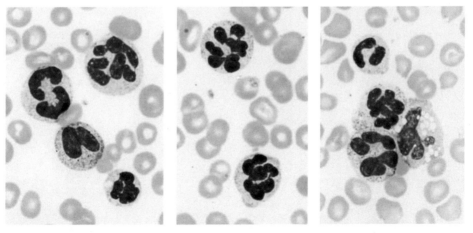

Figure 7.1b Abnormal nuclear hyper-segmentation, but largely preserved cytoplasmic granulation in peripheral blood neutrophils in myelodysplastic syndromes.

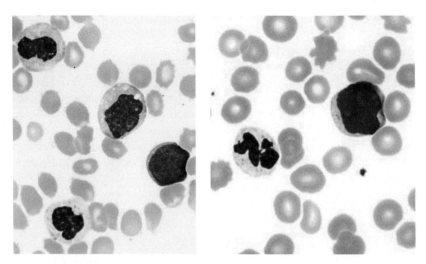

Figure 7.1c Dysplastic neutrophils alongside myeloblasts in peripheral blood in myelodysplastic syndromes.

Table 7.1 Current WHO classification for the myelodysplastic syndromes. The current classification of MDS relies principally upon careful morphological examination, in particular the extent of typical dysplastic changes, the percentage blast cells and the proportion of ring sideroblasts.

Subtype	Peripheral blood	Bone marrow
Refractory cytopenias with unilineage dysplasia (RCUD)	Single lineage cytopenias (most commonly anaemia, but other cytopenias seen), blasts <1%.	Unilineage dysplasia (≥10% of cells) Blasts <5% <15% ringed sideroblasts in erythroid component
Refractory anaemia with ring sideroblasts (RARS)	Anaemia only No blast cells	≥15% ringed sideroblasts in erythroid component Erythroid dysplasia Blasts <5%
Refractory anaemia with multilineage dysplasia (RCMD)	One or more cytopenias Blasts <1% Monocytes $<1\times10^9$/L	≥10% of cells dysplastic in two or more lineages Blasts <5% with no Auer rods
Refractory anaemia with excess blasts-1 (RAEB-1)	One or more cytopenias Blasts <5%, no Auer rods Monocytes $<1\times10^9$/L	One or more lineages dysplastic Blasts 5–9% and no Auer rods
Refractory anaemia with excess blasts-2 (RAEB-2)	One or more cytopenias Blasts 5–19% Monocytes $<1\times10^9$/L Auer rods may be seen	One or more lineages dysplastic Blasts 10–19% Auer rods may be seen
MDS unclassified (MDS-U)	One or more cytopenias Blasts ≤1%	Dysplastic changes in <10% of cell lineage plus cytogenetic evidence of MDS Blasts <5%
MDS associated with isolated del(5q)	Anaemia Normal or increased platelet count Blasts <1%	Typical hypo-lobulated megakaryocytic nuclei Blasts <5% Del(5q) as sole cytogenetic abnormality No Auer rods

Adapted from Swerdlow et al. [4], with permission from Wiley.

Classification of myelodysplastic syndromes

This remains predominantly based upon morphological criteria, with incorporation of some genetic information (i.e. the presence of an isolated del(5q) abnormality) [4] (Table 7.1). The morphological criteria take into account both peripheral blood and marrow findings. As accurate morphological assessment is vital for classification purposes (particularly in terms of blast cell percentage) it is recommended that a 500 cell differential be performed on marrow [4, 5]. Dysplasia is generally considered to be of diagnostic significance when it is present in ≥10% of cells from the lineage in question. The limitations of this system (namely the arbitrary threshold and the subjective criteria for morphological dysplasia) have led to the proposal for an additional subgroup of cases that exhibit cytopenia(s) but no diagnostic dysplastic features (termed idiopathic cytopenia of undetermined significance, or ICUS) [6]. Long-term follow-up is currently suggested for these cases, although it might be hoped that flow cytometry may offer useful diagnostic information in due course.

A detailed discussion of the morphological classification of MDS is outwith the scope of this text; however, a summary of the diagnostic criteria is given in Table 7.1.

Prognosis of myelodysplastic syndromes

As well as exhibiting great morphological heterogeneity, there is great variability in terms of clinical outcomes within this group of disorders, with survival ranging from only a few months to many years. The ability to determine prognosis allows treatment planning. The most widely used prognostic system is the International Prognostic Scoring System (IPSS, shown in Table 7.2), which incorporates blast percentage, karyotype and the number of cytopenias and allocates patients to one of four risk groups [3].

Flow cytometry in myelodysplastic syndromes

Flow has historically been applied in MDS to characterize the blast population(s), in particular those present in transformed disease. While this role remains important, many other abnormalities have been described (within all diagnostic and prognostic groups) and it is anticipated

Table 7.2 The IPSS score for determining prognosis in myelodysplastic syndromes.

Score allocated to each parameter					
Prognostic variable	0	0.5	1.0	1.5	2.0
Bone marrow blasts (%)	<5	5–10	—	11–20	21–30
Karyotype	Good	Intermediate	Poor		
Cytopaenias	0 or 1	2 or 3			

An IPSS score is obtained by adding together the individual scores for the three variables, resulting in stratification of patients into one of four risk groups: low (score 0), Int-1 (score 0.5 to 1.0), Int-2 (score 1.5 to 2.0), or high (score >2.0). Median survival for these groups is 5.7, 3.5, 1.2 and 0.4 years, respectively [3]. Note that the highest category of blast percentage (namely 21–30%) would now be classified as AML. Although the IPSS remains in common use, the new WHO based Prognostic System (WPSS, incorporating karyotype, WHO subgroup and need for transfusion) is more discriminatory and can be applied at any stage during the patient's illness [7].

that flow will become an important adjunct in the diagnosis (and likely prognosis) of the disease. It should be noted that the bulk of published work concerns analysis of marrow material; data on peripheral blood is limited. Detection and interpretation of flow abnormalities in this group of disorders can, however, be challenging for a number of reasons:

1 Marrow cells, in particular granulocytes, remain biologically active after sampling (and therefore sensitive to environmental changes), which may cause alteration in surface antigen expression. Marrow should preferably be collected into heparin and analysed promptly (ideally within 24 hours), as delayed storage in EDTA may alter some antigens in particular CD10, CD11b and CD16 [8, 9] and reduce SSC of granulocytes [10]. Pre-analytical equilibration is recommended at room temperature [8].

2 Many of the abnormalities documented are detected only on a subpopulation of cells and may involve aberrant antigen expression (e.g. lymphoid antigen expression on myeloid cells), asynchronous expression (e.g. CD34 expression persisting as cells mature) and altered intensity of expression. Comparison with the equivalent normal cell type is important to fully characterize these abnormalities (Table 7.3) and by necessity a significant (but arbitrary) 'cut-off' applied (e.g. ≥10% cells exhibiting aberrant antigen expression and antigen intensity increased or decreased by ≥1/3 of a decade on a log scale [11]).

Table 7.3 Summary of the key immunophenotypic features of normal marrow subpopulations which are amenable to assessment in myelodysplastic syndromes.

Myeloblasts	CD34	CD13/33	CD117	HLA-DR	
Type I blast	Pos	Pos	Pos	Pos	
Type 2 blast	Neg	Pos	Pos	Pos	

Myeloid cells	CD11b	CD13	CD15	CD16	CD64
Promyelocyte	Neg	Pos	Dim	Neg	Pos
Myelocyte	Pos	Dim	Dim	Neg	Pos
Metamyelocyte	Pos	Dim	Pos	Dim	Dim
Band cell	Pos	Pos	Pos	Pos	Neg
Neutrophil	Pos	Bright	Bright	Bright	Neg

Monocytes	CD117	CD64	HLA-DR	CD14	
Promonocyte	Dim	Bright	Bright	Dim/Neg	
Monocyte	Neg	Pos	Pos	Bright	

Erythroid series	CD45	CD117	CD71	Glycophorin A	
Early	Neg	Pos	Pos	Neg	
Intermediate	Neg	Neg	Dim	Dim	
Late	Neg	Neg	Neg	Pos	

This table lists the major marrow subpopulations for all lineages at varying stages of development, and highlights their discriminating antigenic profiles. The majority of these normal populations are of interest with regards to direct comparison with equivalent populations in suspected MDS; other populations (such as mature lymphocytes) are uninvolved in the MDS clone and offer a useful internal control population (e.g. for parameters such as CD45 and SSC) with which to compare dysplastic cells.

3 Abnormalities are detected on myeloblasts as well as maturing cell types and different lineages within the same patient will exhibit different abnormalities. Thus, unlike a typical case of ALL or LPD, for example (where a single homogenous neoplastic population is apparent), multiple lineages may exhibit different abnormalities, making gating strategies and antibody panels considerably more complex.
4 Detectable abnormalities may not be specific for MDS; for example similar abnormalities may be observed in reactive conditions (e.g. CD64 expression on granulocytes during sepsis and CD56 expression on myeloid

precursors as a consequence of G-CSF administration) and other myeloid disorders (e.g. aberrant CD7 expression in myeloblasts in AML). CD16 [12] and CD33 [13] (which are often lost on dysplastic myeloid cells) may be lost by constitutional genetic polymorphisms, and CD16 is absent in paroxysmal nocturnal haemoglobinuria (PNH) [14]. Thus, interpretation of flow data must be performed with a full knowledge of the clinical situation. Therefore great variability in findings is possible and reproducibility between laboratories is inevitably difficult. However, considerable efforts in this regard are under way, with attempts to standardize methodology and reporting and develop scoring systems that can aid diagnosis and help predict clinical outcome [9].

The immunophenotypic profile of the normal bone marrow populations is described in detail in Chapter 4. A brief summary of the antigenic acquisition patterns of the cell lineages relevant to myelodysplasia is presented here in Table 7.3.

The possible applications of flow cytometry in MDS are summarized in Figure 7.2, and these are discussed in turn below.

Characterization of Myeloblasts

One of the principal reasons for performing flow cytometry in MDS is to enumerate and characterize the myeloblast population in the marrow. The typical blast cell phenotype in MDS has been meticulously described as $CD34^+$ $CD38^+$ HLA-DR$^+$ $CD13^+$ $CD33^+$, with MPO noted to be absent in >50% of cases by cytochemistry [15]. The latter might suggest a more 'primitive' blast phenotype in MDS than in the majority of *de novo* AML, an observation supported by other studies demonstrating a relative expansion of primitive $CD34^+$ $CD38^{dim}$ primitive precursor cells in MDS as compared to other haematological disorders (including *de novo* AML) and normal cases [15]. Not all of these antigens are positive in all patients, however, and in those occasional cases comprising $CD34^-$ myeloblasts (approximately 4% [15]), CD117 should be used as a progenitor cell marker instead (the blasts may be further characterized using a $CD45^{dim}$ SSC^{low} HLA-DR$^+$ $CD11b^-$ gate [9]). As in some cases of primitive AML, TdT may also be detected in MDS myeloblasts [17]. During normal myeloid maturation CD15 and CD11b first appear on promyelocytes and myelocytes respectively, and continue to be expressed in fully mature neutrophils. Their asynchronous expression on MDS myeloblasts is well documented (in 64% and 48% respectively [15]). In addition, CD10 (present on

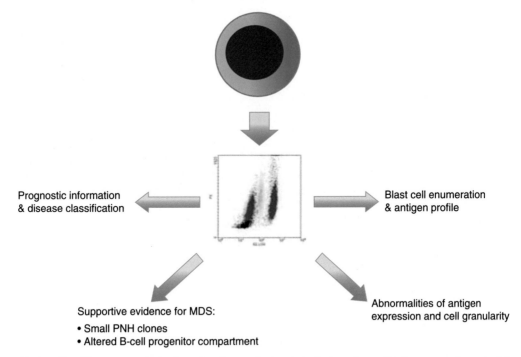

Figure 7.2 The utility of flow cytometry in the diagnosis and prognosis of myelodysplastic syndromes. This figure summarizes potential flow cytometric approaches in MDS. These are each discussed further in the text. PNH, paroxysmal nocturnal haemoglobinuria.

normal neutrophils and B-lymphoblasts) is found on the myeloblasts in almost 20% of cases [14]. Such asynchronous expression of antigens, that is, simultaneous expression of both stem cell antigens and maturation antigens, is also, of course, well documented in *de novo* AML.

In terms of aberrant antigen expression, CD2, CD4, CD5, CD7 and CD56 are described (in 3%, 46%, 3%, 34% and 27% of cases respectively [14]). Interestingly, in this study CD7 was noted to be most prevalent in high risk MDS (conversely the maturation antigens CD10 and CD15 were prevalent in lower risk disease) and was noted to be an independent predictor of poor prognosis. It is worth reinforcing the point that CD7 may be expressed in small subpopulations of normal myeloblasts: any substantial CD7 positive myeloblast population, however, is always abnormal. A summary of the most commonly described flow abnormalities for precursor and maturing cells in MDS is given in Figure 7.3. These abnormalities of asynchronous and/or aberrant antigen expression clearly differentiate an MDS myeloblast population from normal myeloid precursors which do not exhibit any of these findings [18]. To improve diagnostic utility, detection of these and other abnormalities on CD34+ cells have been combined in scoring systems which can aid diagnosis in low risk MDS

in particular, which is especially useful for cases which lack objective markers of dysplasia (e.g. MDS-related karyotypic abnormalities and ring sideroblastosis) [18–20].

Enumeration of myeloblasts

The caveats surrounding enumeration of blast cells by flow are explained in detail in Chapters 3 and 5 and must be borne in mind, as these are also relevant for MDS. In particular, it must be remembered that red cell lysis is performed before antibody staining, and so the blast percentage as defined by flow is calculated using a different denominator to that of a morphological count (which incorporates all nucleated cells). Thus, one might predict the blast percentage to be lower by morphology. One large study found precisely the opposite, likely due to the morphological inclusion of dysplastic myeloid precursors (e.g. hypogranular promyelocytes) and/or promonocytes (blast equivalent cells which are difficult to define by flow) [21]. Furthermore, as mentioned above, not all blasts are CD34+ with, in particular, morphological blast excesses often comprising CD34−, 'type II' blast cells (exhibiting azurophilic granules [22]). Although reasonably good correlations between morphological and flow determined blast counts have been demonstrated [23, 24]

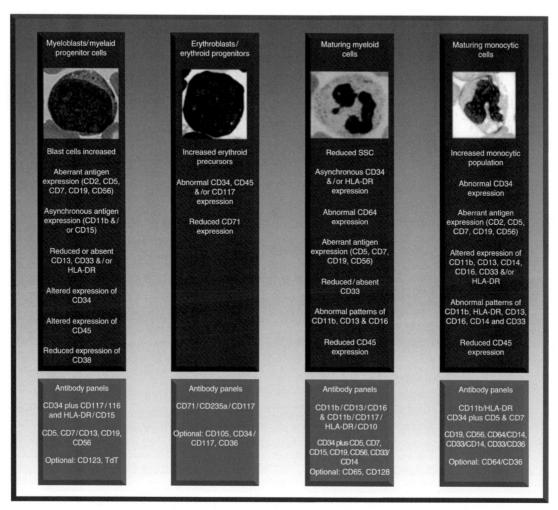

Figure 7.3 A summary of the common lineage-specific immunophenotypic abnormalities in myelodysplastic syndromes and recommended antibody panels. The most widely recognized immunophenotypic abnormalities are highlighted here, alongside the optimal panels for their detection, as recommended by the European LeukaemiaNet [9]. See text for references. Modified from van de Loosdrecht et al. [9], with permission from Wiley.

a recent large MDS registry study of over 600 cases of MDS described significant differences between cytological, flow and histological approaches to blast enumeration. Importantly, all modalities retained predictive relevance in terms of evolution to AML [25]. However, it was notable that the morphological blast count from marrow smears appeared to be the most predictive and this remains the key technique in this regard. Several authors have proposed that a threshold of 3% be introduced as significant for the detection of marrow myeloblasts by flow in MDS, as compared to the traditional 5% used by morphologists [9, 24]. Recent observations also suggest that the detection of circulating myeloblasts in peripheral blood (as opposed to

marrow) likely has prognostic implications, with at least two studies documenting a worse outcome in MDS patients with low levels of circulating blast cells [26, 27].

One circumstance where enumeration of CD34+ cells by flow can be particularly useful is in the separation of hypoplastic MDS from severe aplastic anaemia (SAA). Visual assessment of blast populations in hypocellular specimens can be very difficult and although ICC on a marrow trephine can be useful, accurate counting of stained cells using this technique is laborious and requires experience to do it properly. In one informative study using flow cytometry, only patients with CD34+ cells of 1% or more were subsequently confirmed as

MDS by detection of cytogenetic abnormalities or evolution to higher risk MDS/AML [28]. The mean CD34$^+$ count in these samples was 3.5% of total marrow cells, while those with SAA had a significantly lower mean count of 0.12%.

Lineage related immunophenotypic abnormalities in myelodysplastic syndromes

Abnormalities of erythroblasts and erythroid progenitors

Most patients with MDS are anaemic and many exhibit erythroid dysplasia and an increase in erythroid progenitor cells (both morphologically and by flow, Figure 7.3). The erythroblast population is easily identified (CD45$^-$, SSC^{low}, Glycophorin A/CD235$^+$) [29]. CD117, CD36 and CD105 (endoglin, positive on early erythroblasts) can additionally be used to determine the size of the primitive erythroid compartment [30]. Demonstrating further antigenic abnormalities of erythroid maturation by flow is a challenge, however, largely because of limited commercial availability of specific antibodies. Glycophorin A and CD71 (the transferrin receptor) can be usefully combined; a reproducible finding is that expression of CD71 on erythroblasts from MDS patients is significantly reduced as compared to their normal counterparts [29, 31] (almost three-fold in one study [30]). Two further and intriguing observations have also been made. First, the loss of red cell A, B and H antigens is frequently observed in myeloid disorders (including MDS) by flow cytometric (but not serological) means [32]. Second, flow cytometric detection of mitochondrial ferritin can provide an objective measurement of ring sideroblastosis [30]. These antibodies remain unavailable though, as yet, for routine use.

Abnormalities of maturing myeloid cells and neutrophils

Hypogranularity of neutrophils and their precursors is well described in MDS and is commonly noted morphologically. Flow can aid in this regard, with hypogranular promyelocytes, myelocytes and neutrophils frequently displaying reduced SSC [33] (Figures 7.4a, 7.4b, 7.4c). Some authors recommend expressing SSC as a ratio of granulocyte to lymphoid SSC, which can aid reproducibility [20] (Figure 7.4c).

Screening of peripheral blood for features of neutrophil and perhaps monocyte dysplasia is potentially attractive in the work-up of patients with mild unexplained anaemias, cytopenias or macrocytosis. In addition to quantifying changes in side scatter characteristics, a number of authors

have developed scoring systems for assessing neutrophil dysplasia using a panel of selected antibodies to antigens, such as CD10, CD11a, CD66 and CD116, which can show aberrant expression, even in early stage patients and in those with normal cytogenetics [34, 35]. This approach has shown impressive sensitivity and specificity for MDS when used in this way. A bone marrow examination might therefore potentially be avoided in selected patients.

A further characteristic feature of dysplastic myeloid maturation is the persistence of the precursor cell markers CD34 and HLA-DR into the mature granulocytic population [36, 37]. These antigens are normally both lost by the promyelocyte stage. This was most notable in poorer risk MDS in one study (particularly in cases with multiple cytogenetic abnormalities and treatment related cases) and was often accompanied by reduction of CD10, a marker of neutrophil maturity [36] (Figure 7.5). Increased or decreased expression of other antigens is also noted, including CD11b, CD13, CD16, CD33, CD45 and CD64 [29, 33]. The significance of neutrophil CD64 expression as a marker for MDS is controversial, with an early study detailing increased expression [38] and a more recent study documenting reduced expression [31]. The authors, however, have found this characteristic to appear relatively frequently in MDS, which has been confirmed using standard non-immunophenotypic data (Figure 7.6).

Aberrant expression of CD2, CD7, CD19 or CD56 may also be observed. Myelodysplastic syndrome patients typically demonstrate significantly increased proportions of immature granulocytic cells (CD13$^+$, CD33$^+$, CD45$^+$ and CD16$^-$) and reduced proportions of mature granulocytes (CD13$^+$, CD33$^+$, CD45$^+$, CD16^{++}) [29].

In MDS aberrant expression of precursor related antigens can be detected on myeloid cells beyond the blast cell stage, at a frequency that increases with the degree of dysplasia. This is accompanied by a steady reduction in CD10 expression and fall in the mean neutrophil SSC (data not shown). Data adapted from Xu et al. [36].

Abnormalities of maturing monocytic cells and monocytes

Abnormalities of monocytes and their precursors are well described. Most studies have looked specifically at the monocytes present in chronic myelomonocytic leukaemia (CMML, discussed later in this chapter and now reclassified as a myelodysplastic/myeloproliferative neoplasm) or incorporated these cases within a larger MDS cohort. Observed monocytic abnormalities in MDS

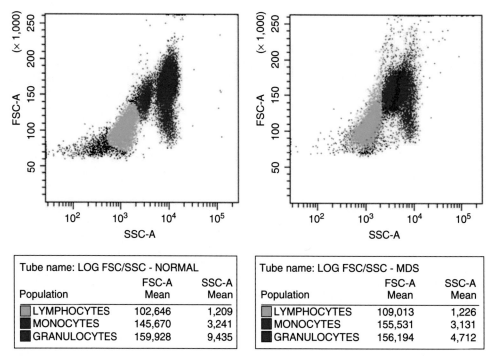

Figure 7.4a A standard FSC/SSC plot of a normal control (left) compared to a patient with confirmed MDS (right). Note how the neutrophil side scatter is shifted towards and overlaps the monocyte population. The mean side scatter value for neutrophils is significantly less than the control.

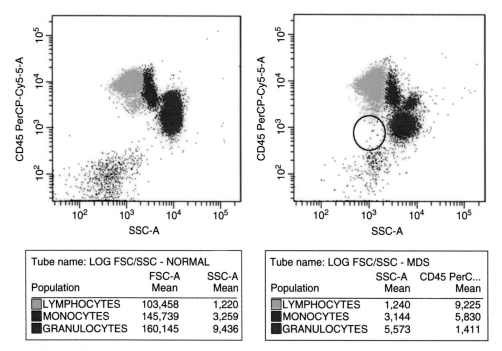

Figure 7.4b A standard CD45 versus SSC plot of the same normal control (left) and patient with confirmed MDS (right). Note how the neutrophil side scatter is shifted left, how the plot identifies two neutrophil populations on the basis of CD45 intensity and how a few events appear in the blast gate (circled) in the patient but not the control.

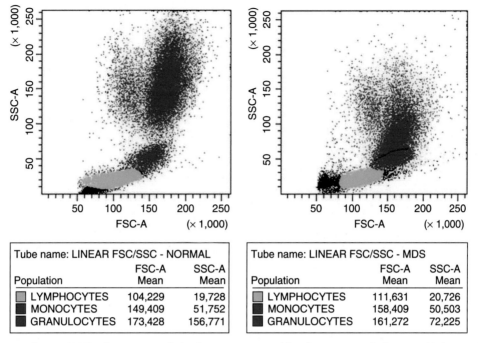

Tube name: LINEAR FSC/SSC - NORMAL		
Population	FSC-A Mean	SSC-A Mean
LYMPHOCYTES	104,229	19,728
MONOCYTES	149,409	51,752
GRANULOCYTES	173,428	156,771

Tube name: LINEAR FSC/SSC - MDS		
Population	FSC-A Mean	SSC-A Mean
LYMPHOCYTES	111,631	20,726
MONOCYTES	158,409	50,503
GRANULOCYTES	161,272	72,225

Figure 7.4c Here the same FSC/SSC plots are presented using linear, rather than logarithmic, axis scales. The reduction in neutrophil side scatter appears more convincing here, and again illustrates how this loss of granularity causes encroachment onto the monocyte zone.

Neutrophils and monocytes are clearly separated in the control sample. It is also possible to calculate a ratio of neutrophil to lymphocyte mean SSC using this approach. The MDS patient ratio is 3.48 compared to 7.94 for the control.

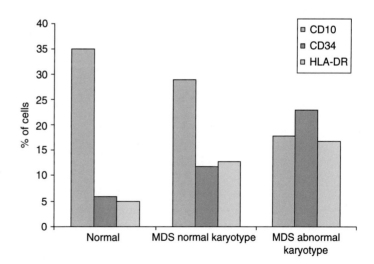

Figure 7.5 Proportion of maturing myeloid cells (including neutrophils) exhibiting aberrant precursor cell antigen expression and loss of CD10. Adapted from [36].

include the asynchronous persistence of CD34 (usually dim) into the mature cell compartment and the presence of aberrant CD56 expression (present in 17% of cases in one study [21]). In two small studies the latter abnormality was significantly more common in the monocytes of

CMML as compared to those analysed from MDS cases [38, 40]. The intensity of any CD56 expression should also be considered; it has been suggested that an intensity of >1 log should be considered as aberrant [21]. Aberrant expression of CD2, CD7 and CD19 on dysplastic mono-

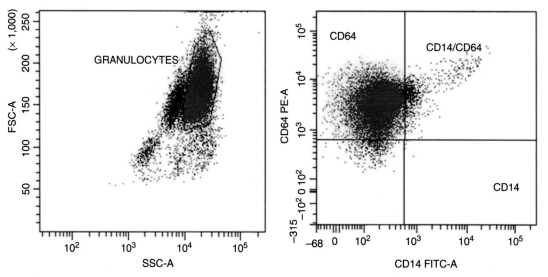

Figure 7.6 Note on the FSC versus SSC plot (left) how the neutrophils again merge with monocytes in this peripheral blood analysis. With neutrophils gated and analysed on a CD14/CD64 plot (right) it is clear that a large proportion of granulocytes are expressing CD64 (an immature myeloid/monocyte antigen) in an aberrant fashion. The gate appears to be contaminated with a few monocytes as indicated by the small dual CD14+/CD64+ population.

cytes is also reported. Further abnormalities are discussed in the CMML section.

Other abnormalities in myelodysplastic syndromes

Detection of paroxysmal nocturnal hemoglobinuria clones in myelodysplastic syndromes

Using high sensitivity flow cytometry, small subclinical PNH clones are not uncommonly detected in MDS patients (<10% of cases, with granulocyte clone sizes <1%) [41]. An ongoing large survey of many thousands of patients in the USA has detected larger clones (median of 16%) in a small proportion of patients (approximately 1%), although again these are not clinically apparent [42]. It has been observed in a number of studies that PNH clones are most frequently found in cases classified as refractory anaemia or other low-blast cell count subtypes [41, 43, 44]. While the clinical utility of detecting small clones remains unclear (although it is possible that it may predict for a response to immuno-suppressive therapy [43]) they provide diagnostic support for a marrow failure syndrome. Their presence raises intriguing questions with regards to the relationship between some cases of apparent MDS and other marrow failure syndromes such as aplastic anaemia [41].

Reduction in B-cell progenitors in myelodysplastic syndromes

A frequent observation is the apparent reduction in marrow B-cell progenitors in MDS patients, although this is not specific to MDS as it is seen in normal elderly marrows and possibly CML [9]. While CD34+ myeloblasts are increased in number in many MDS cases, CD34+ CD19+ B progenitors appear to decrease (<5% was a discriminatory level from control cases in one study [20]).

Conclusions

The introduction of routine flow cytometry in MDS presents considerable challenges, in particular with regards the development of a standardized, reproducible and cost-effective approach. A common theme of many studies is that multiple flow cytometric abnormalities are easily identified in the most dysplastic cases; in other words it is most useful in the cases where the diagnosis is readily apparent using conventional morphology and cytogenetics. Flow could aid the diagnostic process by identifying borderline cases as MDS and refining prognostic scores. The introduction of a scoring system using a limited number of the most discriminatory flow cytometry parameters seems an attractive, but also achievable goal.

Myelodysplastic/myeloproliferative neoplasms

These disorders (abbreviated to MDS/MPN) are characterized by variable degrees of simultaneous ineffective haematopoiesis (most often anaemia) and myeloproliferation (most often a leucocytosis). They comprise CMML, atypical CML (*BCR-ABL* negative), juvenile myelomonocytic leukaemia (JMML), MDS/MPN unclassifiable and the provisional entity refractory anaemia with ring sideroblasts and thrombocytosis (RARS-T) [4]. Outside of its use in CMML and in AML arising from MDS/MPN, flow is not routinely applied in these disorders, which are defined by morphological and molecular criteria.

Chronic myelomonocytic leukaemia

The hallmarks of chronic myelomonocytic leukaemia (CMML) are a peripheral monocytosis $>1 \times 10^9/l$, $<20\%$ bone marrow blasts and the presence of dysplasia in at least one lineage. The percentage of blasts in the marrow allows it to be subdivided into CMML-1 ($<10\%$ blasts) or CMML-2 (11–20%) [4]. On balance, the disease shares more clinical and biological features with MDS (within which it used to be sub-categorized) than with the MPNs. Because of this, reliable incidence data do not exist, as CMML is usually grouped into studies of MDS. One study described CMML as comprising 31% of MDS, where the incidence of the latter was 12.8 cases per 100,000 individuals per year [45].

Clinical features

CMML generally confers a poor prognosis, with a median age at presentation of >65 years. Approximately 20% of CMML will transform to AML, and median survival is approximately 20 months [46]. In addition to the leukaemic presentation some patients develop extramedullary disease, splenomegaly and lymphadenopathy. Many patients presenting with apparent CMML may pose a diagnostic dilemma; for example the common presenting features of cachexia, serous effusions, sweats and raised inflammatory markers can mimic a host of other neoplastic and non-neoplastic conditions. In addition, we have experienced a series of patients with serious haemorrhagic complications (including subdural haematoma) which appear disproportionate to the degree of thrombocytopenia. This may relate to the acquired platelet dysfunction which has been described in this condition [47].

Box. 7.1 The Dusseldorf Prognostic Score for myelodysplastic syndromes.

In this score, one point is allocated to each of the following four parameters:

Bone marrow blasts ≥5%
LDH >200 U/L
Hb ≤9 g/dL
Platelet count ≤100×10⁹/l

Group, score	Survival at 2 years, % p <0.00005	Progression to AML at 2 years, %p <0.05
A, 0	91	0
B, 1 or 2	52	19
C, 3 or 4	9	54

In the original IPSS score for MDS cases with a WCC >12×10⁹/L were excluded from analysis [3]. For proliferative CMML the authors' practice is therefore to use an alternative prognostic score, such as the one proposed by the Dusseldorf Registry derived from a series of 235 untreated patients with primary MDS (including 25 with CMML) The inclusion of LDH may improve assessment of patients with CMML, whose prognosis is viewed too favourably when rated by other scores. The requirement for a specific and discriminatory prognostic score for CMML persists. LDH, lactate dehydrogenase; Hb, haemoglobin.

Source: Malcovati et al. [7].

It has often been divided into 'proliferative' and 'non-proliferative' disease, using an arbitrary WCC cut-off of $13 \times 10^9/L$ [48]. Determination of prognosis in CMML is further complicated by such subdivisions (Box 7.1).

It is important to emphasize that cases exhibiting a leucocytosis manifest both a monocytosis and a neutrophilia (incorporating occasional neutrophil precursor cells), with significant dysgranulopoiesis present in most cases [4]. This often manifests with hypogranularity, but abnormal neutrophil segmentation patterns are common. Peripheral blood monocytes are morphologically abnormal, also showing aberrancies in nuclear shape with loss of vacuoles (Figure 7.7). These abnormalities can generate an indeterminate morphology such that CMML monocytes can often be difficult to differentiate from hypogranular myelocytes, so making bone marrow differential counts difficult (Figure 7.8).

Flow cytometry

A thorough examination of blood and marrow material is required to adequately differentiate neoplastic from reactive myeloid and monocytic proliferations. Considerable

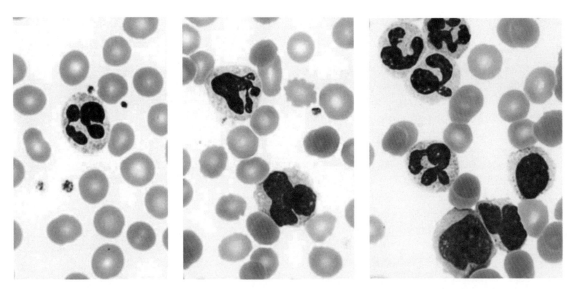

Figure 7.7 A typical blood picture in CMML, showing prominent dysplastic neutrophils, an abnormal monocyte (centre) and an occasional myeloblast (right).

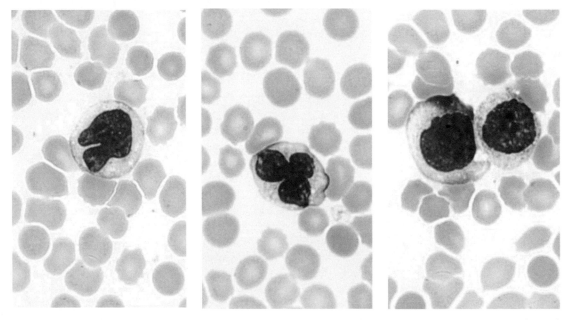

Figure 7.8 Abnormal monocyte morphology in CMML. Cells here are showing abnormal nuclear shape, segmentation and loss of normal vacuolation. Note also in the right hand image how the abnormal monocyte (left) closely resembles the hypogranular myelocyte (right).

difficulty can arise in trying to differentiate between dysplastic, hypogranular myeloid cells and monocytes. Interestingly it is often the granulocytic hyperplasia that is most striking on marrow examination of these cases, with monocytic proliferation being more difficult to appreciate on microscopy alone. In addition, discriminating between the varying morphological stages of monocyte maturation is subject to significant inter-observer variability. Flow cytometry provides useful information in CMML; a sound appreciation of the normal promonocyte and monocyte phenotype is required and an introduction to this has already been given in Chapter 4.

Promonocytes (a comparatively rare component of normal bone marrow) lack CD34, express minimal CD117 and (importantly) exhibit low to absent CD14(15). In addition, they express low levels of CD13, and intermediate levels of CD15 and CD36. Promonocytes are therefore distinguishable from mature forms by their uniformly high expression of HLA-DR, lower CD13 and CD36, higher CD15, and low to absent CD14. Choice of antibody may affect the detection of CD14 in these immature populations, and this is discussed further below. CD64 is a useful monocyte-lineage marker, being expressed at high levels throughout monocytic maturation (while bearing in mind that promyelocytes and myelocytes also express CD64 and that it is found on activated neutrophils during inflammation and sepsis [49]).

The role of flow cytometry in CMML is an important one, and the key points with regards its diagnostic utility are listed below:

1 Detection of an increased proportion of marrow monocytes in CMML. While this may be self- evident they are often difficult to enumerate accurately by morphology alone and ICC can be insensitive in this regard (e.g. staining with CD68 [4]). In one study, enumeration by flow demonstrated a mean of 7.5% monocytes in reactive marrows with a mean of 18% in CMML cases (as a proportion of total nucleated cells analysed) [50]. Normal bone marrow has a median of 3.5% monocytes [51].

2 Demonstration of antigen loss as compared to normal and reactive monocytes. The typical normal monocyte immunophenotype is CD4, CD13, CD14, CD15, CD33, CD36, CD38, CD45, CD64, and HLA-DR+. Reduced expression of CD14 is noted in CMML, with a significantly increased proportion of immature CD14 dim/moderate monocytes than may be seen in reactive cases (over 20% versus 10% respectively [50]). HLA-DR exhibits reduced expression in approximately 50% of cases and occasional cases show reduced CD13, CD15 and CD36 [50].

3 Demonstration of aberrant antigen expression. Several groups have confirmed aberrant CD56 expression on the monocytes of CMML, detectable in at least 80% of cases [21, 40, 52]. It is notable that while some abnormalities of antigen expression are detectable only in the marrow of MDS cases (including CMML), CD56 expression can also be detected on peripheral blood monocytes, making it a potentially useful 'first-pass' test for separation of reac-

tive and neoplastic monocytosis on an initial blood sample [37]. Other less frequent aberrant antigens include CD2 in 10–20% of cases [50, 52] and (very rarely) CD7 [52].

4 Differentiation of CMML from acute monoblastic/monocytic leukaemia (AMoL). This can occasionally give some pause for thought; however, careful morphological and flow cytometric assessment as well as knowledge of the clinical course should avoid difficulties. In CMML, monocytes are generally of a mature appearance, with the presence of ≥20% blasts/promonocytes indicating that the diagnosis is AML. In contrast, in acute monoblastic leukaemia ≥80% of marrow cells are typically of monoblastic appearance, while in acute monocytic leukaemia they are mainly promonocytes [4]. Both AMoL and CMML commonly express aberrant CD56, with CMML apparently more likely to express CD2 and on very rare occasions CD7 [52]. Blasts are increased in AMoL by flow (as defined by CD45dim SSClow parameters) as compared with CMML (18% versus 4% respectively) and there is a striking reduction in granulocytic cells in AMoL (26% versus 52% respectively) [52]. Surprisingly, there were no differences noted in CD14 expression between AMoL and CMML in this study, indicating that this marker does not always distinguish reliably between the chronic monocytosis of CMML and the more acute monoblastosis of AMoL. This is surprising given the immunophenotype of promonocytes (namely CD64 bright, HLA-DR bright and CD14 low or absent [16]) and is possibly due to the CD14 epitope specificity of the antibody used: the MO2 epitope is absent on promonocytes (but present on monocytes) and allows a distinction to be drawn between immature and mature cells [53]. Transforming CMML, usually into an AML of monocytic or myelomonocytic lineage, may well exhibit some features of both disorders. Finally, the presence of an 11q23 cytogenetic abnormality suggests AMoL, as these are rare in CMML [4].

Thus, while CMML remains predominantly a morphological diagnosis, flow cytometry offers very valuable supportive evidence in the majority of cases and should be offered routinely in suspected cases.

Chronic myeloid leukaemia

Chronic phase CML is defined by typical morphological and clinical features (including a neutrophil leucocytosis, thrombocytosis, modest basophilia and eosinophilia,

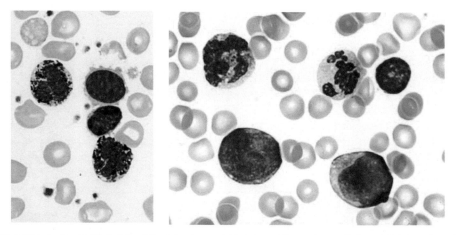

Figure 7.9 Myeloid blast crisis of CML. Peripheral blood showing myeloblasts, one with megakaryocytic features (left image), prominent abnormal basophils and a dysplastic neutrophil.

splenomegaly, night sweats and weight loss) [4]. The diagnosis is established by detection of the *BCR-ABL* translocation using conventional karyotyping, FISH and/or RT-PCR. While flow based methodology has been developed to detect this and other translocations (see Chapter 5) it seems unlikely they will replace these established techniques any time soon. Accelerated phase (AP) and blastic phase (BP) disease are typically characterized by increasing accumulations of blast cells (10–19% and ≥20% in marrow and/or blood respectively), which may also be found in extramedullary tissues. Flow has a limited role in CML, largely confined to the characterization of these blast populations. The authors' practice is to apply an acute leukaemia antibody panel when ≥5% blasts are identified morphologically in blood or marrow (or for any size of population in extramedullary locations such as CSF) (Figure 7.9).

Most cases of BP CML are of myeloid lineage (approximately 70%, including, on occasion, megakaryoblastic, eosinophilic and basophilic lineage blast transformations) with the remaining 20–30% lymphoblastic (usually of B-cell origin and only very rarely T-cell) [54]. Mixed phenotype acute leukaemia (MPAL) has also been reported. The flow characteristics of these precursor cell neoplasms are as described in Chapter 5. Note that it may be impossible to differentiate between a lymphoid blast crisis arising from undiagnosed CML and *de-novo* Ph+ALL, although genetic analysis may help (the p210 *BCR-ABL* transcript is found in the former, with the p190 being most common in the latter). Finally, focal areas of blast accumulation may be observed on trephine specimens that may not be appreciated by flow

or on aspirate smears, and appropriate ICC may be useful here; if significant focal accumulations of blast cells are detected a presumptive diagnosis of BP CML may be made.

Interesting observations in CML patients treated with tyrosine kinase inhibitors (TKI) have recently been made, detailing changes in T and NK cell populations. In a recent study the numbers of CD56+CD57+ (NK-LGL) and CD3+CD57+ (T-LGL) cells increased significantly in dasatinib treated CML patients, implicating such immunomodulatory effects in both the efficacy and toxicity of these agents [55]. Indeed, such phenomenon correlate with a good response to therapy [56], raising the intriguing prospect of utilizing flow cytometry to help predict response to these expensive treatments.

The BCR-ABL negative myeloproliferative neoplasms

These comprise polycythaemia vera, essential thrombocythaemia, primary myelofibrosis, chronic neutrophilic leukaemia and chronic eosinophilic leukaemia, as well as systemic mastocytosis. Apart from the latter (discussed separately below), flow has no routine use in the diagnosis of any of these disorders, which are defined by morphological and genetic criteria. Transformation to AML should of course be confirmed by appropriate flow cytometry; however, there is little data on the use of flow cytometry beyond this setting. A recent study used retrospective flow data to compare primary myelofibrosis

(PMF) cases with myelofibrosis secondary to MDS [57]. Interestingly, aberrant CD56 and altered CD13/CD16 expression was detected with similar frequencies in both situations; for example in PMF CD56 was found in >10% of granulocytes and monocytes in 34% and 69% of cases respectively. A reduction in granulocyte SSC was noted for both situations, although a significant reduction in neutrophil FSC seemed specific for PMF. This further emphasizes the promiscuity of CD56 and clearly indicates its lack of specificity for any particular disorder. An initial report suggesting that numbers of circulating CD34$^+$ cells (as measured by flow cytometry) was independently predictive for outcome in PMF [58] has not been supported by subsequent studies [59].

Mastocytosis

Mast cells develop from multipotent haematopoietic cells in the marrow [60]. Despite their morphological similarities to basophils they develop separately and are both immunophenotypically and functionally distinct. Unlike most other marrow-derived cells, mature mast cells do not circulate but are instead found fixed in a variety of tissues. Similarly, mastocytosis (the umbrella term applied to the clonal disorders of mast cell lineage), generally involves tissue-based accumulations of neoplastic mast cells, with only the rare and aggressive forms (specifically mast cell leukaemia) demonstrating significant numbers of circulating cells. The diagnostic process therefore relies heavily on histopathology, appropriate ICC and detection of activating mutations of *c-KIT* (present in >95% of patients with SM). Bone marrow flow cytometry does, however, have an important role to play, as the aberrant immunophenotype of clonal mast cells is now well described and in systemic disease the marrow is always involved. A detailed description of the rather complex subclassification of mastocytosis (summarized in Table 7.4) is beyond the scope of this book, as is the hugely variable clinical presentation comprising symptoms from both mast cell mediator release and direct tissue infiltration. Interpreting symptoms and signs and embarking on the correct diagnostic pathway is a challenge and clinical suspicion is important in directing appropriate flow cytometry and molecular studies.

Normal marrow mast cells express CD45, CD117, CD33, CD9 and CD68 (and notably lack CD14, CD15 and

Table 7.4 The classification of mastocytosis (WHO 2008 criteria). This table lists the main WHO-defined subtypes of mastocytosis. The clinical behaviour of these disorders varies hugely, ranging from minor skin lesions to aggressive, fulminant malignancies that involve multiple extramedullary sites and blood. Flow cytometry is of particular value in subtypes 2–5 where marrow involvement is expected. This ranges from <1% of total marrow nucleated cells in ISM to >20% in MCL [4].

1 Cutaneous mastocytosis (CM)
2 Indolent systemic mastocytosis (ISM)
3 Systemic mastocytosis with associated clonal haematological non-mast cell lineage disease (SM-AHNMD)
4 Aggressive systemic mastocytosis (ASM)
5 Mast cell leukaemia (MCL)
6 Mast cell sarcoma (MCS)
7 Extracutaneous mastocyoma

Adapted from Swerdlow et al. [4], with permission from Wiley.

Table 7.5 Immunophenotypic profiles of normal and neoplastic mast cells in comparison to basophils. This table illustrates the different expression profiles of key antigens for differentiating neoplastic mast cells from normal marrow equivalents and basophils. CD2/CD25/CD117 is a useful panel in this regard; note that CD2 is less likely to be expressed in aggressive disease (in particular in MCL), whereas CD30 exhibits precisely the opposite pattern, with very weak expression in ISM and strong expression on ASM and MCL. Data summarized from [60, 61]. MC, mast cells.

	Normal MCs	Neoplastic MCs	Basophils
Tryptase	+	+	–/+
CD2	–	+/– to ++	–
CD25	–	+	+
CD30	–	+/– to ++	–
CD117	+	+	–
CD123	–	–	+

CD16) [4]. Note that CD117 may also be detected on myeloid progenitor cells, including basophil precursors. The most common aberrantly expressed antigens in SM are the lymphoid antigens CD2 and CD25, with the latter considered the most sensitive marker for neoplastic mast cells [60]. Immunocytochemistry also reliably detects these antigens. CD30 has recently been described on the surface of cells from ASM and MCL, and it is therefore important to consider these disorders in the differential diagnosis of CD30$^+$ malignancies [531]. These antigen patterns are summarized in Table 7.5. Detection of abnormal mast cells

WORKED EXAMPLE 7.1

A 48-year-old lady was referred for investigation after she was noted to have an abnormal bone marrow signal in an MRI scan of the spine performed because of apparent osteoporosis. She had been attending dermatology for two years with a rash characterized as telangiectasia eruptive macularis perstans (TEMP). She was noted to have a mild normocytic anaemia. A bone marrow aspirate was analysed morphologically and flow cytometry studies were performed. The bone marrow particles were hypercellular and showed a dense population of mast cells trapped within (upper images). Very few mast cells appeared in the smear trails but some clusters are shown in the lower two images.

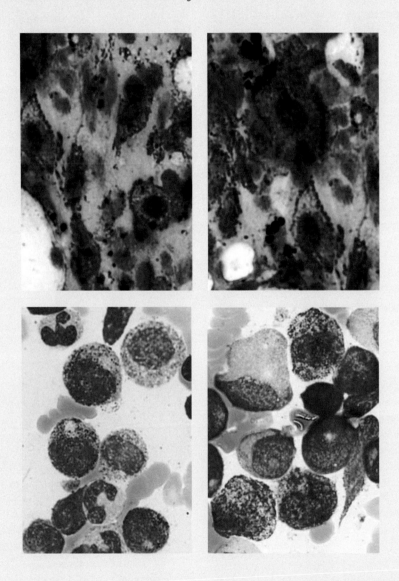

Immunophenotyping studies using a CD117 versus SSC gate identified an aberrant mast cell population demonstrating dual expression of CD2 and CD25.

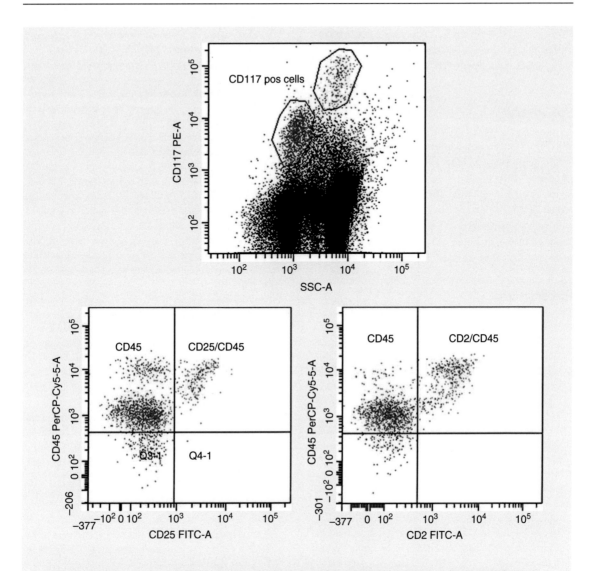

Note the separate populations of CD117 positive cells. The blue population largely represents immature myeloid cells which are CD45dim. The aberrant mast cells (red events) are CD45+ but clearly express CD2 and CD25. The diagnosis was systemic mastocytosis. TEMP is a recognized form of urticaria pigmentosa.

in the marrow can, however, be a challenge for several reasons. First, the disease is often focally distributed and marrow sampling may not be representative. Second, associated reticulin fibrosis may make marrow aspiration difficult. Third, mast cells are most commonly seen in and around aspirate particles and cells outwith these cellular areas are seen to be friable and often disrupted on marrow smears and squashes; cytometry of dilute marrow specimens may

therefore return a low yield of mast cells. In view of this, detection of even a very small population of aberrant mast cells may well be significant; indeed neoplastic marrow mast cells in ISM usually comprise <1% of all nucleated cells. Finally, in the unusual condition SM-AHNMD (where SM co-exists with another non-mast cell lineage haematological disorder, most frequently CMML) the mast cell population may be inadvertently overlooked in favour of the other disorder. Careful correlation between histopathology, cytology, ICC and flow cytometry is required in these cases for proper classification.

Summary

We have illustrated some of the many potential applications of flow cytometry in the diagnosis, classification and prognosis of the myelodysplastic syndromes and myeloproliferative neoplasms. This is an interesting and evolving field. The integration of immunophenotypic data with clinical, cytogenetic and molecular characteristics is likely to further increase our understanding of these diseases and so influence management in the future.

References

1 Paydas S, Zorludemir S, Ergin M. Granulocytic sarcoma: 32 cases and review of the literature. *Leuk Lymphoma* 2006, **47**(12): 2527–41.

2 Sato N, Nakazato T, Kizaki M, Ikeda Y, Okamoto S. Transformation of myelodysplastic syndrome to acute lymphoblastic leukemia: a case report and review of the literature. *Int J Hematol* 2004, **79**(2): 147–51.

3 Greenberg P, Cox C, LeBeau MM, *et al.* International scoring system for evaluating prognosis in myelodysplastic syndromes. *Blood* 1997, **89**(6): 2079–88.

4 Swerdlow SH, Campo E, Harris NL., *et al.* WHO Classification of Tumours of Haematopoietic and Lymphoid Tissues, 4th edn. 2008. *Lyon*, France: IARC Press.

5 Valent P, Horny HP, Bennett JM, *et al.* Definitions and standards in the diagnosis and treatment of the myelodysplastic syndromes: Consensus statements and report from a working conference. *Leuk Res* 2007, **31**(6): 727–36.

6 Wimazal F, Fonatsch C, Thalhammer R, *et al.* Idiopathic cytopenia of undetermined significance (ICUS) versus low risk MDS: The diagnostic interface. *Leuk Res* 2007, **31**(11): 1461–8.

7 Malcovati L, Germing U, Kuendgen A, *et al.* Time-dependent prognostic scoring system for predicting survival and leukemic evolution in myelodysplastic syndromes. *J Clin Oncol* 2007, **25**(23): 3503–10.

8 Elghetany MT, Davis BH. Impact of preanalytical variables on granulocytic surface antigen expression: a review. *Cytometry B Clin Cytom* 2005, **65**(1): 1–5.

9 van de Loosdrecht AA, Alhan C, Bene MC, *et al.* Standardization of flow cytometry in myelodysplastic syndromes: report from the first European LeukemiaNet working conference on flow cytometry in myelodysplastic syndromes. *Haematologica* 2009, **94**(8): 1124–34.

10 Ortolani C. *Flow Cytometry Of Hematological Malignancies.* 2001. Oxford: Wiley-Blackwell.

11 Stachurski D, Smith BR, Pozdnyakova O, *et al.* Flow cytometric analysis of myelomonocytic cells by a pattern recognition approach is sensitive and specific in diagnosing myelodysplastic syndrome and related marrow diseases: emphasis on a global evaluation and recognition of diagnostic pitfalls. *Leuk Res* 2008, **32**(2): 215–24.

12 de Haas M, Kleijer M, van Zwieten R, Roos D, von dem Borne AE. Neutrophil Fc gamma RIIIb deficiency, nature, and clinical consequences: a study of 21 individuals from 14 families. *Blood* 1995, **86**(6): 2403–13.

13 Peiper SC, Ashmun RA, Look AT. Molecular cloning, expression, and chromosomal localization of a human gene encoding the CD33 myeloid differentiation antigen. *Blood* 1988, **72**(1): 314–21.

14 Kwong YL, Lee CP, Chan TK, Chan LC. Flow cytometric measurement of glycosylphosphatidyl-inositol-linked surface proteins on blood cells of patients with paroxysmal nocturnal hemoglobinuria. *Am J Clin Pathol* 1994, **102**(1): 30–5.

15 Ogata K, Nakamura K, Yokose N, *et al.* Clinical significance of phenotypic features of blasts in patients with myelodysplastic syndrome. *Blood* 2002, **100**(12): 3887–96.

16 Monreal MB, Pardo ML, Pavlovsky MA, *et al.* Increased immature hematopoietic progenitor cells CD34+/CD38dim in myelodysplasia. *Cytometry B Clin Cytom* 2006, **70**(2): 63–70.

17 Font P, Subira D, Mtnez-Chamorro C, *et al.* Evaluation of CD7 and terminal deoxynucleotidyl transferase (TdT) expression in CD34+ myeloblasts from patients with myelodysplastic syndrome. *Leuk Res* 2006, **30**(8): 957–63.

18 Ogata K, Kishikawa Y, Satoh C, Tamura H, Dan K, Hayashi A. Diagnostic application of flow cytometric characteristics of CD34+ cells in low-grade myelodysplastic syndromes. *Blood* 2006, **108**(3): 1037–44.

19 Xu F, Li X, Wu L, He Q, Zhang Z, Chang C. Flow cytometric scoring system (FCMSS) assisted diagnosis of myelodysplastic syndromes (MDS) and the biological significance of FCMSS-based immunophenotypes. *Br J Haematol* 2010, **149**(4): 587–97.

20 Ogata K, Della Porta MG, Malcovati L, *et al.* Diagnostic utility of flow cytometry in low-grade myelodysplastic syndromes: a prospective validation study. *Haematologic* 2009, **94**(8): 1066–74.

21 Wells DA, Benesch M, Loken MR, *et al.* Myeloid and monocytic dyspoiesis as determined by flow cytometric scoring in myelodysplastic syndrome correlates with the IPSS and with outcome after hematopoietic stem cell transplantation. *Blood* 2003, **102**(1): 394–403.

22 Oertel J, Huhn D. CD34 immunophenotyping of blasts in myelodysplasia. *Leuk Lymphoma* 1994, **15**(1–2): 65–9.

23 Kanter-Lewensohn L, Hellstrom-Lindberg E, Kock Y. Analysis of CD34-positive cells in bone marrow from patients with myelodysplastic syndromes and acute myeloid leukemia and in normal individuals: a comparison between FACS analysis and immunohistochemistry. *Eur J Haematol* 1996, **56**(3): 124–9.

24 Ramos F, Fernandez-Ferrero S, Suarez D, *et al*. Myelodysplastic syndrome: a search for minimal diagnostic criteria. *Leuk Res* 1999, **23**(3): 283–90.

25 Levis A, Gioia DM, Godio L, *et al*. *Comparison Among Cytology, Histology, and Flow Cytometry in Evaluating Blast values in Myelodysplatic Syndromes (MDS)*. Survey from the Italian "Piedmonte MDS Registry". ASH Annual Meeting Abstracts. 2010, **116**(21): 4028.

26 Knipp S, Strupp C, Gattermann N, *et al*. Presence of peripheral blasts in refractory anemia and refractory cytopenia with multilineage dysplasia predicts an unfavourable outcome. *Leuk Res* 2008, **32**(1): 33–7.

27 Cesana C, Klersy C, Brando B, *et al*. Prognostic value of circulating CD34[+] cells in myelodysplastic syndromes. *Leuk Res* 2008, **32**(11): 1715–23.

28 Matsui WH, Brodsky RA, Smith BD, Borowitz MJ, Jones RJ.Quantitative analysis of bone marrow CD34 cells in aplastic anemia and hypoplastic myelodysplastic syndromes. *Leukaemia* 2006, **20**: 458–62.

29 Malcovati L, Della Porta MG, Lunghi M, *et al*. Flow cytometry evaluation of erythroid and myeloid dysplasia in patients with myelodysplastic syndrome. *Leukemia* 2005, **19**(5): 776–83.

30 Della Porta MG, Malcovati L, Invernizzi R, *et al*. Flow cytometry evaluation of erythroid dysplasia in patients with myelodysplastic syndrome. *Leukemia* 2006, **20**(4): 549–55.

31 Stetler-Stevenson M, Arthur DC, Jabbour N, *et al*. Diagnostic utility of flow cytometric immunophenotyping in myelodysplastic syndrome. *Blood* 2001, **98**(4): 979–87.

32 Bianco T, Farmer BJ, Sage RE, Dobrovic A. Loss of red cell A, B, and H antigens is frequent in myeloid malignancies. *Blood* 2001, **97**(11): 3633–9.

33 Lorand-Metze I, Ribeiro E, Lima CS, Batista LS, Metze K. Detection of hematopoietic maturation abnormalities by flow cytometry in myelodysplastic syndromes and its utility for the differential diagnosis with non-clonal disorders. *Leuk Res* 2007, **31**(2): 147–55.

34 Cherian S, Moore J, Bantly A, *et al*. Flow-cytometric analysis of peripheral blood neutrophils: a simple, objective, independent and potentially clinically useful assay to facilitate the diagnosis of myelodysplastic syndromes. *Am J Hematol* 2005, **79**(3): 243–5.

35 Cherian S, Moore J, Bantly A, *et al*. Peripheral blood MDS score: a new flow cytometric tool for the diagnosis of myelodysplastic syndromes.*Am J Hematol* 2005, **64**(1): 9–17.

36 Xu D, Schultz C, Akker Y, *et al*. Evidence for expression of early myeloid antigens in mature, non-blast myeloid cells in myelodysplasia. *Am J Hematol* 2003, **74**(1): 9–16.

37 Huang M, Li J, Zhao G, Sui X, Zhao X, Xu H. Immunophenotype of myeloid granulocytes: a pilot study for distinguishing myelodysplastic syndrome and aplastic anemia by flow cytometry. *Int J Lab Hematol* 2009, **32**(3): 275–81.

38 Ohsaka A, Saionji K, Igari J, Watanabe N, Iwabuchi K, Nagaoka I. Altered surface expression of effector cell molecules on neutrophils in myelodysplastic syndromes. *Br J Haematol* 1997, **98**(1): 108–13.

39 Lacronique-Gazaille C, Chaury MP, Le Guyader A, Faucher JL, Bordessoule D, Feuillard J. A simple method for detection of major phenotypic abnormalities in myelodysplastic syndromes: expression of CD56 in CMML. *Haematologica* 2007, **92**(6): 859–60.

40 Subira D, Font P, Villalon L, *et al*. Immunophenotype in chronic myelomonocytic leukemia: is it closer to myelodysplastic syndromes or to myeloproliferative disorders? *Transl Res* 2008, **151**(5): 240–5.

41 Wang SA, Pozdnyakova O, Jorgensen JL, *et al*. Detection of paroxysmal nocturnal hemoglobinuria clones in patients with myelodysplastic syndromes and related bone marrow diseases, with emphasis on diagnostic pitfalls and caveats. *Haematologica* 2009, **94**(1): 29–37.

42 Galili N, Ravandi F, Palermo G, *et al*. Prevalence of paroxysmal nocturnal hemoglobinuria (PNH) cells in patients with myelodysplastic syndromes (MDS), aplastic anemia (AA), or other bone marrow failure (BMF) syndromes: Interim results from the EXPLORE trial. *Journal of Clinical Oncology* 2009, **27**(15 s): 7082.

43 Nakao S, Sugimori C, Yamazaki H. Clinical significance of a small population of paroxysmal nocturnal hemoglobinuria-type cells in the management of bone marrow failure. *Int J Hematol* 2006, **84**(2): 118–22.

44 Wang H, Chuhjo T, Yasue S, Omine M, Nakao S. Clinical significance of a minor population of paroxysmal nocturnal hemoglobinuria-type cells in bone marrow failure syndrome. *Blood* 2002, **100**(12): 3897–902.

45 Williamson PJ, Kruger AR, Reynolds PJ, Hamblin TJ, Oscier DG. Establishing the incidence of myelodysplastic syndrome. *Br J Haematol* 1994, **87**(4): 743–5.

46 Germing U, Kundgen A, Gattermann N. Risk assessment in chronic myelomonocytic leukemia (CMML). *Leuk Lymphoma* 2004, **45**(7): 1311–8.

47 Manoharan A, Brighton T, Gemmell R, Lopez K, Moran S, Kyle P. Platelet dysfunction in myelodysplastic syndromes:

a clinicopathological study. *Int J Hematol* 2002, **76**(3): 272–8.

48 Bennett JM, Catovsky D, Daniel MT, *et al.* The chronic myeloid leukaemias: guidelines for distinguishing chronic granulocytic, atypical chronic myeloid, and chronic myelomonocytic leukaemia. Proposals by the French-American-British Cooperative Leukaemia Group. *Br J Haematol* 1994, **87**(4): 746–54.

49 Wood BL. Myeloid malignancies: myelodysplastic syndromes, myeloproliferative disorders, and acute myeloid leukemia. *Clin Lab Med* 2007, **27**(3): 551–75, vii.

50 Xu Y, McKenna RW, Karandikar NJ, Pildain AJ, Kroft SH. Flow cytometric analysis of monocytes as a tool for distinguishing chronic myelomonocytic leukemia from reactive monocytosis. *Am J Clin Pathol* 2005, **124**(5): 799–806.

51 Brooimans R A, Kraan J, van Putten W, Cornelissen J J, Lowenberg B, Gratama JW. Flow cytometric differential of leukocyte populations in normal bone marrow: Influence of peripheral blood contamination. *Cytometry B Clin Cytom* 2008, **76B**(1): 18–26.

52 Kern W, Bacher U, Haferlach C, Schnittger S, Haferlach T. Acute monoblastic/monocytic leukemia and chronic myelomonocytic leukemia share common immunophenotypic features but differ in the extent of aberrantly expressed antigens and amount of granulocytic cells. *Leuk Lymphoma* 2011, **52**(1): 92–100.

53 Yang DT, Greenwood JH, Hartung L, Hill S, Perkins SL, Bahler DW. Flow cytometric analysis of different CD14 epitopes can help identify immature monocytic populations. *Am J Clin Pathol* 2005, **124**(6): 930–6.

54 Silver RT. The blast phase of chronic myeloid leukaemia. *Best Pract Res Clin Haemato* 2009, **22**(3): 387–94.

55 Hayashi Y, Nakamae H, Katayama T, *et al.* Different immunoprofiles in patients with chronic myeloid leukemia treated with imatinib, nilotinib or dasatinib. *Leuk Lymphoma* 2012, **53**(6): 1084–9.

56 Mustjoki S, Ekblom M, Arstila TP, *et al.* Clonal expansion of T/NK-cells during tyrosine kinase inhibitor dasatinib therapy. *Leukemia* 2009, **23**(8): 1398–405.

57 Feng B, Verstovsek S, Jorgensen JL, Lin P. Aberrant myeloid maturation identified by flow cytometry in primary myelofibrosis. *American Journal of Clinical Pathology* 2010, **133**(2): 314–20.

58 Barosi G, Viarengo G, Pecci A, *et al.* Diagnostic and clinical relevance of the number of circulating CD34($^+$) cells in myelofibrosis with myeloid metaplasia. *Blood* 2001, **98**(12): 3249–55.

59 Arora B, Sirhan S, Hoyer JD, Mesa RA, Tefferi A. Peripheral blood CD34 count in myelofibrosis with myeloid metaplasia: a prospective evaluation of prognostic value in 94 patients. *Br J Haematol* 2005, **128**(1): 42–8.

60 Valent P, Cerny-Reiterer S, Herrmann H, *et aln* Phenotypic heterogeneity, novel diagnostic markers, and target expression profiles in normal and neoplastic human mast cells. *Best Pract Res Clin Haematol* 2010, **23**(3): 369–78.

61 Valent P, Sotlar K, Horny HP. Aberrant expression of CD30 in aggressive systemic mastocytosis and mast cell leukemia: a differential diagnosis to consider in aggressive hematopoietic CD30-positive neoplasms. *Leuk Lymphoma* 2011, **52**(5): 740–4.

CHAPTER 8
Disorders of Plasma Cells

Plasma cells are terminally differentiated activated B-cells, which have the ability to produce antibodies against a variety of antigens. These antigens may have been encountered during immunological development (through experience of self and non-self) or exposure to potential and actual pathogens. On re-exposure, plasmablasts and plasma cells are activated and undergo clonal expansion. The antibodies produced are capable of opsonization, whilst cell lysis is mediated through complement or T-cell mediated cytotoxicity.

Plasma cells, like many other important cellular components of the immune system, are susceptible to the development of disordered replication and malignant change. Once a clonal plasma cell population is established it has the potential to behave in a number of different ways: this is translated into the clinically diverse plasma cell disorders which we encounter in everyday practice. Some of these need treatment, but importantly, some do not.

In this chapter we will look at aspects of flow cytometry which can be helpful in plasma cell disorders: in terms of diagnosis, differentiation of plasma cell dyscrasias from lymphoma, determining risk of progression from benign paraproteinaemia, assessing disease prognosis and in monitoring disease response to treatment.

long before any relevant clinical symptoms develop. Notably, a number of lymphoproliferative disorders can also generate paraproteins, so the distinction between the two in clinical and pathological terms is clearly important. A monoclonal gammopathy is defined as any situation in which a clonal paraprotein is present in blood or urine and is indicative of a clonal lymphoid or plasma cell proliferation. Purely reactive proliferations often generate a polyclonal immunoglobulin response, but should not, by definition, generate a paraprotein. The monoclonal gammopathies, in the presence of a clonal plasma cell proliferation can be subdivided into the following possible entities:
- Monoclonal gammopathy of uncertain significance (MGUS)
- Multiple myeloma (MM)
- Isolated plasmacytoma
- Plasma cell leukaemia (PCL)
- Primary amyloidosis
- Immunoglobulin heavy chain and light chain diseases

Flow cytometry studies performed with knowledge of the clinical presentation and background are essential in identifying clonal versus reactive plasma cell proliferations and discriminating them from B-lymphoid lymphoproliferative disorders.

Plasma cell disorders

Polyclonal normal plasma cells generate a spectrum of antibodies according to various heavy chain derivations, IgG, IgA, IgM, IgD and IgE, with a mix of kappa and lambda light chain utilization. A common early finding in plasma cell disorders is the presence of an excess of a heavy and light chain restricted monoclonal serum antibody (a paraprotein, or M protein) which may often be apparent

Current diagnostic criteria

See Table 8.1.

Monoclonal gammopathy of undetermined significance

This is the most common plasma cell disorder. Its incidence rises rapidly with age and affects 3% of the population older than 50 years and 10% of the population

Practical Flow Cytometry in Haematology Diagnosis, First Edition. Mike Leach, Mark Drummond and Allyson Doig.
© 2013 John Wiley & Sons, Ltd. Published 2013 by John Wiley & Sons, Ltd.

Feature	MGUS	Plasma cytoma	Multiple myeloma	PCL	Primary amyloid
Immune paresis	Yes/no	No	Yes	Yes	Yes/no
Hypercalcaemia	No	No	Yes	Yes	No
Renal failure	No	No	Yes	Yes	Yes
Anaemia	No	No	Yes	Yes	Yes/no
Bone lesions	No	Yes, focal	Yes	No	No
Organomegaly	No	No	No	Yes	Yes
BM plasma cells	<10%	<3%	>10%	>10%	Variable
PB plasma cells	Rare	No	Few	Yes	No

Table 8.1 Summary of the clinical features of the plasma cell neoplasms.

older than 70 years [1]. The combination of an increasingly aged population, sensitive laboratory screening methods and frequent inappropriate testing means that these benign paraproteins are now more likely to be discovered. MGUS is characterized by the presence of an M protein in serum not exceeding 30 g/L, with fewer than 10% of plasma cells in the bone marrow [2, 3]. In addition, these patients should not show evidence of bone or end organ damage. About 1% of patients, will progress to myeloma each year, but there remains a significant diversity, in terms of risk of progression.

Smouldering myeloma

Asymptomatic or smouldering myeloma (SM) is characterized by a paraprotein of >30 g/L, with more than 10% plasma cells in bone marrow, in the absence of end organ damage or CRAB symptoms (hypercalcaemia, renal insufficiency, anaemia, bone lesions) [2]. About 10% of patients will progress to multiple myeloma every year.

Multiple myeloma

Multiple myeloma (MM) is characterized by a paraprotein of >30 g/L, greater than 10% plasma cells in bone marrow, evidence of end organ damage and CRAB symptoms [2]. This is a serious disorder that despite modern therapy, including transplant procedures, is virtually impossible to eradicate.

Plasma cell leukaemia

PCL is defined as a clonal plasma cell disorder with a peripheral blood plasma cell population of $>2 \times 10^9$/L, or >20% of circulating leucocytes [4]. It occurs most commonly as a terminal phase of MM (secondary PCL). Primary PCL is an aggressive disorder, which develops de novo; it is often implicated in hypercalcaemia, anaemia and renal failure, has a tendency to cause hepatosplenomegaly and rarely generates bone lesions. The prognosis is poor.

Plasmacytoma

A plasmacytoma is a solid plasma cell tumour which can be encountered in a variety of medullary and extramedullary sites. It often causes local symptoms due to compression of adjacent structures and can produce a paraprotein. It should not cause CRAB symptoms. It is potentially curable with radiotherapy, though some cases do progress to a systemic plasma cell disorder.

Primary amyloidosis

This is a rare plasma cell neoplasm which is categorized by a relative scarcity of bone marrow plasma cells, but with an affinity for the generation of end organ light chain derived amyloid deposition in many tissues. Renal and cardiac amyloid deposition can cause serious organ impairment and death.

It is important to note that some cases of the above clinical disorders can generate an excess of serum free light chains in isolation; such neoplasms appear unable to assemble an intact paraprotein. Furthermore MM, PCL and plasmacytomas are occasionally non-secretory so neither an intact paraprotein or serum free light chains are evident. This often leads to diagnostic confusion or delay and can generate difficulty in assessing response to treatment. The absence of a paraprotein, therefore, should not

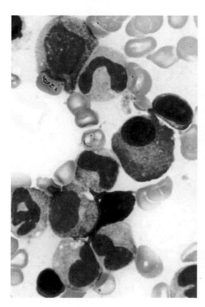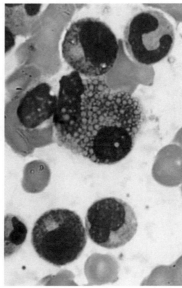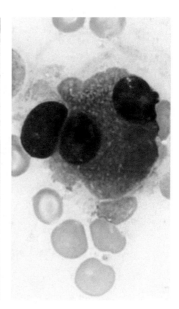

Figure 8.1 Prominent reactive marrow plasma cells, including a mott cell (centre) and binucleate cell (right).

detract from the diagnosis of a plasma cell neoplasm if other clinical and laboratory findings are suggestive.

Plasma cell morphology

It is clear, therefore, that plasma cells can be encountered in a number of neoplastic scenarios both in bone marrow and occasionally peripheral blood. It is important to note that polyclonal, reactive plasma cells are also encountered in a number of different infective, inflammatory and neoplastic conditions. We should be mindful of the fact that a frequent determinant of a raised ESR is a polyclonal increase in serum immunoglobulins with or without a reduction in serum albumin or an adjunctive increase in other high molecular weight proteins such as fibrinogen, factor VIII and von-Willebrand factor. Furthermore, in morphological terms, it can be difficult to differentiate reactive from clonal plasma cells unless plasma cells are present in gross excess, thereby making a clonal proliferation more likely. Reactive plasma cells can show remarkable morphological diversity; the presence of multinucleate, pleomorphic and atypical plasma cells is well recognized in reactive scenarios and cannot be relied upon to indicate neoplasia (Figure 8.1).

Chronic inflammatory conditions such as systemic vasculitis or rheumatoid arthritis, chronic infections like tuberculosis or osteomyelitis, and neoplastic conditions such as Hodgkin lymphoma and renal carcinoma can all generate a florid polyclonal tissue and bone marrow plasma cell response. Flow cytometry studies are very capable at discerning reactive from neoplastic plasma cell proliferations.

In multiple myeloma the plasma cells are typically medium to large ovoid cells with an eccentric nucleus and deep blue, agranular cytoplasm. There is often a perinuclear area of pallor, or hof, which corresponds to the prominent golgi apparatus (Figure 8.2). Cells with multiple nuclei are often evident (Figure 8.3).

The cytoplasmic membrane can appear irregular and fragile as some cells are disrupted by the smear preparation. In some cases the plasma cells appear to have cytoplasmic projections and some patients with IgA myeloma have atypical plasma cells with irregular cytoplasm with apparent eosinophilic inclusions, known as flame cells (Figure 8.4).

The cells seen in PCL are very variable in morphology and can differ enormously between cases (Figure 8.5). It is always important to consider PCL in the differential diagnosis in any patient presenting with atypical non-granular mononuclear cells in peripheral blood, particularly in the presence of renal failure and a monoclonal immunoglobulin. Heavy background blue plasma staining is often a clue to the presence of a substantial paraprotein. If plasma cell leukaemia is not

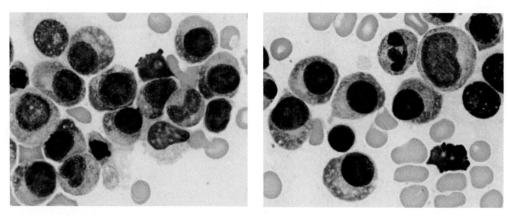

Figure 8.2 An excess of bone marrow plasma cells in multiple myeloma.

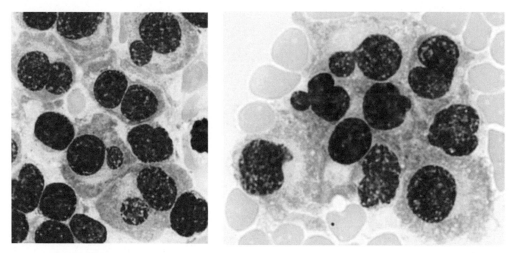

Figure 8.3 Prominent binucleate cells (left) and cells with nuclear convolutions (right).

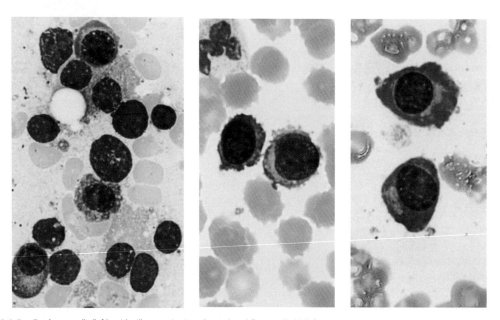

Figure 8.4 Fragile plasma cells (left), with villous projections (centre) and flame cells (right).

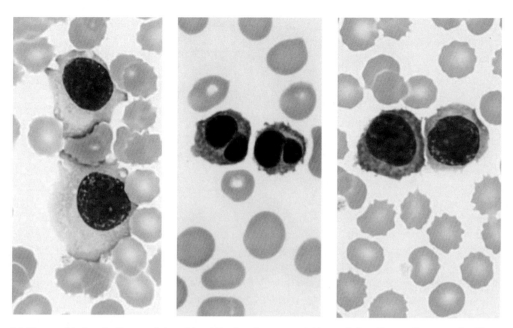

Figure 8.5 Plasma cell leukaemia. Plasma cells in peripheral blood can have very variable morphology. Illustrated here are cells with voluminous cytoplasm, cells with cleaved nuclei and cells with villous cytoplasm.

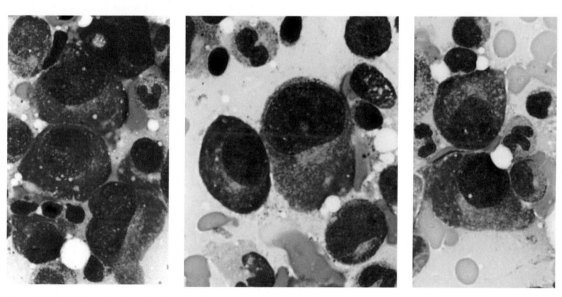

Figure 8.6 Plasmablasts in advanced refractory multiple myeloma.

considered, the diagnosis may be missed and may not be captured by an acute leukaemia or lymphoproliferative type panel of antibodies.

In the presence of disease relapse, and in particular if the malignant plasma cell clone has acquired a TP53 mutation, the plasma cell morphology may take on a further change with the appearance of large pleomorphic nucleolated cells known as plasmablasts. Their appearance often signifies a near terminal stage of disease (Figure 8.6).

The applications of immunophenotyping to plasma cell disorders

Diagnosis

Identification of neoplastic plasma cells

Normal plasma cells express $CD45^{dim}$, CD19, $CD38^{bright}$ and CD138, together with restricted *cytoplasmic* light chain expression. They do not express surface immunoglobulin. As has been discussed in previous chapters, CD38 is a promiscuous marker of cell activation and is seen in a number of other non-plasma cell disorders, including those of mature B-cells, activated T-cells, progenitor cells and haematogones. CD38 and CD138 are also expressed on neoplastic plasma cells, so positivity for these antigens is not discriminatory, but the intensity of expression does change. Generally speaking, CD38 is dimmer and CD138 brighter in malignant plasma cell populations compared to their normal counterpart. Dual staining for CD38/CD138 is a useful mechanism for identifying plasma cells and generates a well-defined gate for subsequent immunophenotypic analysis.

Neoplastic plasma cells often show CD38 and CD138 expression with a larger $CD45^-$ or $CD45^{dim}$ population, together with diminished or absent CD19 (Table 8.2). In contrast most B-cell LPD will express CD19, CD45 and CD20 to variable degree, together with surface light chain restriction. Other informative antigens not typically seen on plasma cells, for example CD5, CD23, CD11c, may also be evident in B-cell LPDs. Neoplastic plasma cells from some patients will express CD19 and/or CD20 and this has been correlated with cyclin D1 positivity (see below). Aberrant CD56 expression is found in most cases of multiple myeloma, but is often absent in plasma cell leukaemia, which may explain the affinity of such neoplasms for extranodal tissues (CD56 being a cell adhesion molecule).

Plasma cell quantification

From the classification systems described above, quantification of neoplastic plasma cells is clearly important for an accurate diagnosis (and prognosis). Flow cytometry is highly sensitive for the detection and characterization of plasma cells and has many advantages over morphological assessment, particularly in the analysis of hypocellular/dilute samples or where plasma cells constitute a low percentage of all cells in a specimen. There is good

Table 8.2 Summary of the basic immunophenotypic characteristics of normal and neoplastic plasma cells.

Antigen	Normal plasma cells	Neoplastic plasma cells
CD45	Dim	Neg
CD38	Bright	Pos
CD138	Pos	Pos
CD19	Pos	Neg
CD56	Neg	Pos/neg

correlation between flow and morphology in the assessment of bone marrow plasma cells [5], but it is important to note that morphological assessment of bone marrow plasma cell percentages is commonly higher than that determined by flow cytometry [6]. There are a number of possible reasons for this:

• Malignant plasma cells are fragile and surface membrane can be disrupted or lost during flow analysis.

• Differences in plasma cell enrichment if serial rather than single pull marrow aspirations are taken.

• Plasma cells often form clusters in bone marrow which are not freed up for single cell analysis in the cytometer.

Although morphological bone marrow plasma cell percentages are the accepted gold standard for diagnosis some studies have suggested that bone marrow plasma cell percentages as determined by flow cytometry, but not by morphology, are an independent prognostic factor for overall survival [5]. Given the caveats above, our own practice is to utilize ICC +/− ISH on marrow aspirate sections or trephine biopsies when accurate enumeration of plasma cells is required.

Differential diagnosis of myeloma from lymphoplasmacytoid lymphoma

Certain non-Hodgkin lymphomas, particularly marginal zone and lymphoplasmacytoid lymphoma, commonly show a degree of lymphoplasmacytic differentiation in association with a serum paraprotein. These conditions may cause confusion with a plasma cell dyscrasia; however, flow cytometry can reliably differentiate between them. Plasmacytoma and plasma cell myeloma cells have a $CD19^-$, $CD56^+$, $CD45^{dim/-}$ phenotype, whereas the lymphomas are normally $CD19^+$, $CD56^-$, $CD45^+$. Other important phenotypic differences are summarized in Table 8.3 (and are further discussed in Chapter 5).

WORKED EXAMPLE 8.1

A 64-year-old male presented with bone pain, lethargy, anorexia and thirst. He was found to have a normocytic anaemia, hypercalcaemia and renal failure. He had a serum paraprotein (IgG of 40 g/L) and elevated serum free light chains. A bone marrow aspirate showed a large population of pleomorphic plasma cells. Flow cytometry, which is not essential for diagnosis with such a classic presentation, generated the following profile. Plasma cells were identified using a CD138 versus SSC gate. Note the presence of CD138, CD38 and CD56, and the absence of CD19 expression. This is a typical malignant plasma cell phenotype in multiple myeloma.

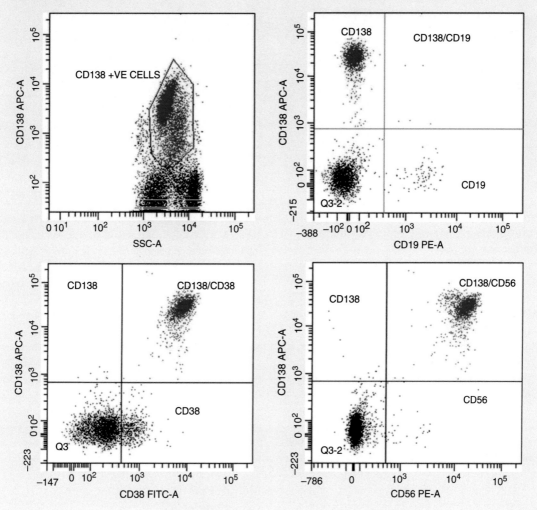

In 15–20% of multiple myeloma cases the cells express CD20 and show cyclin D1 and PAX5 expression by immunohistochemistry [7, 8]. In addition, these cases often show lymphoplasmacytoid morphology so this is a potential trap for the unwary [9].

As CD20 and PAX5 are normally lost from B-cells undergoing final plasma cell differentiation, it is likely that CD20+ myeloma has arisen from a mutation in a cell undergoing this process. There does not, however, appear to be any impact of CD20 positivity on prognosis, though there

Table 8.3 Summary of the basic immunophenotypic differences between the cells of plasmacytoid lymphomas and multiple myeloma.

Character	Plasmacytoid lymphoma	Plasma cell neoplasms
CD45	Pos	Neg
CD38	Pos/neg	Pos
CD138	Neg	Pos
CD19	Pos	Neg
CD20	Pos	Pos/neg
CD56	Neg	Pos/neg
CD23	Pos/neg	Neg
Surface Ig	Pos	Neg

Table 8.4 The risk of progression to multiple myeloma from MGUS and smouldering myeloma (SM) stratified according to the percentage of residual normal bone marrow plasma cells in each entity at the time of diagnosis.

Entity	Normal plasma cells >5%	Normal plasma cells <5%
MGUS	5%	25%
SM	8%	64%

Table 8.5 The prognostic significance of CD28 and CD117 expression in multiple myeloma.

Immunophenotype	Survival at 5 years
CD28⁻, CD117⁺	72%
CD28⁻, CD117⁻ or CD28⁺, CD117⁺	57%
CD28⁺, CD117⁻	43%

exists the potential to evaluate anti-CD20 monoclonal antibody therapy in these relatively rare disorders.

Differential diagnosis of myeloma from monoclonal gammopathy of undetermined significance

As noted above there are standard criteria to assist in the differential diagnosis of myeloma and MGUS. We have noted, though, some of the difficulties encountered in bone marrow plasma cell enumeration, whether using morphology or flow cytometry. Furthermore, the immunophenotype of the malignant plasma cell population in MGUS and myeloma is essentially the same. Another approach is to assess the proportion of residual normal plasma cells as a means of discriminating between MGUS and myeloma. Over 98% of MGUS patients have more than 3% residual normal plasma cells as a percentage of the total bone marrow plasma cell compartment. In symptomatic myeloma only a minority of myeloma patients have any residual normal plasma cells. Finally the proportion of residual normal plasma cells in MGUS is also prognostically important in terms of risk of progression (see below).

Prognosis
Monoclonal gammopathy of undetermined significance, smouldering myeloma and risk of progression

Approximately 1% of MGUS patients will progress to symptomatic myeloma each year [10] compared to 10% per year with SM [11]. A different follow-up strategy is

therefore necessary for these patients. A number of parameters are known to influence the risk of progression, including the size of the M component, the Ig isotype (IgA) and abnormal serum free light chain ratio [12]. As noted above, the proportion of polyclonal plasma cells remaining carries prognostic significance in terms of risk of progression in MGUS patients. In one study a cut-off of 5% residual normal plasma cells was most discriminatory. In the MGUS group with <5% normal plasma cells 24% of patients progressed at a median of 107 months. In the group with >5% plasma cells only 4% of patients progressed [13]. In smouldering myeloma (SM) patients a threshold of 5% normal plasma cells was also predictive; the rate of progression for cases with more or less than 5% normal plasma cells was 10% versus 63%, respectively. The risk of progression at five years in each condition is summarized in Table 8.4.

Antigenic profile of malignant plasma cells in myeloma

CD28 is an antigen normally expressed on T lymphocytes and is involved in cytokine secretion and clonal expansion. It is not expressed by normal plasma cells and is infrequently seen on malignant plasma cells of MGUS. It is frequently expressed in symptomatic myeloma and appears to correlate with disease proliferative activity, advanced stage and progression free survival [14]. CD28 expression is also associated with TP53 mutation and t(4;16).

WORKED EXAMPLE 8.2

A 55-year-old male presented with low back, rib and pelvic pain. He had a 45 g/L IgG serum paraprotein and multiple bony lucencies throughout the skeleton. A bone marrow aspirate was hypercellular. The smears showed an apparent lymphoplasmacytoid cell infiltrate that was not typical of the working diagnosis of multiple myeloma. The cells were smaller than typical plasma cells, with less cytoplasm; some resembled small mature lymphocytes.

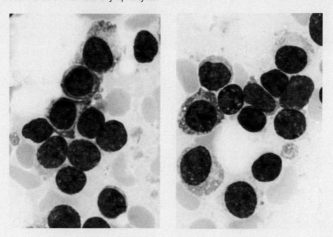

Flow cytometry studies were informative in this case. The malignant cells were gated using a CD138 versus SSC approach. The neoplastic population was CD138$^+$, CD19$^-$, CD45$^-$, but in addition showed dim CD20 positivity. This is therefore CD20 positive multiple myeloma, in contrast with a lymphoplasmacytic lymphoma, which should show a CD45$^+$, CD19$^+$, CD20$^+$, CD38$^{+/-}$, sIg$^+$ phenotype. Immunohistochemistry on the bone marrow trephine (bottom panel) confirmed cyclin D1 overexpression, in keeping with this entity.

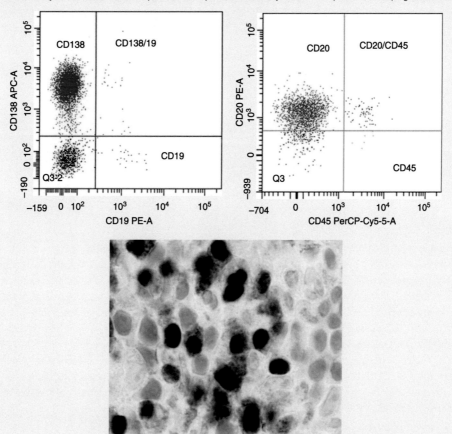

WORKED EXAMPLE 8.3

An 80-year-old male presented with a confusional state, renal failure and anaemia. An FBC showed Hb 80 g/L, WBC 25×10⁹/L, platelets 80×10⁹/L. He had a 20 g/L IgA paraprotein. The blood film showed prominent acanthocytes, rouleaux and pleomorphic abnormal plasma cells. Flow cytometry studies confirmed these cells to be malignant plasma cells, CD138⁺, CD45dim, CD19⁻ and CD56⁻, with an immunophenotype typical of plasma cell leukaemia.

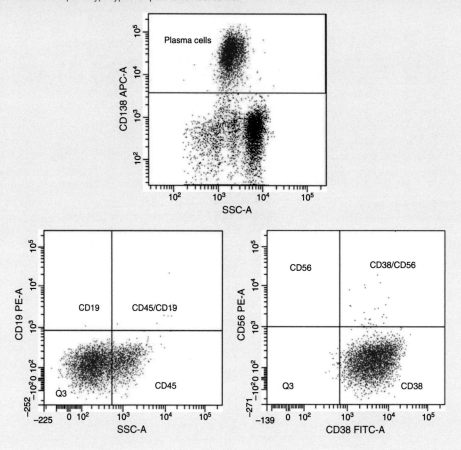

CD117 is not expressed on normal plasma cells but in myeloma it appears to confer a better prognosis in terms of progression free and overall survival. When the two antigens are combined there is synergism in terms of prognostic power (Table 8.5).

CD56 (NCAM) is an adhesion molecule involved in anchoring myelomatous plasma cells to bone marrow stroma. It is expressed in the majority of myeloma cases. The absence, or loss of, CD56 is associated with aggressive disease, relapse and extramedullary or leukaemic progression [15]. It is frequently absent in *de novo* plasma cell leukaemia [4].

Circulating plasma cells

Plasma cells can be detected in peripheral blood in MGUS, SM, MM and, of course, PCL. These circulating plasma cells are predictive of disease progression. In MGUS circulating plasma cells are present in a minority of patients, but their presence increases the risk of progression to myeloma two-fold [16]. In newly diagnosed MM 75% of patients have circulating malignant plasma cells [17]. The circulating plasma cell load appears to carry prognostic significance [18], but correlates only weakly with tumour mass, suggesting that plasma cell circulation is a reflection of disease biology.

Minimal residual disease and prognosis post transplant

Autologous stem cell transplant is now established as a standard of care for myeloma patients <65 years of age, on achieving first remission. Although a complete remission by standard criteria is the norm in many patients, all will eventually relapse due to residual disease. The presence, or not, of malignant plasma cells in peripheral blood of myeloma patients in the two weeks prior to stem cell harvest is important prognostically and is associated with a shortened interval to disease progression (14.1 versus 22 months) and overall survival (33.2 and 58.6 months), respectively. Not surprisingly, progression free survival is also shortened in patients with heavy malignant plasma cell contamination of the stem cell harvest [19]. Finally, patients with a flow cytometric complete remission on a day 100 bone marrow aspirate have a longer progression free and overall survival than those with detectable disease [20]. The potential benefit of tandem autologous transplant, generating lower residual plasma cell levels, as assessed using flow cytometry, appears to correlate with overall survival post procedure [21]. In the setting of allogeneic transplantation for multiple myeloma, persistent MRD positivity may influence patient management in terms of decisions on donor lymphocyte infusions. This is an area in which the application of flow cytometry studies will continue to evolve.

References

1 Kyle RA, on behalf of the IMWG Criteria for the classification of monoclonal gammopathies, multiple myeloma and related disorders: a report of the International Myeloma Working Group. *Br J Haematol* 2003, **121**(5): 749–57.

2 Rajkumar, SV. MGUS and smoldering multiple myeloma: update on pathogenesis, natural history, and management. *Hematology Am Soc Hematol Educ Program* 2005, 340–5.

3 Kyle RA, Rajkumar SV. Monoclonal gammopathy of undetermined significance. *Clin Lymphoma Myeloma* 2005, **6**(2): 102–14.

4 Sher T, *et al.* Plasma cell leukaemia and other aggressive plasma cell malignancies. *Br J Haematol* 2010, **150**(4): 418–27.

5 Paiva B, *et al.* Multiparameter flow cytometry quantification of bone marrow plasma cells at diagnosis provides more prognostic information than morphological assessment in myeloma patients. *Haematologica* 2009, **94**(11): 1599–602.

6 Rawstron AC, *et al.* Report of the European Myeloma Network on multiparametric flow cytometry in multiple myeloma and related disorders. *Haematologica* 2008, **93**(3): 431–8.

7 Lin P, *et al.* Expression of PAX5 in CD20-positive multiple myeloma assessed by immunohistochemistry and oligonucleotide microarray. *Mod Pathol* 2004, **17**(10): 1217–22.

8 Robillard N, *et al.* CD20 is associated with a small mature plasma cell morphology and t(11;14) in multiple myeloma. *Blood* 2003, **102**(3): 1070–1.

9 Heerema-McKenney A, *et al.* Clinical, immunophenotypic, and genetic characterization of small lymphocyte-like plasma cell myeloma: a potential mimic of mature B-cell lymphoma. *Am J Clin Pathol* 2010, **133**(2): 265–70.

10 Kyle RA, *et al.* A long-term study of prognosis in monoclonal gammopathy of undetermined significance. *N Engl J Med* 2002, **346**(8): 564–9.

11 Kyle RA, Rajkumar SV. Monoclonal gammopathy of undetermined significance and smouldering multiple myeloma: emphasis on risk factors for progression. *Br J Haemato* 2007, **139**(5): 730–43.

12 Rajkumar SV, *et al.* Serum free light chain ratio is an independent risk factor for progression in monoclonal gammopathy of undetermined significance. *Blood* 2005, **106**(3): 812–7.

13 Perez-Persona E, *et al.* New criteria to identify risk of progression in monoclonal gammopathy of uncertain significance and smoldering multiple myeloma based on multiparameter flow cytometry analysis of bone marrow plasma cells. *Blood* 2007, **110**(7): 2586–92.

14 Mateo G, *et al.* Prognostic value of immunophenotyping in multiple myeloma: a study by the PETHEMA/GEM cooperative study groups on patients uniformly treated with high-dose therapy. *J Clin Oncol* 2008, **26**(16): 2737–44.

15 Sahara N, Takeshita A. Prognostic significance of surface markers expressed in multiple myeloma: CD56 and other antigens. *Leuk Lymphoma* 2004, **45**(1): 61–5.

16 Kumar S, *et al.* Prognostic value of circulating plasma cells in monoclonal gammopathy of undetermined significance. *J Clin Oncol* 2005, **23**(24): 5668–74.

17 Rawstron AC, *et al.* Circulating plasma cells in multiple myeloma: characterization and correlation with disease stage. *Br J Haematol* 1997, **97**(1): 46–55.

18 Nowakowski GS, *et al.* Circulating plasma cells detected by flow cytometry as a predictor of survival in 302 patients with newly diagnosed multiple myeloma. *Blood* 2005, **106**(7): 2276–9.

19 Kopp HG, *et al.* Contamination of autologous peripheral blood progenitor cell grafts predicts overall survival after high-dose chemotherapy in multiple myeloma. *J Cancer Res Clin Oncol* 2009, **135**(4): 637–42.

20 Paiva B, *et al.* Multiparameter flow cytometric remission is the most relevant prognostic factor for multiple myeloma patients who undergo autologous stem cell transplantation. *Blood* 2008, **112**(10): 4017–23.

21 Johnsen HE, *et al.* Multiparametric flow cytometry profiling of neoplastic plasma cells in multiple myeloma. *Cytometry B Clin Cytom* 2010, **78**(5): 338–47.

CHAPTER 9
Minimal Residual Disease

Introduction

For most neoplastic haematological entities assessment of treatment response has historically been based on the following criteria:

1 Resolution of presenting symptoms
2 Reduction in the degree of lymphadenopathy, hepatomegaly or splenomegaly
3 Recovery of blood counts toward normal
4 Clearance of diseased cells from blood, bone marrow, effusions or CSF

The relative importance of these criteria will vary according to the disease entity in question; for example nodal resolution is clearly important in lymphoma, whereas bone marrow recovery and remission status are of utmost importance in the acute leukaemias (AL). Regarding the latter, remission status is assessed with respect to the clearance of disease cells below a defined threshold.

For AL this threshold is accepted as a reduction of leukaemic blasts to a level of less than 5% of all nucleated marrow cells. This is a relatively arbitrary definition that has been established on the basis of what is reproducibly discernible through routine morphological examination of marrow aspirates. Light microscopy lacks sensitivity, however; the ability to detect one AL blast in 20–30 cells using morphological criteria translates into a sensitivity of 3–5%. Furthermore, this is not an all or nothing phenomenon (which the setting of a threshold might suggest); we have all encountered scenarios where a patient has achieved a morphological remission but adjunctive studies such as cytogenetics, FISH or molecular studies have indicated that the disease burden is still substantial. This disease load, quantifiable using ultra- sensitive techniques but which is not identifiable through standard methods, is known as minimal residual disease (MRD). The principle of MRD analysis within the context of modern treatment protocols is illustrated in Figure 9.1.

MRD assessment can be applied to a number of leukaemic diseases, both during and after standard treatment; MRD status is predictive of likely outcome and can influence decisions on the duration, type and intensity of treatment likely to be necessary for any individual patient. A number of techniques are available for assessing MRD, in a quantifiable way. The two main methodologies of relevance here are:

1 Sensitive polymerase chain reaction (PCR) based MRD detection methods
2 Flow cytometric analysis using sequential gating and detection of low level events in relation to an aberrant disease-specific and/or patient-specific immunophenotype.

Each methodology has its advantages and disadvantages, and each requires dedicated technical expertise. Such techniques clearly require careful validation and evaluation in parallel to normal controls. As a rough guide, MRD analysis is capable of detecting one leukaemic cell in 10,000: the power of the methodology is remarkable, but the results it generates can only be interpreted with full knowledge of the limitations and sensitivity of the methods it employs. Furthermore the application of these data to the clinical management of patients must be rigorously tested in prospective, randomized clinical trials.

Some general principles apply to any leukaemia where flow cytometry is used for MRD quantitation:

1 The target disease needs to have a unique immunophenotype (either disease specific or patient specific).
2 Large numbers of events (500,000+) need to be analysed to gain the degree of sensitivity required.

Practical Flow Cytometry in Haematology Diagnosis, First Edition. Mike Leach, Mark Drummond and Allyson Doig.
© 2013 John Wiley & Sons, Ltd. Published 2013 by John Wiley & Sons, Ltd.

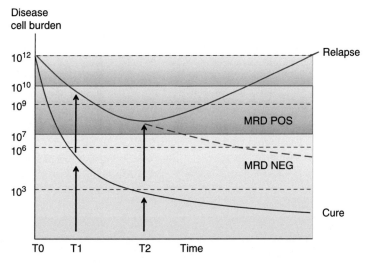

Figure 9.1 The principle and prognostic significance of minimal residual disease status. Disease burden in terms of cell number, response assessment and MRD is shown. A patient presents with an acute leukaemia at time T0 with an arbitrary cell burden of 10^{12} cells. As treatment commences cells are killed and the burden falls. The rate of fall, which is proportional to the chemosensitivity of the cells, varies between patients as illustrated in the profiles of patient 1 (red line) and patient 2 (blue line). Both patients achieve a morphological remission, having reduced the cell burden a hundred-fold from 10^{12} to 10^{10}, but a substantial cell load still exists. The actual cell load can be measured by MRD evaluation following induction chemotherapy at time T1. Patient 1 is MRD positive (low level disease detectable) and despite continued treatment shows eventual relapse, whereas patient 2 is MRD negative (low level disease undetectable) and remains in remission. A further assessment, following completion of chemotherapy at time T2, shows a lower MRD load for both patients, but persisting positivity in patient 1. This is predictive of future relapse in this patient. Had additional therapy, such as stem cell transplant, been offered to patient 1 at T2 or earlier, then it might be possible to achieve MRD negativity, so preventing relapse (dashed red line). Additional therapy is clearly not necessary for patient 2, who might have been harmed in the process.

3 The operating laboratory needs to be familiar with the technical aspects of MRD flow.

4 Consensus protocols need to be followed.

5 EQA participation is essential.

Despite these caveats, there is now good evidence that MRD status (either using flow or PCR-based techniques) carries substantial weight in terms of optimal disease management and treatment outcome in a number of diseases, including acute lymphoblastic leukaemia (ALL), acute myeloid leukaemia (AML, particularly APML), chronic myeloid leukaemia (CML) , chronic lymphocytic leukaemia (CLL) and hairy cell leukaemia (HCL).

In this chapter we will ultimately focus on the experience in ALL where the sequential gating approach is illustrated and where the assessment of MRD status using flow cytometry is most established [1–5]. In this setting the predictive power of MRD is powerful, and independent of other clinically relevant risk factors, such as age, blast count, presence of informative cytogenetics and response to steroids. Before embarking on the ALL MRD story we will briefly address two other diseases where the importance of MRD assessment using flow has been established: these are CLL and AML.

Chronic lymphocytic leukaemia

Chronic lymphocytic leukaemia (CLL) is the commonest leukaemia of the Western world. Unlike the acute leukaemias, which are uniformly fatal without treatment, CLL is a curious entity that shows very variable behaviour. Some patients never require therapy, whereas others need aggressive treatment at the outset and may have a very short survival without resort to stem cell transplant. Our increased understanding of the biology of CLL (in terms of IgVH gene mutation status, Zap 70 expression and cytogenetics) has added much to assist us in defining prognosis [6, 7]. This disorder is covered in more detail in Chapter 6. Chronic lymphocytic leukaemia is essentially a disease of the elderly, with a median age at presentation of 67 years. For many patients, therefore, the priority is to control the condition, to relieve symptoms and improve quality of life without unduly increasing the ever-present risk of infection. Up to 30% of patients, however, are given a diagnosis of CLL before their 55th year [8]. The priorities here might be somewhat different in these young patients, in particular those with progressive symptomatic disease, adverse prognostic parameters, autoimmune complications and serious infections. Treatments capable of influencing the natural history of the disease and potentially modifying outcome are increasingly important for these young poor risk patients. Furthermore, the historical criteria for assessing response to therapy in CLL are based on traditional light microscopy methods which, we now know, are somewhat crude assessments of residual disease status; they did, however, recognize that depth of response was an important principle in response criteria [9]. With the introduction of highly effective monoclonal antibody therapies and transplant techniques, residual disease burdens commonly fall below a detectable level using conventional techniques. Using MRD assessment of response, outcome can be predicted even in high risk patients [10–12]. Most recently, the MRD status of patients receiving front-line therapy (German CLL Group CLL8 study evaluating FC versus FCR therapy) was demonstrated to be highly predictive for both progression free and overall survival [13]. Importantly, this study showed that MRD negativity was predictive of a good prognosis regardless of the treatment that achieved it; MRD negative patients in the FC and FCR arms did equally well, although more patients reached this goal in the FCR group. It is likely that MRD status will increasingly be viewed as a valuable surrogate marker for outcome, as an alternative to progression free survival, particularly in conditions where improved overall survival may be difficult to demonstrate due to the chronicity of the disorder.

Polymerase chain reaction based techniques have been generally considered to be the most sensitive method of MRD assessment in CLL. However, they can only be applied to a proportion of patients (70–80%), where mutations in the IgVH genes allow binding of consensus primers. In addition, the ability of these primers to demonstrate a disease specific product is limited by the presence of normal lymphocytes so limiting the sensitivity. This interference by normal B-cells can be overcome by the development of patient specific consensus primers, a technique known as allele specific oligonucleotide PCR (ASO-PCR). This approach is highly sensitive

but needs considerable expertise, is labour intensive and is slow to deliver results. It is not ideally suited, therefore, to guiding patient therapy in 'real time'. With continued advances in flow cytometry methodology, including the use of sequential gating strategies, multiple colour analysis in a single tube and the ability to analyse hundreds of thousands of events it is possible to detect very low levels of disease cells (as few as one CLL cell in 10^5 normal leucocytes). Despite the varying methodologies applied, it is consistently observed that patients who achieve an MRD-negative remission have significantly longer progression free and overall survival.

Chronic lymphocytic leukaemia has a unique immunophenotype which is quite unlike that of other B-cell lymphoproliferative disorders; it is therefore a disorder that seems eminently suitable for MRD analysis by flow. An important caveat, however, is to be aware of low levels of normal cells with a similar phenotype that might exist in blood or bone marrow [14], a principle that applies to any leukaemia where MRD flow technology is applied. The typical CLL immunophenotype is $CD19^+$, $CD20^{dim}$, $CD5^+$, $CD79a^{dim/neg}$, $CD22^{dim/neg}$, $CD23^+$, $CD43^+$, $FMC7^{neg}$, $CD81^-$, sIg^{dim}. This offers ample opportunity for sequential gating strategies in flow cytometry for CLL cell isolation, allowing the detection of one cell in 10^4 to 10^5. By selecting a series of antigens which show maximal sequential differentiation between normal cells and CLL cells, flow is able to identify small discrete disease cell populations. An approach using CD19, SSC, CD5, CD20, CD79b and CD38 is highly discriminatory. This MRD flow technique was pioneered by the Leeds group [15] and has since been adopted by many other centres worldwide following agreement on a standardized approach [16]. The technical principles of flow in this setting are similar to those in ALL, and are discussed in detail later in this chapter.

Acute myeloid leukaemia

Despite achieving remission rates in excess of 80% following intensive induction chemotherapy, less than 40% of all patients with AML will survive for five years. The relapse that many patients experience with AML is thought to be generated from the residual disease cell population [17, 18], and many patients with relapse are incurable. Much attention has therefore been directed at methods of assessing MRD in AML. PCR based quantification has a role in MRD analysis, but such techniques are currently only applicable to AML with a specific gene fusion, for example PML-RARα, AML1-ETO or CBFβ-MYH11. Together these leukaemias comprise less than 30% of patients with AML.

Multi-parameter flow cytometry appears to be a valuable tool for predicting relapse [18–20]. The detection of MRD in AML, however, poses a number of difficulties, predominantly due to phenotypic heterogeneity requiring determination of the leukaemia-associated immunophenotype (LAIP) at diagnosis. As we have seen AML cells have a very variable phenotype depending on the disease biology and degree of differentiation. A standard CD34+ CD117+ CD13+ CD33+ AML profile does not lend itself to MRD flow monitoring as this is also the phenotype of normal marrow myeloblasts. Furthermore, the monocytic leukaemias are often CD34− and CD117−; these are potentially very difficult to track and to differentiate from normal monocytic cells which are so prevalent in recovering bone marrow. In contrast, the immunophenotype and light scatter characteristics in ALL are much more consistent and this explains why the role of flow in MRD assessment is established in this disease as compared to AML (see below).

The LAIP in AML is a patient specific phenotype that may be characterized on the basis of one or more of the following:
• Asynchronous antigen expression, for example CD34/CD117 with CD15
• Aberrant antigen expression, such as CD19, CD7 and CD56
• Antigen over expression
• Aberrant scatter properties
• Antigen loss
The identification of an LAIP may require the use of multiple additional antibodies, utilizing four or five colours or more. The proportion of cases where an LAIP can be determined is generally in the range of 60–90% [21] though some centres using extensive panels and five-colour flow can achieve this in 94% of cases [22]. Aberrant antigen expression remains the most robust characteristic for the separation of residual leukaemic cells from normal myeloblasts, with expression of CD2, CD56, CD11b, CD7 and CD19 being the most useful [22].

The quality of LAIP for MRD tracking depends on the following:
• Specificity of the antigen combination and the scarcity of that phenotype in normal bone marrow cells

• Sensitivity in terms of:
  – the proportion of AML blasts showing the LAIP
  – the cellularity of specimens obtained
  – the number of events analysed
• Stability of the LAIP due to changes in immunophenotype during disease course
Appropriate matched isotype controls are essential to identify baseline background fluorescence and no fewer than 250,000 events need to be analysed. In the presence of a robust LAIP one abnormal cell in 10,000 can be detected [23].

The application of flow cytometry for MRD quantitation in AML therefore continues to evolve, but is not nearly as well established compared to ALL because of the issues covered above. Its role continues to be explored in large AML trials, such as the current AML17 trial in the UK.

Minimal residual disease analysis in the management of acute lymphoblastic leukaemia

Levels of MRD, as assessed using flow cytometry, are strongly correlated with outcome in both paediatric and adult ALL. For example, MRD monitoring of paediatric ALL allows risk stratification, use of appropriate therapy and perhaps avoidance of late toxicities from over treatment in good risk patients. The prognosis in most cases is good with modern therapy but even so 20% of children with ALL will relapse [24, 25].

There have been several large-scale studies during recent years demonstrating that the absence of MRD in BM predicts good outcome, and that the risk of relapse is proportional to the level of MRD detectable [26–30]. These studies have included both B and T-cell disease. Reduced rates of early blast clearance during induction therapy are a particularly important indicator of high risk ALL. Indeed there is significant support for replacement of morphological analysis of early disease response with flow cytometric analysis (as is currently happening in the United States [1, 2]).

Monitoring minimal residual disease in acute lymphoblastic leukaemia

Any methodology for detection of MRD, and its clinical applicability, must be defined with regards the following:

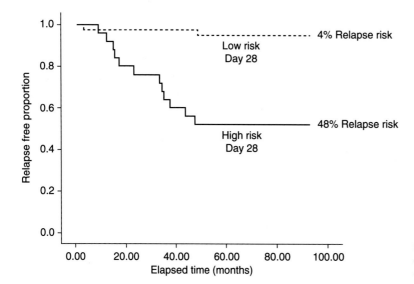

Figure 9.2 Kaplan Meier survival curve according to flow MRD status at day 28 (UKALL97 Study [31]).

1 The threshold that is used for clinical decision making

2 Proportion of patients for whom this level of quality can be achieved

3 Sensitivity of technique

4 Specificity of technique

Another important issue is that sensitivity and specificity of the relevant techniques may vary from patient to patient as they depend on the quality of the LAIP being used for flow cytometry, or the copy numbers of the leukaemia associated genes that are used for PCR analysis.

Currently, the most sensitive method to track disease in ALL is by PCR, followed closely by flow cytometric analysis:

1 Molecular techniques (PCR) 10^{-5}

2 Immunophenotyping (flow) 10^{-4}

3 Cytogenetics 10^{-1} to 10^{-2}

4 Fluorescent *in situ* hybridization 10^{-1} to 10^{-2}

The current clinical applications of MRD analysis include the assessment of early response and prognosis, direction of therapy intensity (intensification or reduction) and monitoring for relapse after conventional chemotherapy and pre- and post-allogeneic stem cell transplant (ASCT).

The value of MRD analysis in ALL is best illustrated by a study reported by van Dongen *et al.* (1998) on behalf of the International BFM Study Group [31]. The authors showed that information on the kinetics of the tumour load reduction at two consecutive time points (after induction treatment and before consolidation treatment) discrimi-

nated between MRD low-risk (five-year relapse rate of 2%), MRD high-risk (five-year relapse rate of 80%) and MRD intermediate-risk patients (five-year relapse risk of 22%). As a result of this and other such studies risk grouping based on the speed of clearance of MRD is now an integral part of most modern treatment protocols for both childhood and adult ALL. This has been evaluated in numerous trials, in particular those used by the Children's Oncology Group (COG) and St Judes, but also by the International-BFM Study group and in UK studies performed at Birmingham Children's Hospital (Figure 9.2) [24, 25, 27–29].

In summary, these studies show:

1 Flow MRD >0.01% at end of induction therapy is associated with 40–50% relapse risk.

2 Flow MRD <0.01% at end of induction therapy is associated with <5% relapse risk.

3 Flow MRD at early time-points (day 8 or day 15 of treatment) can identify patients with very high risk of relapse (>10% MRD-relapse risk ~50%) in whom novel therapy or early stem cell transplant would be appropriate.

4 Flow MRD at early time points (day 8 or day 15 of treatment) can identify patients with very low risk of relapse (<0.01%, relapse risk <5%, in UK data set 0%) in whom treatment reduction may be possible.

Multivariate analysis in the recent COG study [32] showed that morphological analysis of blast percentage at day 8 was not predictive of outcome; however day 8 flow MRD assessment was predictive of risk of relapse. It is

Table 9.1 Day 8/15 UK flow MRD result and relapse risk (70 samples analysed at day 8/15).

% MRD	Relapse risk (%)	Number
<0.01%	0	5
0.01–1%	14	33
1–10%	25	20
>10%	40	12

Reproduced from Borowitz et al. [32], with permission from Wiley.

Table 9.2 Guidelines for clinical interpretation [28].

Clinical interpretation	MRD% (and total events counted)
High risk	0.01% or above with minimum of 50 clustered events. Total events counted >100,000.
Low risk	<0.01% total events counted >500,000–1000.000 in at least two MRD markers.
POQR	0.001–0.01% with a cluster of events identifiable as MRD (positive outside quantifiable range).
Indeterminate	<0.01% but impaired sensitivity due to one or combination of the following: 1 Total events counted <500,000 2 Markers non-informative 3 Only one MRD marker analysed

Reproduced from Jesson et al. [28], with permission from Ferrata Storti Foundation.

anticipated that analysis at day 8/day 15 may be used in future to predict risk (Table 9.1).

Within clinical trial protocols there are strict guidelines as to how flow data is interpreted. An example is shown in Table 9.2 (as used in the UKALL97 trial) [28].

Minimal residual disease flow immunophenotyping versus molecular polymerase chain reaction analysis

The results of molecular and flow cytometric analyses are not interchangeable as they measure different things (i.e. DNA versus intact cells). While most studies have demonstrated good concordance between the two methodologies, there are also discordant measurements. However, both are equally predictive of outcome, as has been shown for patients treated on UK protocols [28]. If both

techniques are available flow MRD could be used for risk stratification in those children where no molecular marker is identified or indeed the reverse (as used by the St Jude group) where molecular analysis is used if no flow markers are identified.

Current UKALL National Trials use molecular MRD techniques to risk stratify patients during treatment. However, flow cytometric analysis of MRD has several advantages and current trials offer the ideal opportunity to prospectively compare these two techniques. Comparisons are ongoing, but to date show an overall concordance of 85% between the two techniques (Table 9.3).

Technical aspects of minimal residual disease flow assessment in acute lymphoblastic leukaemia

When considering the advantages or disadvantages of this technique it is useful to compare findings with other methods available. Advantages might include:
- Applicability >90%: similar to molecular techniques, although flow requires a minimum of two 'markers' to track, whereas with molecular only one is necessary.
- Accessibility: flow cytometers are routinely used in many laboratories in contrast to real time PCR analysers.
- Turnaround times: relatively quick compared with molecular analysis.
- Cost: estimated at £300 per patient for MRD ALL screen at diagnosis and follow-up time-points (day 8, day 28 and week 11). This is significantly less than the cost of a molecular screen which is between £2000–3000 per patient.

Disadvantages may include:
- Detailed analysis: required for all LAIPs and subpopulations at diagnosis/relapse.
- Phenotypic shifts: some patients show shifts in mean fluorescent intensity up to day 28.
- Sensitivity: less sensitive than molecular (10^{-4} compared with 10^{-5}).

Standardized quality assured MRD protocols were developed during the UKALL2003/2007 Studies to monitor both B-cell and T-cell ALL and are in current use in laboratories throughout the UK [10]. The key issues for any flow-based MRD protocol are considered below [33, 34].

Use of Controls

Positive and negative controls for each monoclonal antibody should be used to monitor the validity of the immune-staining and the lysing procedures. This is essential when a new monoclonal antibody and/or batch

Day 28	PCR HR	PCR LR
Flow HR	64	33
Flow LR	25	128

Day 28	N = 250
Concordant	77%
Discordant	23%

Wk 11	PCR HR	PCR LR
Flow HR	1	5
Flow LR	0	96

Wk 11	N = 102
Concordant	95%
Discordant	5%

Combined	PCR HR	PCR LR
Flow HR	65	38
Flow LR	25	224

Combined	N = 352
Concordant	82%
Discordant	18%

Table 9.3 Immunophenotyping versus PCR comparison (1998–2008). At day 28 and week 11 330 B-cell and 22 T-cell leukaemia samples were analysed by flow and molecular with six UK labs participating. Results at day 28 and week 11 were compared for both techniques using multivariate analysis. For the discordant samples, MRD levels were between 0.001% and 0.05%, thus close to the borderline of positivity. HR, high risk; LR, low risk.

of reagents is introduced, after an instrument service or calibration and/or when a new technique is applied. Positive and negative controls should be either leukaemic or normal cells on which the antigen is known to be expressed or not expressed. Normal residual cells within the sample may also act as an internal control. Additional controls are incorporated within the panel for positive MRD markers only. These can be used to adjust the MRD percentage for any background events falling within the MRD regions.

Normal bone marrow templates

It is crucial that all laboratories performing MRD establish normal marrow templates to assess the patterns of staining seen in normal BM progenitors. Trackable MRD appears in 'empty spaces' when comparing diagnostic marrow to normal templates. Acid citrate dextrose (ACD) or EDTA anticoagulants are suitable for sample collection and ammonium chloride whole marrow lysis is recommended for sample preparation prior to immunostaining. A minimum of five normal marrow samples should be analysed in each laboratory to determine the normal expression for all antigens of interest in the screening panel. Samples should be analysed, preferably within 24 hours and ideally within six hours. Samples are considered positive for an antigen when >20% of cells are positive for a surface antigen (Figure 9.3).

Selection of leukaemia associated immunophenotype and antibody panels

A panel is run to identify one or more LAIPs at diagnosis. Diagnostic phenotypes are then compared to normal BM using 'empty spaces' to determine the most suitable phenotypes to monitor for each patient. Patient specific panels are then used to track the relevant LAIPs. A minimum acquisition of 500,000 cells is required for at least two LAIPs. It is useful to track as many combinations as possible to gain experience; however, there are cost implications to consider. In B-cell ALL a hierarchy has been established to assist with selection of the most appropriate LAIPs to follow [28]. For any given patient the best LAIPs to track would be those that do not overlap normal marrow templates. It is recommended that for a suitable antigen the abnormal population is at least half a log decade away from the median of the cell distribution seen in normal template to be considered suitable.

Hierarchy for LAIPs used to monitor B-cell ALL:
1 CD45 under expression
2 CD38 under expression
3 CD58 over expression
4 CD123 over expression
5 CD13/CD33/CD66c aberrant expression
6 CD20 usually weak or negative
7 CD10/CD34 over expression
8 CD34+/CD22+ asynchronous antigen expression

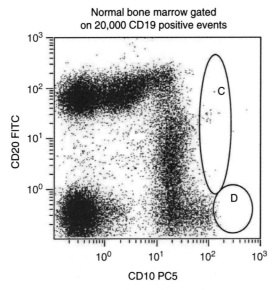

Figure 9.3 These composite plots have been gated on CD19+ events and represent normal marrow template for CD20 and CD10 expression. C+D represent 'empty spaces' and could be used to track disease.

Table 9.4 Four colour MRD B-cell ALL panel. The first five combinations (highlighted) have been found to be the most informative.

CD45	CD34	CD10	CD19
CD38	CD34	CD10	CD19
CD58	CD34	CD10	CD19
CD123	CD34	CD10	CD19
CD66c	CD34	CD10	CD19
CD20	CD34	CD10	CD19
CD13	CD34	CD10	CD19
CD33	CD34	CD10	CD19
CD22	CD34	CD10	CD19

A4 colour antibody panel consists of a common 'spine' (CD34/CD10/CD19) plus the additional marker of interest. Coulter and Becton Dickinson panels used are slightly different due to fluorochromes available (Table 9.4).

Table 9.5 highlights the most informative B-cell markers evaluated in the UKALL2007 Study [28]. CD123 was not included in the original panel but has been assessed and replaces CD66c in the hierarchy.

Table 9.5 Most informative markers for B-ALL. The columns refer to the numbers and percentages of cases in which the marker in question was informative.

Marker	Number on follow-up	Percentage
CD45	57	80
CD38	52	73
CD58	36	51
CD66c	25	35
CD13	9	13
CD33	8	11
CD20	8	11
CD22	3	4

Table 9.6 Technical applicability was increased due to the incorporation of CD123. Clinical applicability increased as no week 11 samples to fail on for low risk arm of the UKALL2007 Trial. Results are based on 109 patients.

	Sept 2007–2008 (8 tubes)	Sept 2008–2009 (4 tubes)
% Technical applicability	92	97
% Clinical applicability	76	93
% HR at day 28	41	47
% LR at day 28	40	46
% IND at day 28	19	7
% >1% at day 8/15	58	61

A reduced 4×4 colour tube panel using the first four combinations was compared with an eight tube panel for technical/clinical applicability (Table 9.6). Results indicate no loss in applicability/sensitivity, with the advantage of reduced costs and operator time.

Analysis of minimal residual disease flow data in B-ALL

Guidelines utilise the agreed four-colour panel developed by the UK Flow MRD working group for use with Becton Dickinson and Beckman Coulter instrument platforms. The panels have been developed with reference to the published work of the European Biomed Consortium [27] and Dario Campana [1, 2]. A systematic gating strategy

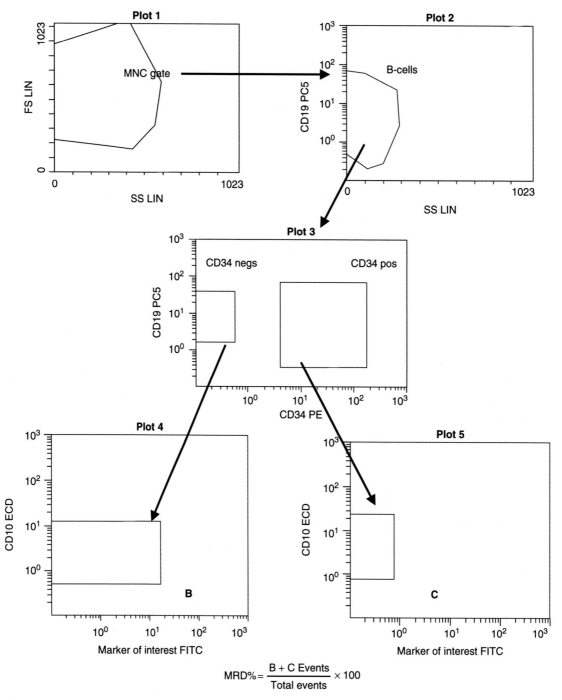

$$MRD\% = \frac{B + C \text{ Events}}{\text{Total events}} \times 100$$

Figure 9.4 Gating strategy for assessing minimal residual disease in B-cell acute lymphoblastic leukaemia.

Logical Gating Strategy

Plot 1, gate blast region on basis of FSC/SSC.

Plot 2, Gate CD19+ low side scatter events.

Plot 3, CD19+ CD34– and CD19+ CD34+ events gated separately.

Plot 4, CD19+, CD34– CD10 versus marker of interest.

Plot 5, CD19+ CD34+ CD10 versus marker of interest.

is used to monitor MRD in B-Cell ALL (Figure 9.4). An initial analysis gate is drawn around the blast population based on FSC/SSC properties. A further gate is used to define CD19 positive events derived from the blast gate. A further two gates are used to separate CD19$^+$ CD34$^-$ events and CD19$^+$ CD34$^+$ events as this will help to identify any subpopulations which must also be tracked. Another gate is then created: 'CD10 versus marker of interest':

- CD10 versus CD45
- CD10 versus CD38
- CD10 versus CD58
- CD10 versus CD123

The formula used to calculate the results (Figure 9.4) must also include a correction factor if required, to account for inclusion of any non-specific binding events in isotype controls which are an integral part of any screening panel. MRD positive events are expressed as a percentage of total events counted minus any events occurring in the MRD background control. An example of gating on an LAIP at diagnosis and at follow-up is shown in Figure 9.5 and Figure 9.6 respectively.

Analysis of minimal residual disease flow data in T-ALL

The four-colour T-cell panel consists of a common CD3/CD7 spine plus combinations of markers of interest. Coulter and Becton Dickinson panels used are slightly different due to fluorochromes available (Table 9.7).

As with B-ALL, the guidelines are based on compliance with the agreed four-colour panel developed by the UK Flow MRD Working Group for use with the Becton Dickinson and Coulter Instruments. Notes regarding the use of specific antigens are highlighted in Table 9.8. The methodology for T-ALL is shown in Figure 9.7 and is as follows:

1 On an FSC/SSC ungated data plot define a region of analysis for the lymphoid/blast region (region 1).

2 Based on this gate define an SS versus CD7 plot. Gate the CD7$^+$ low side scatter (region 2).

3 Based on the combined data from region 1 and 2 define a two-colour fluorescent dot plot of CD3 versus CD7 plot.

4 Define two analysis regions to analyse separately the CD7$^+$CD3$^+$ cells and the CD7$^+$CD3$^-$ cells (region 3 and 4).

5 Define a dot plot for each analysis region 3 and region 4. The following analyses may further assist in defining the blast population

a CD4 versus CD8
b CD5 versus CD56
c CD5 versus CD2
d CD34 versus CD38
e HLA-DR versus CD10
f CD1a versus CD2
g CD13 versus CD5
h CD33 versus CD5
i CD99 versus CD5
j TDT versus CD99
k CytCD3 versus CD3

T-cell Analysis Guidance Notes
See Table 9.8.

The following dot plots (Figure 9.7) illustrate gating strategy described above to monitor disease in a patient who presented with T-cell ALL and subsequently relapsed. The LAIPs identified at relapse were the same as those found at diagnosis:

- CD5 CD2 CD3 CD7
- CD56 CD2 CD3 CD7
- CD1a CD2 CD3 CD7
- CD5 CD99 CD3 CD7

This patient was treated on ALL2003 protocol regimen A throughout induction and was a good early responder morphologically with 7% blasts at day 8. This patient was risk stratified as 'high risk' for ALL 2003 by flow cytometry.

Technical challenges

Low cell counts/small sample volume
For flow cytometric analysis to be sufficiently sensitive to detect low levels of residual leukaemia, large numbers of cells need to be analysed in follow-up samples. The aim is to acquire 10^6 cells for each antibody combination in the follow-up panel. Unfortunately, this is not always possible if the samples received for analysis are of low count (especially for day 28 samples) and/or small volume. If the sample size is limited, panel selection should be according to the hierarchy of LAIPs previously defined.

Sample preparation
There are variations in methods used to prepare samples for analysis. Previous studies [1, 2] have used a lymphoprep technique for sample preparation which enriches

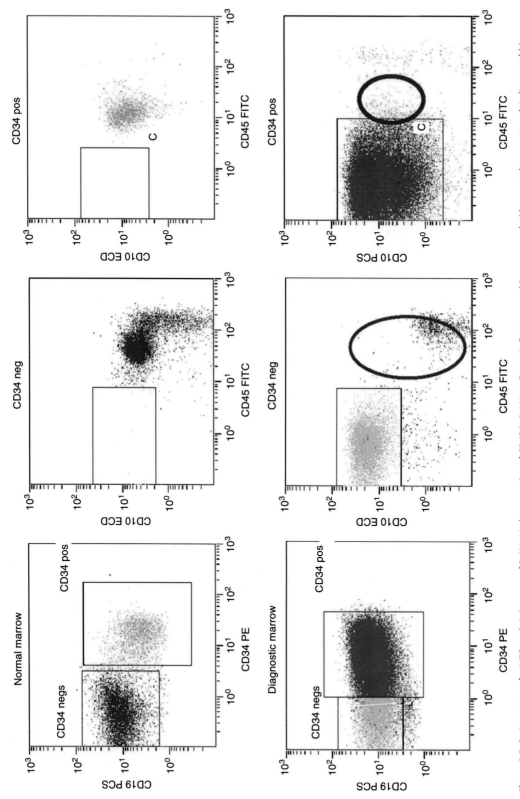

Figure 9.5 Gating strategy for MRD analysis in a case of B-ALL. Under expression of CD45 in B-ALL at diagnosis (bottom panels) as compared with a normal marrow template (top panels) is illustrated. The blue ellipses correspond to the position of normal marrow cells in the diagnostic marrow. Under expression of CD45 (for both CD34neg and CD34pos cells) in diagnostic marrow compared to normal CD45 expression indicates that this LAIP is a suitable marker to monitor disease for this patient. The leukaemic population does not overlap the normal maturation templates.

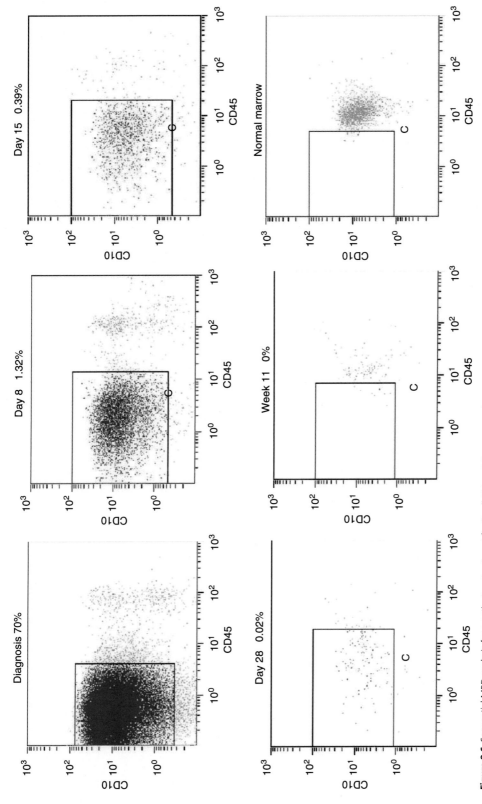

Figure 9.6 Sequential MRD analysis for a patient on treatment for B-cell ALL and the amount of residual disease found at various time-points (figures in brackets) using under expression of CD45 to monitor. A normal marrow (bottom right hand panel) is included for reference.

Table 9.7 UKALL 2007 four-colour T-cell panel.

CD8	CD4	CD3	CD7
CD5	CD2	CD3	CD7
CD5	CD56	CD3	CD7
CD38	CD34	CD3	CD7
CD1a	CD2	CD3	CD7
CD5	CD33	CD3	CD7
CD5	CD13	CD3	CD7
HLA-DR	CD10	CD3	CD7
TdT	CD34	cytCD3	CD7

Table 9.8 Antigens useful in the assessment of MRD in T ALL.

CD34+	T precursors follow all positive cases.
CD5/CD2	Follow aberrant T-cell marker expression as compared to normal templates. Relies on good CD3 pos/neg separation.
CD5/CD56	Follow aberrant T-cell marker expression as compared to normal templates. Relies on good CD3 pos/neg separation.
CD13/CD33	Only follow when positive.
CD10	Only follow when positive.
CD8/CD4	T precursors follow all dual positives only. Shifts to 8+/4− overlap with NK cell population and yield false + MRD results.
CD1a	Only follow when positive.
CD38	Follow over expression only. Under expression becomes uninformative at later time-points. Natural killer cells are CD38 dim.
CD99	Follow over expression
TDT	T precursors not seen in normal bone marrow.

the blast population. The UK Flow MRD study uses an ammonium chloride red cell lysis technique, which is a method used routinely for diagnostic flow analysis. Comparative studies using both techniques have been evaluated showing a strong correlation. Lymphoprep samples showed a higher result above 1% but no clinical risk bias was found. (Figure 9.8).

Phenotypic shifts

Some patients show shifts in mean fluorescent intensity up to day 28. The antigens most commonly affected are:
- Increase in intensity: CD20, CD45, CD19
- Decrease in intensity: CD10, CD34, CD66c, CD58, TdT
- Stable: CD123, CD22, CD38.

Sensitivity

All laboratories should assess the sensitivity of their MRD panel by performing serial dilution experiments to confirm a sensitivity of 10^{-4} for all antibody combinations used in their protocols (Figure 9.9).

Red cell/debris correction

Syto 13 is a nucleic acid stain that can be used to stain RNA and DNA in both live and dead cells. When patients are on treatment, on occasion the red cells show an increased resistance to red cell lysis. Red cell contamination will interfere with scatter plots and reduce overall MRD percentage. Excessive lysis will result in changes to FSC/SSC, causing the cells to shrink. Syto 13 can be used to correct the dilution factor due to incomplete/variable red cell lysis or dilution factor due to incorrect threshold for FSC/SSC settings (Figure 9.10).

Haematogones

Haematogones in normal and especially regenerative marrow may influence MRD results, especially for MRD markers relying on over/under expression of normal antigens (in particular CD20, TdT, CD34, CD10, CD19, CD38 and CD22). At early time-points there is an increase in mature B-cells which increases the reliability of these MRD phenotypes. Later time-points show an increase in immature lymphoid precursor cells that morphologically resemble leukaemic cells. This may reduce the sensitivity of some MRD phenotypes.

Quality assurance

To ensure the accuracy and precision of the data generated, the performance of the flow cytometer must be rigorously monitored and controlled. The laboratory must establish a standardized robust internal quality assurance scheme (IQAS) to confirm that the flow cytometer performs to its expected standard, thus ensuring instrument settings are optimized prior to acquisition and analysis. A flow MRD NEQAS scheme has been established and is evolving [35]. A pilot scheme was developed during the course of the

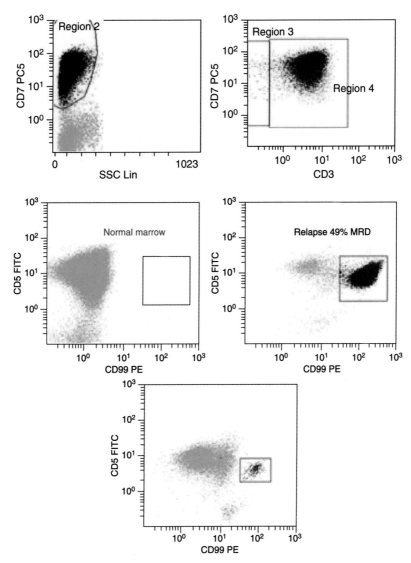

Figure 9.7 An illustration of the ability of a CD5 CD99 CD3 CD7 analysis to discriminate blasts (purple) from normal marrow cells (upper images). A normal marrow CD5 versus CD99 analysis is shown for comparison (middle image, left). The predictive MRD assessment at day 8 is shown (lower image) together with the disease events at relapse in the middle right plot.

Figure 9.8 Comparison regression analysis of Lymphoprep versus red cell lysis (log scale). Cohort of 41 samples, split and analysed by both methods: Lymphoprep versus red cell lysis technique. A Good correlation is demonstrated (R=0.98). Reproduced from Jesson et al. [28], with permission from Ferrata Storti Foundation.

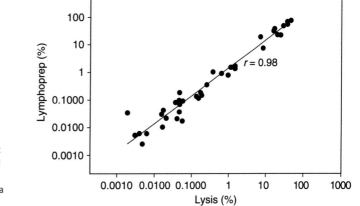

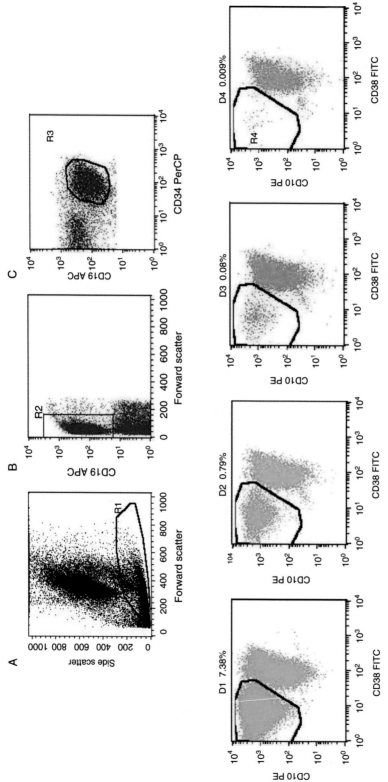

Figure 9.9 Assessment of sensitivity by serial dilution analyses. Dot plots D1–4 show plots for the serial dilutions; blast region identified as R4. Dot plots A–D represent the sequential gating strategy, that is, B is gated on a lymphoid gate (R1) derived from A. C is gated on R1 and a region 2 (R2) which defines CD19+ cells. Finally, D dot plots are gated for R1 and R2 and a region 3 (R3) containing CD19 and CD34 dual positive cells defined in C. Dot plots D1–4 show the final analyses plots for the serial dilutions, with the blast region identified as R4. This confirms the sensitivity for CD38. This experiment should be repeated to confirm sensitivity for all antibody combinations used in protocol.

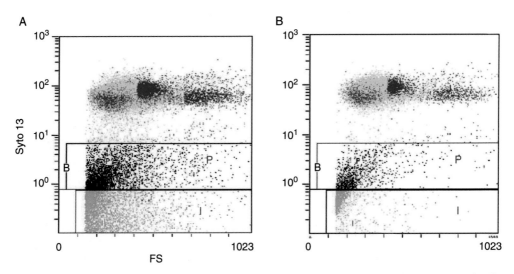

Figure 9.10 Example of the effect of unlysed red cell precursors on MRD quantitation. These plots relate to an NEQAS exercise, analysed by two independent operators. Events in region P+I (red cell precursors) in sample A are greater than events in region P+I in sample B. Correction in sample A increases MRD from 0.17% to 0.20%. Minimal correction required in sample B, MRD remains at 0.22%.

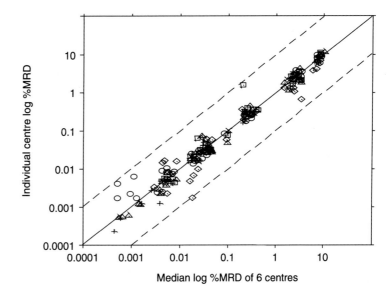

Figure 9.11 Cumulative correlation of a single centre performance against that of all other centres registered with the UK MRD NEQAS Pilot Study.

UKALL2007 study, with six UK laboratories participating in the programme and the results to date show excellent consensus (Figure 9.11).

The scheme has now been rolled out across Europe and the USA (I-BFM/NOPHO/Campana), with 50 laboratories registered to date.

Conclusions

Flow-based MRD is an immensely powerful but technically demanding technique. Ongoing prospective clinical trials are testing its applicability to direct risk-adapted therapy for patients with AL in particular.

Acknowledgements

UKALL FLOW MRD Working Party.

The authors wish to thank Linda Knotts, Chief Biomedical Scientist at Haematology Laboratories, Yorkhill Hospital, Glasgow, for her contribution to Chapter 9, in particular the role of MRD assessment in acute lymphoblastic leukaemia.

References

1 Campana D. Minimal residual disease studies in acute leukemia. *Am J Clin Pathol* 2004, **122**(Suppl): S47–57.

2 Campana D, Coustan-Smith E. Minimal residual disease studies by flow cytometry in acute leukemia. *Acta Haematol* 2004, **112**(1–2): 8–15.

3 Ciudad J, San Miguel JF, Lopez-Berges MC, *et al.* Prognostic value of immunophenotypic detection of minimal residual disease in acute lymphoblastic leukemia. *J Clin Oncol* 1998, **16**(12): 3774–81.

4 Coustan-Smith E, Sancho J, Hancock ML, *et al.* Clinical importance of minimal residual disease in childhood acute lymphoblastic leukemia. *Blood* 2000, **96**(8): 2691–6.

5 Dworzak MN, Froschl G, Printz D, *et al.* Prognostic significance and modalities of flow cytometric minimal residual disease detection in childhood acute lymphoblastic leukemia. *Blood* 2002, **99**(6): 1952–8.

6 Dohner H, Stilgenbauer S, Benner A, *et al.* Genomic aberrations and survival in chronic lymphocytic leukemia. *N Engl J Med* 2000, **343**(26): 1910–6.

7 Orchard JA, Ibbotson RE, Davis Z, *et al.* ZAP-70 expression and prognosis in chronic lymphocytic leukaemia. *Lancet* 2004, **363**(9403): 105–11.

8 Oscier D, Fegan C, Hillmen P, *et al.* Guidelines on the diagnosis and management of chronic lymphocytic leukaemia. *Br J Haematol* 2004, **125**(3): 294–317.

9 Cheson BD, Bennett JM, Grever M, *et al.* National Cancer Institute-sponsored Working Group guidelines for chronic lymphocytic leukemia: revised guidelines for diagnosis and treatment. *Blood* 1996, **87**(12): 4990–7.

10 Bosch F, Ferrer A, Lopez-Guillermo A, *et al.* Fludarabine, cyclophosphamide and mitoxantrone in the treatment of resistant or relapsed chronic lymphocytic leukaemia. *Br J Haematol* 2002, **119**(4): 976–84.

11 Cargo CA, Westerman DA, Gambell P, Juneja S, Szer J, Ritchie D. Flow-cytometric minimal residual disease monitoring for chronic lymphocytic leukaemia in the post-allogeneic transplant period. *Leuk Lymphoma* 2011, **52**(11): 2185–7.

12 Moreton P, Kennedy B, Lucas G, *et al.* Eradication of minimal residual disease in B-cell chronic lymphocytic leukemia after alemtuzumab therapy is associated with prolonged survival. *J Clin Oncol* 2005, **23**(13): 2971–9.

13 Bottcher S, Ritgen M, Fischer K, *et al.* Minimal Residual Disease Quantification Is an Independent Predictor of Progression-Free and Overall Survival in Chronic Lymphocytic Leukemia: A Multivariate Analysis From the Randomized GCLLSG CLL8 Trial. *J Clin Oncol* 2012, **30**(9): 980–8.

14 Durrieu F, Genevieve F, Arnoulet C, *et al.* Normal levels of peripheral CD19($^+$) CD5($^+$) CLL-like cells: toward a defined threshold for CLL follow-up – a GEIL-GOELAMS study. *Cytometry B Clin Cytom* 2011, **80**(6): 346–53.

15 Rawstron AC, Kennedy B, Evans PA, *et al.* Quantitation of minimal disease levels in chronic lymphocytic leukemia using a sensitive flow cytometric assay improves the prediction of outcome and can be used to optimize therapy. *Blood* 2001, **98**(1): 29–35.

16 Rawstron AC, Villamor N, Ritgen M, *et al.* International standardized approach for flow cytometric residual disease monitoring in chronic lymphocytic leukaemia. *Leukemia* 2007, **21**(5): 956–64.

17 van Rhenen A, Feller N, Kelder A, *et al.* High stem cell frequency in acute myeloid leukemia at diagnosis predicts high minimal residual disease and poor survival. *Clin Cancer Res* 2005, **11**(18): 6520–7.

18 Kern W, Voskova D, Schoch C, Hiddemann W, Schnittger S, Haferlach T. Determination of relapse risk based on assessment of minimal residual disease during complete remission by multiparameter flow cytometry in unselected patients with acute myeloid leukemia. *Blood* 2004, **104**(10): 3078–85.

19 Al-Mawali A, Gillis D, Lewis I. The use of receiver operating characteristic analysis for detection of minimal residual disease using five-color multiparameter flow cytometry in acute myeloid leukemia identifies patients with high risk of relapse. *Cytometry B Clin Cytom* 2009, **76**(2): 91–101.

20 Al-Mawali A, To LB, Gillis D, Hissaria P, Mundy J, Lewis I. The presence of leukaemia-associated phenotypes is an independent predictor of induction failure in acute myeloid leukaemia. *Int J Lab Hematol* 2009, **31**(1): 61–8.

21 Al-Mawali A, Gillis D, Lewis I. The role of multiparameter flow cytometry for detection of minimal residual disease in acute myeloid leukemia. *Am J Clin Pathol* 2009, **131**(1): 16–26.

22 Al-Mawali A, Gillis D, Hissaria P, Lewis I. Incidence, sensitivity, and specificity of leukemia-associated phenotypes in acute myeloid leukemia using specific five-color multiparameter flow cytometry. *Am J Clin Pathol* 2008, **129**(6): 934–45.

23 Campana D, Coustan-Smith E. Detection of minimal residual disease in acute leukemia by flow cytometry. *Cytometry* 1999, **38**(4): 139–52.

24 Kersey JH. Fifty years of studies of the biology and therapy of childhood leukemia. *Blood* 1998, **92**(5): 1838.

25 van der Velden VH, Boeckx N, van Wering ER, van Dongen JJ. Detection of minimal residual disease in acute leukemia. *J Biol Regul Homeost Agents* 2004, **18**(2): 146–54.

26 Biondi A, Valsecchi MG, Seriu T, *et al.* Molecular detection of minimal residual disease is a strong predictive factor of relapse in childhood B-lineage acute lymphoblastic leukemia with medium risk features. A case control study of the International BFM study group. *Leukemia* 2000, **14**(11): 1939–43.

27 Borowitz MJ, Pullen DJ, Winick N, Martin PL, Bowman WP, Camitta B. Comparison of diagnostic and relapse flow cytometry phenotypes in childhood acute lymphoblastic leukemia: implications for residual disease detection: a report from the children's oncology group. *Cytometry B Clin Cytom* 2005, **68**(1): 18–24.

28 Jesson J. Establishment and validation of a standard protocol for the detection of minimal residual disease in B-lineage acute lymphoblastic leukaemia by flow cytometry in a multi-center setting; on behalf of the UKALL Flow MRD group and UK MRD steering group. *Haematologica* 2009, **94**(6).

29 Knechtli CJ, Goulden NJ, Hancock JP, *et al.* Minimal residual disease status before allogeneic bone marrow transplantation is an important determinant of successful outcome for children and adolescents with acute lymphoblastic leukemia. *Blood* 1998, **92**(11): 4072–9.

30 Neale GA, Coustan-Smith E, Stow P, *et al.* Comparative analysis of flow cytometry and polymerase chain reaction for the detection of minimal residual disease in childhood acute lymphoblastic leukemia. *Leukemia* 2004, **18**(5): 934–8.

31 van Dongen JJ, Seriu T, Panzer-Grumayer ER, *et al.* Prognostic value of minimal residual disease in acute lymphoblastic leukaemia in childhood. *Lancet* 1998, **352**(9142): 1731–8.

32 Borowitz MJ, Devidas M, Hunger SP, *et al.* Clinical significance of minimal residual disease in childhood acute lymphoblastic leukemia and its relationship to other prognostic factors: a Children's Oncology Group study. *Blood* 2008, **111**(12): 5477–85.

33 Borowitz MJ, Pullen DJ, Shuster JJ, *et al.* Minimal residual disease detection in childhood precursor-B-cell acute lymphoblastic leukemia: relation to other risk factors. A Children's Oncology Group study. *Leukemia* 2003, **17**(8): 1566–72.

34 Weir EG, Cowan K, LeBeau P, Borowitz MJ. A limited antibody panel can distinguish B-precursor acute lymphoblastic leukemia from normal B precursors with four color flow cytometry: implications for residual disease detection. *Leukemia* 1999, **13**(4): 558–67.

35 Barnett D, Granger V, Storie I, *et al.* Quality assessment of CD34+ stem cell enumeration: experience of the United Kingdom National External Quality Assessment Scheme (UK NEQAS) using a unique stable whole blood preparation. *Br J Haematol* 1998, **102**(2): 553–65.

CHAPTER 10

Red Cells, Leucocytes and Platelets

Flow cytometry offers a large number of applications suitable for use in the diagnosis of non-neoplastic phenomena. As always, the clinical circumstances should guide its utility as the results so encountered need interpretation with the full knowledge of patient circumstances. The diagnostician should know what they are looking for, why it is relevant and how the results should be interpreted in a particular clinical scenario. Immunophenotypic analysis of red cells, leucocytes and platelets can generate very useful clinical information in non-neoplastic disorders. Some of the many potential applications are discussed in this chapter.

Paroxysmal nocturnal haemoglobinuria

Paroxysmal nocturnal haemoglobinuria (PNH) is a rare stem cell disorder characterized by the following triad:
• Intravascular haemolysis
• Peripheral blood cytopenias due to bone marrow failure
• Predisposition to venous thrombosis
It is a rare acquired disease with an estimated prevalence of 2–6 per million. It can present at any age and causes premature death through the consequences of thrombosis, often involving unusual sites, and bone marrow failure [1]. It is worth noting that diagnosis is often delayed as it is a clinically heterogenous condition where not all the features necessarily present together, so vigilance is always necessary on behalf of the investigating clinician.

The acquired defect in PNH is the loss of glycosyl phosphatidylinositol (GPI) anchored protein expression by haemopoietic stem cells. A classification scheme that takes into account the clinical circumstances in which the PNH clone is identified has been proposed by the International PNH Interest Group [2], as follows:

1 Classical PNH, where patients have large clones and intravascular haemolysis
2 PNH in the setting of another bone marrow disorder (aplastic anaemia (AA) or myelodysplastic syndromes (MDS))
3 Subclinical PNH where small clones are detected in the absence of haemolysis

The appearance of a number of cluster differentiation (CD) related epitopes is influenced by mutations in the X-linked gene (PIG-A) which controls development of normal GPI anchored proteins. Sequencing studies have shown that mutations in this gene are identified in all patients with a PNH phenotype [3, 4]. The nature of this mutation also influences the acquired defect in the GPI biosynthetic pathway, resulting in partial or complete loss of antigen. This translates into the clinical phenotype, which in turn influences clinical manifestations (see below). The acquisition of a PNH clone allows the development of a subset of stem cells lacking in the expression of these antigens. This clone appears to develop a survival advantage, particularly in the presence of bone marrow hypoplasia, possibly because the GPI anchor itself allows recognition by autoreactive T-cells. The autoimmune process damaging bone marrow stem cells is cytotoxic T-cell driven [5] and PNH stem cells appear to escape this activity, resulting in a survival advantage, though other studies appear to cast doubt on this notion [6]. The consequences of the loss of these GPI anchored antigens are only partially understood, but CD55 (decay accelerating factor, DAF) and CD59 (membrane inhibitor of reactive cell lysis, MIRL) are both complement regulatory proteins and their loss from red cells allows uncontrolled complement activation and

Practical Flow Cytometry in Haematology Diagnosis, First Edition. Mike Leach, Mark Drummond and Allyson Doig.
© 2013 John Wiley & Sons, Ltd. Published 2013 by John Wiley & Sons, Ltd.

intravascular haemolysis. The release of free haemoglobin results in nitric oxide scavenging, which in turn contributes to the many physiological consequences, such as fatigue, impotence, abdominal pain and oesophageal spasm. Although the haemostatic pathophysiology is currently not clear, loss of GPI linked proteins is also implicated in venous thrombosis and thromboembolism [7]. These thromboses frequently affect hepatic, splenic, portal, mesenteric and cerebral vessels, causing serious morbidity or death [1, 8].

These GPI linked epitopes are easily detected on peripheral blood cells. PNH, therefore, lends itself perfectly to accurate diagnosis by flow cytometric analysis of red cells or leucocytes by evaluating expression of GPI associated CD antigens. Flow cytometry has become the gold standard for diagnosis and has completely replaced the traditional Ham's test, which relied on the demonstration that PNH red cells show enhanced lysis in the presence of fresh complement and acidified serum. The latter test often failed to identify non-haemolysing patients with small clones and was influenced by the effect of red cell transfusions.

A selection of relevant antigens which are evaluable and the cells on which they are expressed, is presented in Table 10.1 (adapted from [9]).

The early approach to flow cytometric diagnosis was through the assessment of CD55 and CD59 as these were the first antigens reported to be regularly lost on the red cells, leucocytes and platelets of PNH patients [10, 11]. With the continued development of new monoclonal fluorochrome-linked antibodies a spectrum of other GPI linked epitopes can now be analysed.

Peripheral blood is eminently suitable for PNH diagnosis as it is easily obtained, provides a number of cell types for analysis and avoids the complexity of bone marrow populations which show maturation dependent expression of antigens, particularly CD16 and CD15, which appear later in maturation on neutrophils and monocytes, respectively [12]. In addition, CD55 expression appears to increase sequentially with maturation in bone marrow myeloid precursors [13]. Peripheral blood neutrophils and monocytes should show uniform bright expression of these antigens: their expression can however be reduced in the MDS so this is worth noting in any analysis performed on patients presenting with cytopenias but without haemolysis [14, 15]. It is also recommended that at least two GPI

Table 10.1 Summary of accessible GPI linked antigens evaluable by flow cytometry.

Antigen	Name/function	Cellular expression
CD14	Lipopolysaccharide receptor	Monocytes
CD16	FCγIII receptor	Neutrophils
CD24	Cellular adhesion	Neutrophils, B lymphocytes
CD52	Campath-1 antigen	Monocytes, lymphocytes
CD55	Decay accelerating factor	Haemopoietic cells
CD58	LFA-3 lymphocyte function associated Ag	Haemopoietic cells
CD59	Membrane inhibitor of reactive lysis	Haemopoietic cells
CD66	Cellular signalling and adhesion	Neutrophils, eosinophils
CD87	UPAR cell signalling molecule	All leucocytes

linked antigens be assessed in each cell line as rare cases of inherited antigen deficiency and antigen polymorphism have been reported [16–18].

Aerolysin is a channel-forming toxin produced by the *Aeromonas hydrophilia* bacteria that has the remarkable ability to bind directly with high affinity to the cell membrane GPI anchor, rather than the antigens which are associated with it. It is unable to bind to PNH cells which have lost the GPI anchor and these cells are therefore far less susceptible to lysis as a result [19]. Biological modification of these aerolysins (such that they still bind to the anchor but without lysing normal cells) and their linking to a fluorescent chromophore has led to the availability of a proaerolysin variant (FLAER) suitable for use in the diagnostic laboratory [20]. FLAER is more reliable than anti-CD59 in the detection of PNH clones when assessing peripheral blood leucocytes; it shows a high sensitivity and specificity in defining GPI deficient cells and is able to detect very small clones in patients with aplastic anaemia [21, 22]. Because it binds to the GPI anchor, and not to the antigens linked to it, its activity is less dependent on the maturational stage of myeloid cells. Most diagnostic laboratories therefore currently use FLAER as part of their PNH screening profile on leucocytes [23].

Indications for paroxysmal nocturnal haemoglobinuria screening

Patients with PNH clones can present with a wide variety of symptoms, signs and laboratory abnormalities. It is useful, therefore, to have a set of criteria which are good indications for PNH screening. The first consensus guideline on PNH diagnosis and monitoring [24] has set out the circumstances in which screening for PNH clones is important, summarised as follows:

1 Intravascular haemolysis with haemoglobinuria
2 Thrombosis involving unusual sites:
   a hepatic, portal, splanchnic or splenic veins
   b dermal veins
   c cerebral veins
3 Bone marrow failure with:
   a marrow hypoplasia
   b unilineage dysplasia
   c unexplained peripheral cytopenias

The age of the peripheral blood specimen is important in that alteration in scatter and antigen expression can change in granulocyte populations on storage. Our experience, and that of others, suggests that specimens should be processed within 48 hours [24]. As the sample ages some antigen expression is lost, for example CD16, and as neutrophil cells die they can show non-specific antibody adsorption. It is recommended that PB samples are collected into EDTA, that ammonium chloride red cell lysis be utilized for leucocyte assessment and that at least 5000 events, analysing the appropriate cell lineage, are recorded. Note that a large number of events require to be collected in situations where a high sensitivity is required, such as in the detection of very small PNH clones.

Analysis of red cells

Red cells are easily assessed by flow cytometry for defective antigen expression, the most frequently studied being CD55 and CD59. Cells may show normal expression (type I cells), partial deficiency (type II cells) or complete deficiency (type III cells) of the relevant antigen, illustrated schematically in Figure 10.1.

The relative proportions of each deficient population can be quantified as this is relevant to the presenting features and to potential future clinical consequences of the disease for the patient. Notably, all patients with haemolytic PNH have type III red cells and the majority of cases have more than 20% [1]. In contrast, hypoplastic PNH patients are more likely to have small type III populations and so are much less inclined to haemolysis. Type II cells

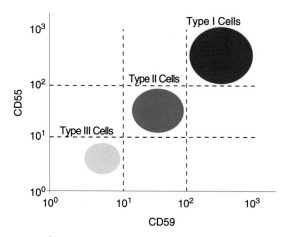

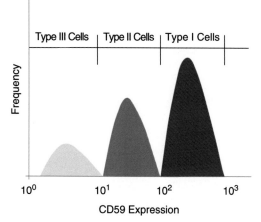

Figure 10.1 Schematic representation of normal, partial loss and complete loss of GPI anchor related antigen expression in PNH.

show some preservation of CD55 and CD59, so haemolysis, if present, tends to be mild. Furthermore, the risk of thrombotic complications also appears to be related to clone size; in one study no patients with less than 61% PNH phenotype granulocytes (type II or type III together) developed a thrombosis compared to half of those with a clone above this level. For each 10% change in total clone size the risk of thrombosis increased by a ratio of 1.64 [8], thrombosis being the major cause of death in PNH [1, 25]. It is important, therefore, to not only accurately define the total PNH clone but to quantify the subsets of type II and type III cells as this is closely correlated with clinical phenotype [1]. Note that type II cells are more easily defined on red cells than they are on granulocytes [24]. As the size of the PNH clone can change over time, appropriate monitoring can influence

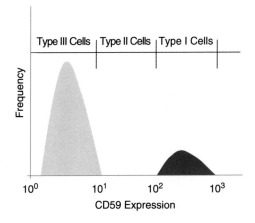

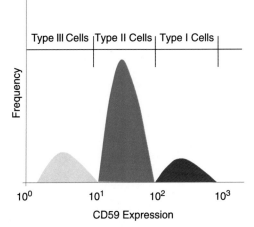

Figure 10.2 Plot illustrating how the PNH clone size and type influences clinical phenotype. A large type III clone (upper example) (left) is associated with severe intravascular haemolysis and high thrombotic risk. A large total clone, but small type III clone is seen in patients with modest or minimal haemolysis but still a high thrombotic risk (lower image).

decisions on appropriate prophylactic anti-thrombotic treatment [2].

A schematic illustration of how cell type influences phenotype is presented in Figure 10.2 above.

The apparent size of the abnormal red cell population, however, is always likely to be less than that quantified on granulocytes in haemolytic PNH due to the preferential loss of susceptible red cells through complement mediated haemolysis and from the restorative effect of blood transfusion [13]. The difference in deficient populations when comparing red cells with granulocytes can be up to three-fold [1]. As PNH red cells are constantly being lost in haemolytic patients, it has been reported that reticulo-

cyte analysis is more reliable in accurately defining clone size and gives estimations higher than red cells and closer to those on leucocytes [26]. The size of the PNH clone can therefore be easily underestimated if red cell analysis is performed in isolation, and this is one of the main reasons why most laboratories prefer granulocyte analysis.

Analysis of granulocytes

A number of antigens are suitable for assessment on granulocytes as noted above. As with red cells, it is recommended that deficiency of more than one antigen is demonstrated. Granulocytes can be gated by using a FSC/SSC approach or by using CD15, CD33 or CD45 versus SSC, for example, prior to analysis for the potentially deficient antigens (Figure 10.3). It is clearly important not to use an antigen that is GPI linked for the selection of the neutrophil gate. If side scatter properties are being used for gating alongside a lineage specific antigen it is important to be aware of hypogranular neutrophils which might be encountered in myelodysplastic syndromes.

Antibodies to CD16, CD24, CD55, CD59 and CD66 are all suitable for PNH screening on granulocytes [13], but blood samples should ideally be fresh, as a degree of antigen loss and non-specific antibody binding can occur with cells undergoing apoptosis [27]. Particularly valuable, as discussed above, is the semisynthetic fluorochrome linked proaerolysin, FLAER. It is often used in combination with CD16, CD24 or CD66 when screening granulocytes. The use of FLAER typically produces tight and better defined populations, allowing more accurate clone quantitation compared to traditional antibodies (Figures 10.4, 10. 5 and 10.6).

Analysis of monocytes

Monocyte analysis is generally less popular in the screening and evaluation of PNH. It does, however, give equivalent results to granulocyte analysis. Monocytes can be gated using a CD33, CD64 or CD4 versus SSC strategy. CD14 cannot be used to define lineage as it is GPI linked, but gives good discrimination of PNH clones once the monocytes are accurately gated. A combination of CD45, CD33, CD24 and FLAER allows the simultaneous screening of peripheral blood granulocytes and monocytes in one tube [18].

Monocytes might be preferred as the screening cell of choice in the following circumstances:
• Patients with severe neutropenia, where granulocytes are scarce

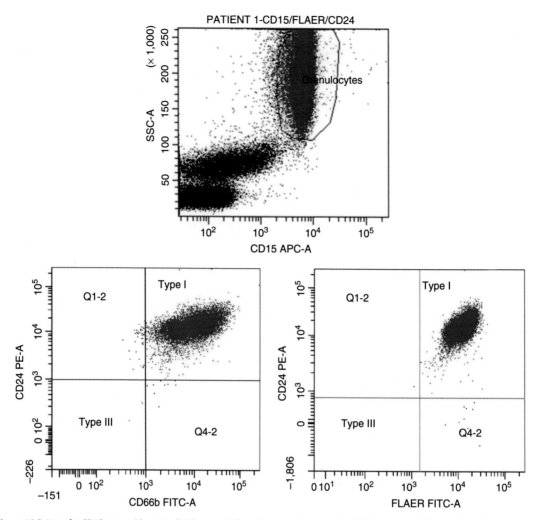

Figure 10.3 Use of a CD15 versus side scatter (SSC) approach for gating granulocytes and a CD24 versus CD66b, together with a CD24 versus FLAER analysis showing normal antigen expression. Note how tightly clustered the events are with FLAER compared to CD66b.

• Patients with relative excess of eosinophils (CD13+ CD16−) to neutrophils

• Patients with prominent myeloid left shift (CD13+ CD16dim) in peripheral blood

As with granulocytes, there are multiple possible approaches to monocyte evaluation.

Analysis of lymphocytes

Even though PNH is a stem cell disorder, screening of peripheral blood lymphocytes and NK cells is not routinely recommended. Lymphocytes are long-lived cells and in patients acquiring a PNH clone it may take a while

to become evident in lymphocyte populations. Conversely, PNH clones may still be detectable in lymphocytes long after the disease has remitted and where a granulocyte clone is no longer present [28]. In addition, lymphocyte subset analysis is often itself abnormal in PNH, so further complicating the issue [29].

Analysis of platelets

As thrombosis is a major feature of PNH, being responsible for significant morbidity and mortality, the analysis of platelets appears attractive. The implications of GPI anchor deficiencies on platelet function are not well

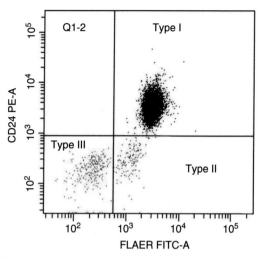

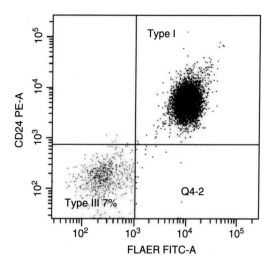

Figure 10.4 Illustration of the value of FLAER in characterization of PNH clones. Note relatively discrete normal population (black), type II cells (blue) and type III cells (red) using FLAER with CD24. By using CD24 alone the type II and type III cells could not be separated.

Figure 10.6 A small type III clone (7%) in a patient with aplastic anaemia.

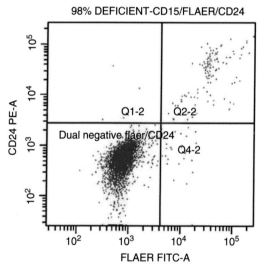

Figure 10.5 Identification of a large type III PNH clone (98%) in a patient with classic haemolytic PNH and a history of thrombosis, using FLAER/CD24.

understood but may relate to the marked pro-thrombotic tendency in this disease and the peculiar affinity of thrombosis for unusual sites. PNH clones have been reliably identified on platelets and their size seems to correlate with those on granulocytes [30, 31], but platelets are notoriously difficult to handle in the laboratory

as compared to leucocytes or red cells and currently do not provide any additional diagnostic data at the present time.

Paroxysmal nocturnal haemoglobinuria clones in myelodysplastic syndromes

This issue is discussed in more depth in Chapter 7. Suffice to say, PNH clones are not infrequently present in patients with bone marrow failure due to MDS and can be encountered in up to 18% of cases [32, 33]. As in AA, they may prosper due to lack of immune surveillance within a defective bone marrow environment. It is interesting to consider whether MDS patients with a PNH clone may have more of an immune dysfunctional pathogenesis to their disease similar to that of AA and whether immune suppression, may be therapeutically useful. Figure 10.7 shows a small PNH clone identified in a patient with apparent MDS who was initially blood and platelet transfusion dependent (Hb 80 g/L, platelets $<20 \times 10^9$/L). Treatment with ciclosporin for six months generated significant improvement in peripheral counts (Hb > 11 g/L, platelets >80 × 10^9/L).

In a number of studies, MDS patients with PNH clones appeared to have a disease with more favourable behaviour in terms of MDS subtype (all had refractory anaemia (RA)), risk of progression to acute leukaemia,

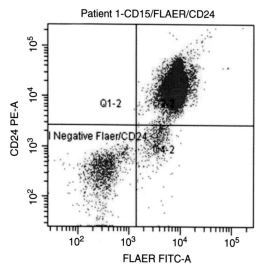

Patient 1-CD15/FLAER/CD24

Figure 10.7 Significant PNH clone (1.5% type III, 0.5% type II) in a patient with MDS.

prevalence of cytogenetic abnormalities and response to ciclosporin [33–35]. Other studies have found PNH populations in a more favourable group of RA patients but have highlighted the technical difficulties due to intrinsic altered antigen expression in MDS and neutrophil hypo-granulation influencing accurate gating of neutrophils and monocytes, making interpretation difficult in some cases [36].

Summary

Despite much interest in the value of flow cytometry in PNH diagnosis and the availability of new diagnostic antibodies there is still a requirement for consensus as to the optimal approach. Some notable recent publications have assisted in this respect. While the guideline of Borowitz *et al.* [24] has clarified some of these issues there is no real consensus as to what constitutes a significant clone, though most agree that 1% is a reasonable cut-off. Most normal populations can have clones up to this level, though the majority are much less than 0.5% [32]. The findings have always to be considered in relation to the clinical circumstances; a 1% clone could well be important in establishing the diagnosis and potential treatment options in favourable-risk MDS, but is very unlikely to be causal in a patient presenting with intravascular haemolysis. High sensitivity flow protocols for PNH clone screening are under development [23], so the

exact significance of low-level populations still remains to be determined.

It is important that the methodology is standardized as PNH is a rare disease and the quantitation of nature and size of clones can have important clinical implications. The United Kingdom National External Quality Assessment Scheme for leucocyte immunophenotyping (UK NEQAS LI) now distributes stabilized peripheral blood specimens for PNH EQA analysis [37, 38]. This is generating important feedback on the varied approaches to PNH screening and might further aid recommendations for the optimal approach in terms of cell choice and antibody profiles in various clinical scenarios.

Red cell membrane disorders

Hereditary spherocytosis (HS) is the most common inherited membrane disorder causing haemolytic disease among people of Northern European descent. Spherocytic red cells show decreased deformability within the microcirculation, premature sequestration in the spleen, extravascular haemolysis and a shortened red cell lifespan. Patients present with varying degrees of anaemia, jaundice, splenomegaly and pigment gall stones. The disorder, however, is rather heterogenous in that there are a number of genes, both dominant and recessive, controlling the production of several membrane proteins, all of which can be implicated in its pathogenesis.

The red cell membrane consists of two main layers, an outer lipid bilayer and an inner spectrin based cytoskeleton layer. These two layers have no direct contact but dynamically relate to each other to allow the fluid deformability and elasticity shown by normal cells. Deficiency or dysfunction in one or more of the cytoskeletal proteins results in disruption of the vertical interaction with the lipid bilayer, formation of spherocytes lacking deformability and subsequent premature splenic removal. Hereditary spherocytosis may result from inherited deficiencies of one or more of the following cytoskeletal proteins:

• Band 3
• Protein 4.2
• Ankyrin
• α and β spectrins

Furthermore, a number of different mutations in genes encoding each protein are encountered, so adding further

Table 10.2 Summary of the main features of the hereditary spherocytic disorders.

Defective protein	Mutation type	Blood film	Prevalence	Clinical picture
Beta spectrin	Dominant	Spherocytes Acanthocytes	15 to 20%	Mild/moderate haemolysis
Ankyrin	Dominant (or recessive)	Regular spherocytes	50%	Mild to severe haemolysis
Band 3	Dominant	Mushroom or pincered cells	20%	Mild haemolysis
Protein 4.2	Recessive	Stomatocytes Spherocytes	5%	Mild haemolysis
Alpha spectrin	Recessive	Variable	<5%	Variable

Table 10.3 Summary of the morphological features, cell volume characteristics and EMEA binding behaviour of the common inherited red cell membrane disorders (plus CDA type II).

Disorder	Membrane defect	MCV	Morphology	EMEA binding
Hereditary spherocytosis	Band 3 Spectrin Ankyrin Protein 4.2	N	Spherocytes Acanthocytes Pincered cells	Reduced
Hereditary elliptocytosis	Spectrin variants Partial protein 4.1 defect	N	Elliptocytes Ovalocytes	Normal
Hereditary pyropoikilocytosis	Band 3 Rh protein Rh Ag CD47	↓	Pleomorphic Spherocytes Micro-poikilocytes	Much reduced
South East Asian ovalocytosis	Band 3 defect (qualitative)	N	Ovalocytes Stomatocytes No anaemia	Reduced
Hereditary stomatocytosis	Stomatin deficiency	N/↑	Stomatocytes	Increased
Dehydrated stomatocytosis	Cation channel defect	N/↑	Pleomorphic Ovalocytes Stomatocytes	Increased
Cryohydrocytosis	Stomatin Protein 7.2	N/↑	Stomatocytes	Reduced
Congenital dyserythropoiesis type II	Band 3 defect (qualitative)	↑	Oval macrocytes Tear drop cells	Normal/ reduced

to the clinical and laboratory heterogeneity. Some patients have a severe chronic haemolytic anaemia whereas others only experience significant haemolysis during intercurrent infection. The nature of the membrane defect has a clear correlation with the clinical severity and laboratory parameters associated with HS in any given patient. Spectrin deficiencies, for example, tend

to cause more severe haemolysis and so are more likely to be diagnosed in childhood. Band 3 deficiency tends to cause a milder phenotype with more subtle red cell changes and is more likely to be diagnosed in adulthood [39] or even in the elderly. Hereditary spherocytosis may cause neonatal jaundice and in some cases requires exchange transfusion, but diagnosis can be difficult due to pleomorphic neonatal red cells. The presence of an MCHC over 360 g/L may be a useful pointer to this diagnosis in these circumstances [40].

A broad summary of the main features of HS according to type of mutation is presented in Table 10.2.

Many cases of HS present no diagnostic difficulty in the context of a family history of the disorder, clear haemolytic parameters and a typical blood film. Up to 25% of patients, however, do not report a family history of the disorder and have atypical or non-specific morphology. Reliable labora-

tory screening tests are therefore valuable in these cases. The traditional osmotic fragility test was cumbersome to perform, requires very accurate hypotonic dilutions and is not specific for HS, giving positive results in acquired spherocytic red cell disorders. False negative results can also be encountered in patients with coexistent iron deficiency and it is not a reliable test in neonates. This test is no longer recommended for use in HS diagnosis [41].

Flow cytometry has been successfully applied to the screening of patients for HS [42]. It is able to quantify

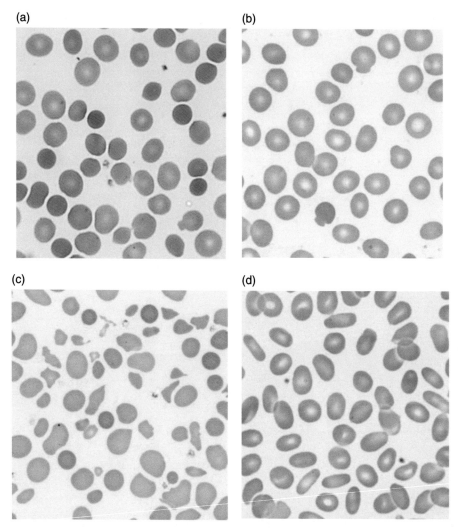

Figure 10.8 Typical morphological features which can assist in the diagnosis of inherited red cell membrane disorders. (a) Hereditary spherocytosis due to spectrin deficiency. (b) Hereditary spherocytosis due to band 3 deficiency. (c) Hereditary pyropoikilocytosis. (d) Hereditary elliptocytosis.

the fluorescence intensity of intact red cells labelled with the dye eosin-5-maleimide (EMEA), which reacts with cytoskeletal band 3 protein, Rh protein, Rh glyco-protein and CD47 [43]. HS patients show a distinct reduction in dye binding as compared to normal controls. Furthermore, the test is relatively easy to perform, gener-ates rapid results, has a high sensitivity and specificity and outperforms the osmotic fragility test [44–46]. In addition, the reduction in EMEA fluorescence appears to correlate with clinical severity of the underlying HS dis-order [43, 47] and the nature of the membrane protein defect as identified using polyacrylimide gel electropho-resis (SDS-PAGE) [47].It cannot, however be used in iso-lation as results have to be interpreted in the light of family history, clinical presentation and blood film mor-phology [48]. A number of non-HS inherited red cell disorders will also show reduction in in EMEA bind-ing, summarized in Table 10.3.

Notably, most cases of hereditary elliptocytosis show normal or mildly reduced binding [34, 41], but in the majority of patients the diagnosis of this condition is straightforward without the need for supplementary tests. A group of membrane disorders affecting cation exchange channels are characterized by excessive cation leak and in some cases pseudo-hyperkalaemia [42]. They are known collectively as hereditary stomatocytoses (HST) and actu-ally show increased EMEA fluorescence, so further improving the diagnostic utility of this investigation. The overhydrated and dehydrated forms of stomatocytosis show increased EMEA uptake, whilst that of cryohydro-cytosis [43] (a form of stomatocytosis with accelerated cation loss at 4 °C and sometimes neurodevelopmental disorders) is reduced [37]. It is important that HS is con-firmed and clearly defined from HST, in that splenectomy often benefits the former but not the latter, by signifi-cantly increasing the risk of thromboembolic complica-tions [44]. The typical morphological features of a selection of membrane disorders, is shown in Figure 10.8.

The coexistence of other haematological disorders, such as beta thalassaemia and sickle cell trait, or the effects of haematinic deficiency can all have variable effects on pres-entation and blood indices in HS, but EMEA absorption should not be altered. In selected cases, SDS PAGE might still be necessary and will assist diagnosis in equivocal cases.

It is important that each flow laboratory using this test develops an operating procedure in accordance with the protocols suggested in the defining publications [42, 45, 46] and evaluates the 'in-house' sensitivity and specificity by analysing cells from patients with an established HS diagnosis and other membrane disorders, alongside nor-mal controls. It is recommended that the EMEA MFI val-ues for test and controls are expressed as a ratio as the reagent fluorescence intensity deteriorates rapidly on storage [42]. Our practice is to freeze aliquots of new rea-gent at −40 °C and to thaw a sufficient amount at the time of each new diagnostic request. We also recommend using age-matched controls alongside the test sample. There is no published data to indicate that EMA binding is influenced by patient age, but we have noted a trend toward reduced binding in children less than one year of age. We therefore require six age-matched controls for testing alongside patient samples on all diagnostic requests (unpublished data) until this observation is veri-fied or refuted.

Foetal maternal haemorrhage

Haemolytic disease of the newborn (HDN) is the result of the passive transplacental transfer of maternal IgG alloantibodies, which are directed against foetal red cell antigens. It can result in varying degrees of anaemia and at worst intrauterine death due to hydrops foetalis. These maternal antibodies are produced following sensitization due to bleeding of foetal red cells, into the maternal cir-culation, across the placental barrier. The most serious HDN results in mothers with high titre anti-D directed against the D antigen of the Rhesus blood group system, the foetus having inherited the D antigen from the father. Once these antibodies are present they affect each subse-quent pregnancy where the foetus carries the D antigen. Such pregnancies are high risk, need careful monitoring in specialist centres and often require intervention with repeated intra-uterine transfusions. It is therefore pre-ferable in all cases to try and prevent the formation of maternal alloantibodies in pregnancy and anti-D pro-phylactic therapy has been highly successful in this respect [49]. Current UK practice is to give doses of 500iu anti-D at 28 weeks, 34 weeks and delivery [50]. This adopted antibody remains in the maternal circula-tion through the third trimester and peri-delivery, when trans-placental bleeds are most common, and it causes clearance of D positive foetal cells before a maternal immune response is activated. More than 99% of women

WORKED EXAMPLE 10.1

A 21-year-old female with a mild chronic anaemia, intermittent jaundice and a family history of an undefined red cell disorder was referred for investigation. The blood film showed prominent spherocytes, polychromasia and notably acanthocytes.

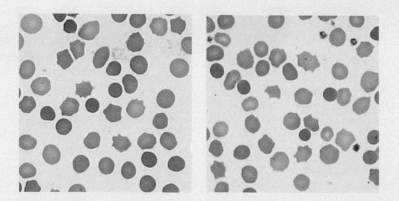

She had an absolute reticulocyte count of 220 ×10⁹/L, mild elevation of serum bilirubin and LDH and serum haptoglobin was absent. Her red cell EMEA binding study is illustrated below.

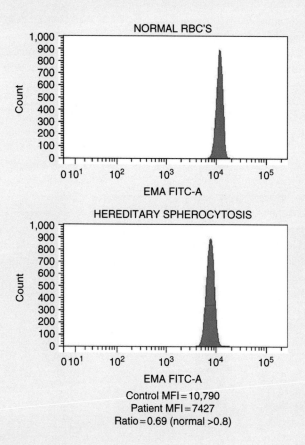

Control MFI = 10,790
Patient MFI = 7427
Ratio = 0.69 (normal >0.8)

These findings and morphology are consistent with hereditary spherocytosis; the presence of acanthocytes in addition to spherocytes might indicate a beta spectrin deficiency.

WORKED EXAMPLE 10.2

Illustrated below are three examples of FMH quantitation post delivery using an FITC labelled anti-D where the infant was confirmed to be Rh D positive. The red cells are gated on the FSC/SSC plot.

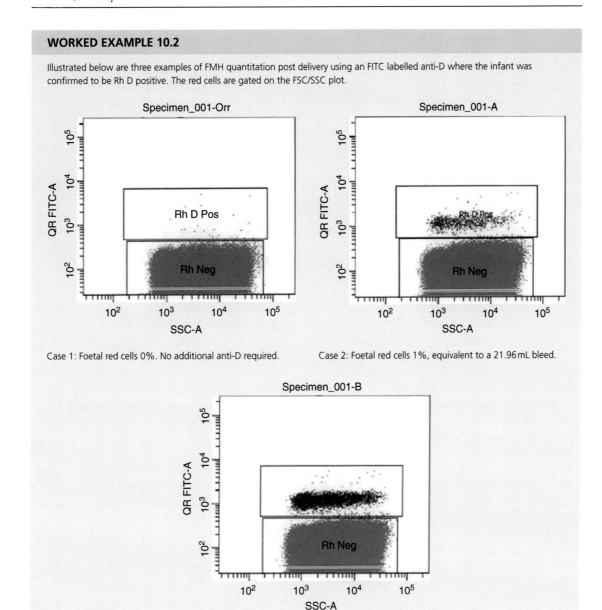

Case 1: Foetal red cells 0%. No additional anti-D required.

Case 2: Foetal red cells 1%, equivalent to a 21.96 mL bleed.

Case 3: Foetal red cells 2%, equivalent to a 43.92 mL bleed.

will have a foetomaternal haemorrhage of less than 4 mL at delivery. A 500iu dose of anti-D is capable of removing 4 mL of foetal RhD positive cells from the maternal circulation and so is adequate in most cases [50]. Additional doses might be necessary at other times during pregnancy, for example following abdominal trauma or invasive pre-natal tests or if a larger bleed is encountered at delivery. The quantitation of any potential FMH is necessary at these times to allow adequate anti-D prophylaxis, as large bleeds will require appropriate larger anti-D doses to allow rapid clearance. Historically, the Kleihauer-Betke (KB) method was the first method reported that was able to do this reliably [51]. It depends on the differential resistance to acid elution of red cells in maternal blood smears containing Hb A and Hb F; the former (the maternal cells) are eluted and appear as ghosts, whilst the latter (the foetal cells) are resistant and stain positively with eosin. The test, however, is technically difficult and subject to inter-operator variation in reporting. In addition, in mothers with high levels of Hb F due to a coexistent haemoglobinopathy or hereditary persistence of Hb F, it can be extremely difficult to define foetal from maternal cells and provide accurate FMH quantitation. Furthermore, the maternal level of HbF normally increases in pregnancy, further increasing the heterogeneity of staining [52].

Flow cytometry offers an alternative method for quantifying the magnitude of FMH [53] and the results it provides appear to be more accurate and reproducible [54, 55]. It allows the analysis of a large number of red cell events (500,000+) which further improves sensitivity and accuracy [56]. Two main types of antibody have been employed, either directed at HbF or the Rh D antigen. A limitation of the anti-D approach is that the foetal D type needs to be known so its use during the antenatal period is limited. For this reason the anti HbF antibody approach has been preferred [54, 57] and provides a simple, convenient, rapid and reproducible method which is particularly able to discriminate foetal cells from adult cells with increased Hb F [58, 59]. The method employs a brief red cell fixation followed by permeabilization, to allow access of the single antibody to intracellular Hb F [54]. Because of its relative simplicity the method shows excellent reproducibility between laboratories [60] and has allowed accurate quantitation of FMH following invasive prenatal tests [61].

Many laboratories still use the Kleihauer test to identify the small proportion of cases with a FMH of potentially greater than 4 mL. Flow cytometry is then performed on the same sample and the size of FMH is quantified as percentage of foetal red cells. This can then be transposed into an actual volume of foetal red cells using the formula [62]:

$$\left(\text{Percentage foetal cells} \times 1800 \times 1.22\right)\text{mL}$$

Where 1800 represents the maternal red cell volume and 1.22 corrects for cord blood MCV.

An additional 500 iu of anti-D are required to clear each 4 mL of foetal blood over 4 mL. In other words, an 8 mL

haemorrhage requires an additional 500 iu to the standard 500 iu dose given at delivery (total 1000 iu). Further assessment of the maternal sample for remaining foetal red cells is recommended at 72 hours to confirm clearing. If foetal red cells persist (again quantified by flow cytometry) then further doses of anti-D, in proportion to the residual volume of foetal cells, should be administered [62].

More recently, a combined two-colour dual antibody method utilizing anti-HbF and anti-D, has been described [63]. The method was calibrated by spiking non-pregnant D negative donor samples with foetal red cells and showed a high degree of accuracy. In addition to quantifying FMH this method has the ability to ascertain the foetal D type, which is clearly of additional benefit in managing the pregnancy.

Lymphocyte subset analysis and immunodeficiency

See also Chapter 4.

One of the commonest applications of flow cytometry in non-neoplastic conditions is in lymphocyte subset analysis, particularly in the context of the inherited and acquired immunodeficiency disorders. For example, CD4$^+$ lymphocyte counts are commonly used to assess response to treatment in patients infected with HIV and the degree of T-cell depletion in patients undergoing treatment with fludarabine, alemtuzumab and bone marrow transplant.

The following subsets, expressed as relative and absolute values, are commonly assessed:
- Total CD3$^+$ T-cells
- CD3$^+$ CD4$^+$ T helper subset
- CD3$^+$ CD8$^+$ T suppressor subset
- CD5$^+$ T-cells
- CD19$^+$ B-cells
- CD3$^-$ CD16$^+$ CD56$^+$ NK cells

There are specific guidelines for CD4 enumerations in HIV infected patients using a single platform [64].

Haemopoietic stem cell enumeration

Autologous or allogeneic haemopoietic stem cell transplant is commonly used in the treatment of patients with relapsed and refractory leukaemias and lymphomas. It is essential that a minimum number of CD34$^+$ cells are harvested, processed and reinfused if the bone marrow is to be successfully repopulated following chemoradiotherapy conditioning [65]. The timing of stem cell harvesting from patients and donors is carefully guided by peripheral blood CD34+ cell counts, which accurately predict the likelihood of satisfactory peripheral blood leucapheresis. A number of different approaches to CD34 quantitation have been described, including the Milan/Mulhouse, single platform (flow cytometer alone) and dual platform (haematology analyser and flow cytometer) ISHAGE (International Society for Haematotherapy and Graft Engineering) protocols. These methods seem to give comparable results [66]. The ISHAGE protocol, which identifies stem cells in the CD45^{dim}, CD34+, SSC^{low} compartment, is described in more detail in Chapter 2. A number of recommendations, including the use of bright fluorochrome anti-CD34 monoclonals able to detect all glycoforms of CD34, counterstaining with CD45, careful exclusion of platelets, unlysed red cells and debris and utilization of low side scatter properties were made by the European Working Group on Clinical Cell Analysis [67]. Standardization of any flow cytometry protocol is clearly essential, but even more so in protocols for CD34 cell enumeration where the aim is to produce a therapeutic cell product for patient haemopoietic rescue.

Granulocyte disorders

Some selected inherited disorders of granulocyte function are assessable using flow cytometric techniques.

A full discussion of these rare and complex disorders is outside the scope of this text, but some basic principles are presented here for completeness. Comprehensive investigation of suspected granulocyte disorders should be performed in recognized reference centres.

These disorders are characterized by recurrent bacterial or fungal infections involving skin, soft tissues, sinuses, middle ear and lung, often starting in childhood. The most prevalent of these disorders, chronic granulomatous disease (CGD), which is a disorder of phagocyte oxidase activity, shows X-linked inheritance and is variable in clinical severity between families. Some studies have used the ability of neutrophils to generate peroxidase dependent green fluorescence, after pre-treatment with dihydrorhodamine 123, as a tool in diagnosis in CGD [68], alongside the standard nitroblue tetrazolium test and genetic profiling. The other disorders are all rare but flow cytometry studies may assist if certain conditions are being considered (Table 10.4).

Finally, it is worth noting congenital myeloperoxidase (MPO) deficiency. Myeloperoxidase is a haem protein localized in the azurophilic granules of neutrophils and the lysosomes of monocytes and is involved in killing of several microorganisms. Myeloperoxidase deficiency is a relatively common anomaly, which affects approximately 1 in 2000 individuals, with the degree of enzyme loss ranging from partial to complete [74]. It can be noted incidentally, in affected individuals, when using automated analysers which incorporate myeloperoxidase staining in determining the leucocyte differential count [75]. Many individuals are asymptomatic, but some

Table 10.4 Summary of inherited functional granulocyte disorders that might be assessed using flow cytometry.

Disorder	Defect/features	Antigen assessable
Chronic granulomatous disease [69]	Peroxide/NADPH oxidase killing, X-linked or autosomal recessive, granuloma formation	Cytoplasmic peroxidase
Leukocyte adhesion disorder type I [70]	Impaired tissue migration, neutrophilia Lack of tissue inflammation	CD11 expression CD18 expression
Leukocyte adhesion disorder type II [71]	Neutrophilia Impaired growth Mental retardation	CD15s expression
Neutrophil specific granule deficiency [72, 73]	Impaired migration, phagocytosis and intracellular killing Deficiency of type I/II granules Abnormal neutrophil morphology	CD15 expression CD16 expression CD66 expression

WORKED EXAMPLE 10.3 NEUTROPHIL SPECIFIC GRANULE DEFICIENCY

A young adult male presented with a chronic external malleolar soft tissue infection, which had been present for many months and had failed to clear with repeated courses of broad-spectrum antibiotics and previous attempts at skin grafting. He gave a history of repeated bacterial infections (mainly staphylococcal and streptococcal species) from infancy; his sister and mother were similarly affected.

In contrast to the other inherited granulocyte disorders his neutrophils showed abnormal morphology; the neutrophils were hypogranular with abnormal nuclear segmentation. Some neutrophils were difficult to differentiate from monocytes because of the relative absence of granules.

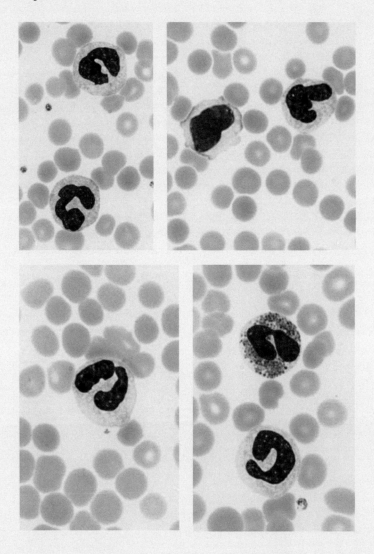

This abnormal granulation leads to a misidentification of neutrophils as monocytes by automated analysers as the reduced side scatter superimposes the neutrophils onto the monocyte zone (FSC/SSC plot), not only falsely elevating the monocyte count but also indicating an apparent neutropenia. Previous investigations in other hospitals had been directed toward the investigation of an inherited neutropenia syndrome rather than a granulocyte function disorder. Note also that the patient eosinophils also show a degree of reduced side scatter.

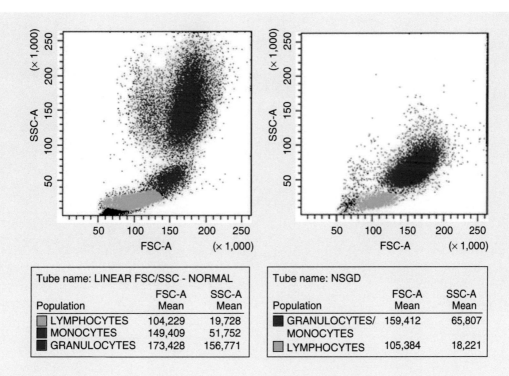

Tube name: LINEAR FSC/SSC - NORMAL		
Population	FSC-A Mean	SSC-A Mean
▨ LYMPHOCYTES	104,229	19,728
■ MONOCYTES	149,409	51,752
■ GRANULOCYTES	173,428	156,771

Tube name: NSGD		
Population	FSC-A Mean	SSC-A Mean
■ GRANULOCYTES/ MONOCYTES	159,412	65,807
▨ LYMPHOCYTES	105,384	18,221

FSC/SSC plot: abnormal side scatter of neutrophils in NSGD, normal control left, patient right (neutrophils red, monocytes blue, lymphocytes green).

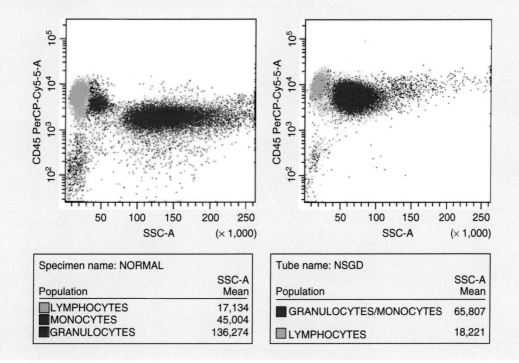

Specimen name: NORMAL	
Population	SSC-A Mean
▨ LYMPHOCYTES	17,134
■ MONOCYTES	45,004
■ GRANULOCYTES	136,274

Tube name: NSGD	
Population	SSC-A Mean
■ GRANULOCYTES/MONOCYTES	65,807
▨ LYMPHOCYTES	18,221

CD45/SSC plot: abnormal side scatter of neutrophils in NSGD, normal control left, patient right (neutrophils red, monocytes blue, lymphocytes green). Note in both SSC plots above how the monocyte population is obscured by the hypogranular neutrophils.

Flow cytometric studies of the patient's granulocytes indicated a significant reduction in surface CD15 and CD66 (shown below, normal control left, patient right) together with reduced CD16 expression (not shown).

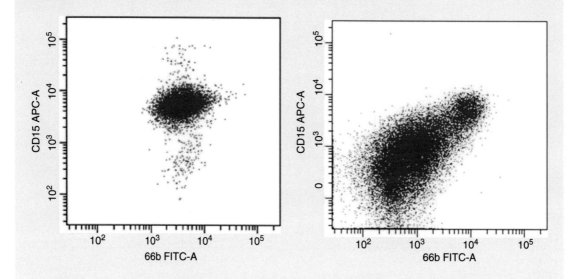

Cytoplasmic lactoferrin and myeloperoxidase expression was also significantly reduced.

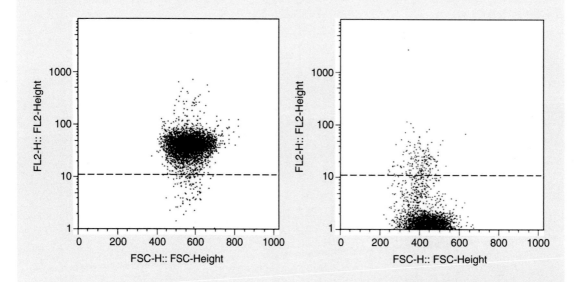

Lactoferrin plot: cytoplasmic lactoferrin expression (y axis) in a normal control (left) and the patient (right). Courtesy of Dr G. Sandilands, University of Glasgow.

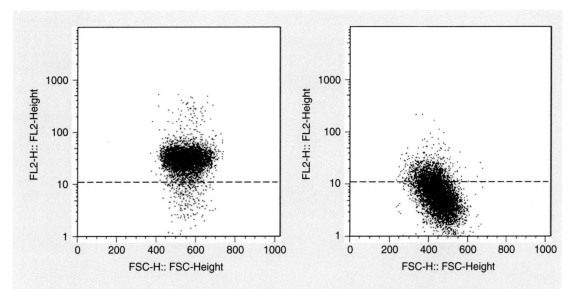

Myeloperoxidase plot: cytoplasmic myeloperoxidase expression (y axis) in a normal control (left) and the patient (right). Courtesy of Dr G. Sandilands, University of Glasgow.

These findings are all in keeping with a diagnosis of neutrophil specific granule deficiency. Neutrophil specific granule deficiency neutrophils show multiple functional abnormalities, including abnormal migration, phagocytosis and intracellular microbial killing.

series have shown a definite increase in the frequency of infections and prevalence of inflammatory disorders. Notably, candida species infections, sometimes invasive, have been observed, particularly in patients who also have diabetes. It has been postulated that total MPO deficiency might predispose to solid tumours as affected granulocytes *in vivo* show reduced lytic activity against malignant cells and may be partially implicated in the pathophysiology of atherosclerosis, Alzheimer's disease and multiple sclerosis [76]. Of course, we should also remember that anti-MPO diagnostic antibodies will not be useful in the flow cytometric determination of lineage in MPO deficient patients with acute leukaemia.

Platelet disorders

A variety of inherited and acquired platelet disorders can also be assessed using flow cytometry, but current applications are still limited or subject to development in the research environment [77]. The availability of new commercial antibodies has extended the potential

applications, but FCM diagnosis has been far less important than that seen in WBC analysis. Similar to above, the more complex investigations are best coordinated by reference laboratories. Platelets can be difficult to handle *in vitro* and unfixed samples are subject to inadvertent spontaneous activation when being handled in the lab. They also vary significantly in size ranging from 1 μm to 5 μm in diameter, with corresponding marked variation in volume: this has implications for identifying platelets in scatter plots during flow studies. Platelets also have a tendency to adhere to leucocytes *in vitro*, further confusing the situation. Finally, platelet fixatives might alter the antigenic profile of apparent resting steady state platelets. The availability of new fixatives, which are able to stabilize the antigenic profile, may at least partially address this situation [78].

Inherited disorders

A number of inherited qualitative platelet disorders can be identified using FCM studies. Detection of defective platelet receptors in these conditions is relatively straightforward and follows principles similar to those for assessing

Table 10.5 Summary of the inherited platelet disorders amenable to diagnosis using flow cytometry.

Disorder	Defect	Antigen (ref)
Von-Willebrand disease	Von-Willebrand factor	VWF Ag [79]
Glanzmann's thrombasthaenia	Deficiency GPIIb/IIIa	CD41, CD61 [80, 81]
Bernard Soulier syndrome	GPIb-IX-V complex	CD42b, CD42a, CD42d [82]
Storage pool disease	Defective dense granules	Serotonin [83]

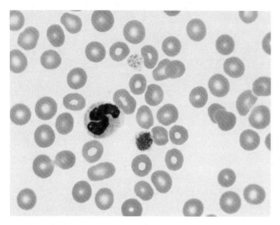

Figure 10.9 Large platelets and thrombocytopenia in Bernard Soulier syndrome.

leucocytes. The disorders where membrane or granule antigen expression can be quantified are summarized in Table 10.5. Bernard Soulier syndrome is one of the most easily characterized inherited platelet disorders, in that in addition to platelet dysfunction, these patients also show thrombocytopenia with macroplatelets (Figure 10.9).

More recently, a subgroup of autosomal dominant inherited thrombocytopenias without macro-platelets, has been shown to have a reduced expression of the GPIa/IIa complex (major collagen receptor) [84]. This is clearly an area for future development in terms of further classifying the inherited qualitative and quantitative platelet disorders.

Acquired disorders

A number of acquired platelet disorders, which are much more frequently encountered in clinical practice,

are also amenable to assessment using flow. There is much interest in the potential role of activated platelets in the pathophysiology of arterial thrombotic disease [70]. A number of studies have been directed at the quantitation of platelet activity in the context of cardiovascular risk, analysing expression of markers of *in vivo* activation such as CD40L, CD62P (P selectin) and CD63. Increased platelet activation, as quantified by flow cytometry, has been documented in a wide variety of vascular disorders including acute ischaemic stroke, coronary thrombosis, pre-eclampsia, diabetic retinopathy and peripheral vascular disease [85–89]. Platelet activation is also common post surgery [90], particularly cardiac bypass surgery [91].

Furthermore, activated platelets adhere to neutrophils and monocytes to form aggregates as well as generating platelet microparticles: these phenomena can be assessed by flow using combinations of antibodies to assess cell type, together with markers of platelet activation and gating according to cell scatter properties [92]. Platelet microparticles (PMP) are vesicles released during *in vivo* platelet activation. They generate platelet activating factor (PAF), express high affinity receptors for factor VIII and receptors for endothelial adhesion, such as P selectin (CD62P) [93]. They also promote endothelial tissue factor release and encourage leucocyte endothelial adhesion at sites of high shear stress and have been directly implicated in the pathogenesis of arteriosclerosis [94]. They are easily quantified and characterized using flow cytometric methods [95, 96].

Finally, there is some evidence that increased platelet membrane expression of CD154 (CD40 ligand) is able to activate auto-reactive B lymphocytes and may at least partially be implicated in the pathogenesis of immune thrombocytopenia [97].

Monitoring of antiplatelet drug therapy

Antiplatelet agents are commonly used for prophylaxis or treatment of a wide spectrum of arterial diseases. Aspirin is the oldest and still most frequently used drug in cardiovascular disorders. It impairs prostaglandin synthesis and so protects from *in vivo* platelet adhesion/activation. Thus, the aspirin effect on platelets can be assessed using flow cytometric quantitation of markers of activation such as CD62P [98]. It may be clinically important to quantify aspirin effect as patients show variable responses to a fixed dose. In patients with aspirin resistance and unstable cardiovascular syndromes a higher dose might be appropriate to generate the desired effect and so protect from progressive thrombus formation over an atherosclerotic plaque or coronary stent [99]. In contrast, aspirin hyper-responders might be more at risk of bleeding during surgical [100] or percutaneous stenting procedures. Flow cytometric analysis, therefore, might allow individualized aspirin dosing.

The thienopyridine drugs, clopidogrel and ticlopidine act by blocking *in vivo* ADP mediated platelet activation. Clopidogrel is commonly used to reduce platelet activation around the time of an acute coronary event and for secondary prophylaxis. It is often used in combination with aspirin as the two are synergistic and act through different mechanisms. This synergism can be demonstrated using flow studies by quantifying platelet activation [101, 102].

Finally, the GPIIb/IIIa receptor antagonists, such as abciximab, are also used to inhibit platelet reactivity in acute coronary syndromes, sometimes in combination with aspirin or clopidogrel. Their effect can be quantified by assessing receptor occupancy by drug [103] or by features of activation as before. These studies might allow more rational choice of drug combinations and methods of drug delivery in order to achieve fast and effective platelet blockade in patients with acute coronary syndromes.

References

1 Hillmen P, *et al.* Natural history of paroxysmal nocturnal hemoglobinuria. *N Engl J Med* 1995, **333**(19): 1253–8.

2 Parker C, *et al.* Diagnosis and management of paroxysmal nocturnal hemoglobinuria. *Blood* 2005, **106**(12): 3699–709.

3 Bessler M, *et al.* Mutations in the PIG-A gene causing partial deficiency of GPI-linked surface proteins (PNH II) in patients with paroxysmal nocturnal haemoglobinuria. *Br J Haematol* 1994, **87**(4): 863–6.

4 Bessler M, *et al.* Paroxysmal nocturnal haemoglobinuria (PNH) is caused by somatic mutations in the PIG-A gene. *EMBO J* 1994, **13**(1): 110–7.

5 Karadimitris A, *et al.* Abnormal T-cell repertoire is consistent with immune process underlying the pathogenesis of paroxysmal nocturnal hemoglobinuria. *Blood* 2000, **96**(7): 2613–20.

6 Karadimitris A, *et al.* PNH cells are as sensitive to T-cell-mediated lysis as their normal counterparts: implications for the pathogenesis of paroxysmal nocturnal haemoglobinuria. *Br J Haematol* 2000, **111**(4): 1158–63.

7 Almeida AM, *et al.* Hypomorphic promoter mutation in PIGM causes inherited glycosylphosphatidylinositol deficiency. *Nat Med* 2006, **12**(7): 846–51.

8 Moyo VM, *et al.* Natural history of paroxysmal nocturnal haemoglobinuria using modern diagnostic assays. *Br J Haematol* 2004, **126**(1): 133–8.

9 Richards SJ, Hillmen P. Advances in the laboratory diagnosis of paroxysmal nocturnal haemoglobinuria. *Clinical and Applied Immunology Reviews* 2001(Rev 1): 315–30.

10 van der Schoot CE, *et al.* Deficiency of glycosyl-phosphatidylinositol-linked membrane glycoproteins of leukocytes in paroxysmal nocturnal hemoglobinuria, description of a new diagnostic cytofluorometric assay. *Blood* 1990, **76**(9): 1853–9.

11 Nicholson-Weller A, Spicer DB, Austen KF. Deficiency of the complement regulatory protein, 'decay-accelerating factor', on membranes of granulocytes, monocytes, and platelets in paroxysmal nocturnal hemoglobinuria. *N Engl J Med* 1985, **312**(17): 1091–7.

12 Thomason RW, *et al.* Identification of unsuspected PNH-type cells in flow cytometric immunophenotypic analysis of peripheral blood and bone marrow. *Am J Clin Pathol* 2004, **122**(1): 128–34.

13 Olteanu H, *et al.* Differential usefulness of various markers in the flow cytometric detection of paroxysmal nocturnal hemoglobinuria in blood and bone marrow. *Am J Clin Pathol* 2006, **126**(5): 781–8.

14 Stetler-Stevenson M, *et al.* Diagnostic utility of flow cytometric immunophenotyping in myelodysplastic syndrome. *Blood* 2001, **98**(4): 979–87.

15 Xu Y, *et al.* Flow cytometric analysis of monocytes as a tool for distinguishing chronic myelomonocytic leukemia from reactive monocytosis. *Am J Clin Pathol* 2005, **124**(5): 799–806.

16 Yamamoto K, *et al.* Evidence for a novel polymorphism affecting both N-linked glycosylation and ligand binding of the IgG receptor IIIB (CD16). *Tissue Antigens* 2001, **57**(4): 363–6.

17 Wu J, *et al.* A novel polymorphism of FcgammaRIIIa (CD16) alters receptor function and predisposes to autoimmune disease. *J Clin Invest* 1997, **100**(5): 1059–70.

18 Yamashina M, *et al.* Inherited complete deficiency of 20-kilodalton homologous restriction factor (CD59) as a cause of paroxysmal nocturnal hemoglobinuria. *N Engl J Med* 1990, **323**(17): 1184–9.

19 Brodsky RA, *et al.* Resistance of paroxysmal nocturnal hemoglobinuria cells to the glycosylphosphatidylinositol-binding toxin aerolysin. *Blood* 1999, **93**(5): 1749–56.

20 Brodsky RA, *et al.*, Improved detection and characterization of paroxysmal nocturnal hemoglobinuria using fluorescent aerolysin. *Am J Clin Pathol* 2000, **114**(3): 459–66.

21 Sutherland DR, *et al.* Use of a FLAER-based WBC assay in the primary screening of PNH clones. *Am J Clin Pathol* 2009, **132**(4): 564–72.

22 Sutherland DR, *et al*. Diagnosing PNH with FLAER and multiparameter flow cytometry. *Cytometry B Clin Cytom* 2007, **72**(3): 167–77.

23 Battiwalla M, *et al*. Multiparameter flow cytometry for the diagnosis and monitoring of small GPI-deficient cellular populations. *Cytometry B Clin Cytom* 2010, **78**(5): 348–56.

24 Borowitz MJ, *et al*. Guidelines for the diagnosis and monitoring of paroxysmal nocturnal hemoglobinuria and related disorders by flow cytometry. *Cytometry B Clin Cytom* 2010, **78**(4): 211–30.

25 Socie G, *et al*. Paroxysmal nocturnal haemoglobinuria: long-term follow-up and prognostic factors. French Society of Haematology. *Lancet* 1996, **348**(9027): 573–7.

26 Hochsmann B, Rojewski M, Schrezenmeier H. Paroxysmal nocturnal hemoglobinuria (PNH): higher sensitivity and validity in diagnosis and serial monitoring by flow cytometric analysis of reticulocytes. *Ann Hematol* 2011, **90**(8): 887–99.

27 Dransfield I, *et al*. Neutrophil apoptosis is associated with a reduction in CD16 (Fc gamma RIII) expression. *J Immunol* 1994, **153**(3): 1254–63.

28 Nakakuma H, *et al*. Persistence of affected T lymphocytes in long-term clinical remission in paroxysmal nocturnal hemoglobinuria. *Blood* 1994, **84**(11): 3925–8.

29 Richards SJ, *et al*. Lymphocyte subset analysis and glycosylphosphatidylinositol phenotype in patients with paroxysmal nocturnal hemoglobinuria. *Blood*, 1998, **92**(5): 1799–806.

30 Jin JY, *et al*. Glycosylphosphatidyl-inositol (GPI)-linked protein deficiency on the platelets of patients with aplastic anaemia and paroxysmal nocturnal haemoglobinuria: two distinct patterns correlating with expression on neutrophils. *Br J Haematol* 1997, **96**(3): 493–6.

31 Vu T, *et al*. Aplastic anaemia and paroxysmal nocturnal haemoglobinuria: a study of the GPI-anchored proteins on human platelets. *Br J Haematol* 1996, **93**(3): 586–9.

32 Maciejewski JP, *et al*. Relationship between bone marrow failure syndromes and the presence of glycophosphatidyl inositol-anchored protein-deficient clones. *Br J Haematol* 2001, **115**(4): 1015–22.

33 Wang H, *et al*. Clinical significance of a minor population of paroxysmal nocturnal hemoglobinuria-type cells in bone marrow failure syndrome. *Blood* 2002, **100**(12): 3897–902.

34 Nakao S, Sugimori C, Yamazaki H. Clinical significance of a small population of paroxysmal nocturnal hemoglobinuria-type cells in the management of bone marrow failure. *Int J Hematol* 2006, **84**(2): 118–22.

35 Sugimori C, *et al*. Minor population of CD55⁻CD59⁻ blood cells predicts response to immuosuppressive therapy and prognosis in patients with aplastic anemia. *Blood* 2006, **107**(4): 1308–14.

36 Wang SA, *et al*. Detection of paroxysmal nocturnal hemoglobinuria clones in patients with myelodysplastic syndromes and related bone marrow diseases, with emphasis on diagnostic pitfalls and caveats. *Haematologica* 2009, **94**(1): 29–37.

37 Richards SJ, Barnett D. The role of flow cytometry in the diagnosis of paroxysmal nocturnal hemoglobinuria in the clinical laboratory. *Clin Lab Med* 2007, **27**(3): 577–90, vii.

38 Richards SJ, *et al*. Development and evaluation of a stabilized whole-blood preparation as a process control material for screening of paroxysmal nocturnal hemoglobinuria by flow cytometry. *Cytometry B Clin Cytom* 2008, **76B**(1): 47–55.

39 Mariani M, *et al*. Clinical and hematologic features of 300 patients affected by hereditary spherocytosis grouped according to the type of the membrane protein defect. *Haematologica* 2008, **93**(9): 1310–7.

40 Christensen RD, Henry E. Hereditary spherocytosis in neonates with hyperbilirubinemia. *Pediatrics* 2010, **125**(1): 120–5.

41 Bolton-Maggs PH, *et al*. Guidelines for the diagnosis and management of hereditary spherocytosis. *Br J Haematol* 2004, **126**(4): 455–74.

42 King MJ, *et al*. Rapid flow cytometric test for the diagnosis of membrane cytoskeleton-associated haemolytic anaemia. *Br J Haematol* 2000, **111**(3): 924–33.

43 King MJ, *et al*. Detection of hereditary pyropoikilocytosis by the eosin-5-maleimide (EMA)-binding test is attributable to a marked reduction in EMA-reactive transmembrane proteins. *Int J Lab Hematol* 2011, **33**(2): 205–11.

44 Kar R, Mishra P, Pati HP. Evaluation of eosin-5-maleimide flow cytometric test in diagnosis of hereditary spherocytosis. *Int J Lab Hematol* 2010, **32**(1 Pt 2): 8–16.

45 King MJ, Smythe JS, Mushens R. Eosin-5-maleimide binding to band 3 and Rh-related proteins forms the basis of a screening test for hereditary spherocytosis. *Br J Haematol* 2004, **124**(1): 106–13.

46 King MJ, *et al*. Using the eosin-5-maleimide binding test in the differential diagnosis of hereditary spherocytosis and hereditary pyropoikilocytosis. *Cytometry B Clin Cytom* 2008, **74**(4): 244–50.

47 Crisp RL, *et al*. A prospective study to assess the predictive value for hereditary spherocytosis using five laboratory tests (cryohemolysis test, eosin-5'-maleimide flow cytometry, osmotic fragility test, autohemolysis test, and SDS-PAGE) on 50 hereditary spherocytosis families in Argentina. *Ann Hematol* 2011, **90**(6): 625–34.

48 Bolton-Maggs PH, *et al*. Guidelines for the diagnosis and management of hereditary spherocytosis – 2011 update. *Br J Haematol* 2012, **156**(1): 37–49.

49 Hartwell EA. Use of Rh immune globulin: ASCP practice parameter. American Society of Clinical Pathologists. *Am J Clin Pathol* 1998, **110**(3): 281–92.

50 Lee D, *et al*. Recommendations for the use of anti-D immunoglobulin for Rh prophylaxis. British Blood Transfusion Society

and the Royal College of Obstetricians and Gynaecologists. *Transfus Med* 1999, **9**(1): 93–7.

51 Kleihauer E, Braun H, Betke K. (Demonstration of fetal hemoglobin in erythrocytes of a blood smear). *Klin Wochenschr* 1957, **35**(12): 637–8.

52 Duguid JK, Bromilow IM. Laboratory measurement of feto-maternal hemorrhage and its clinical relevance. *Transfus Med Rev* 1999, **13**(1): 43–8.

53 Johnson PR, *et al*. Flow cytometry in diagnosis and management of large fetomaternal haemorrhage. *J Clin Pathol* 1995, **48**(11): 1005–8.

54 Davis BH, *et al*. Detection of fetal red cells in fetomaternal hemorrhage using a fetal hemoglobin monoclonal antibody by flow cytometry. *Transfusion* 1998, **38**(8): 749–56.

55 Savithrisowmya S, *et al*. Assessment of fetomaternal hemorrhage by flow cytometry and Kleihauer-Betke test in Rh-negative pregnancies. *Gynecol Obstet Invest* 2008, **65**(2): 84–8.

56 Lloyd-Evans P, *et al*. Use of a directly conjugated monoclonal anti-D (BRAD-3) for quantification of fetomaternal hemorrhage by flow cytometry. *Transfusion* 1996, **36**(5): 432–7.

57 Mundee Y, *et al*. Simplified flow cytometric method for fetal hemoglobin containing red blood cells. *Cytometry* 2000, **42**(6): 389–93.

58 Bromilow IM, Duguid JK. Measurement of feto-maternal haemorrhage: a comparative study of three Kleihauer techniques and tow flow cytometry methods. *Clin Lab Haematol* 1997, **19**(2): 137–42.

59 Chen JC, *et al*. Multicenter clinical experience with flow cytometric method for fetomaternal hemorrhage detection. *Cytometry* 2002, **50**(6): 285–90.

60 de Wit H, *et al*. Reference values of fetal erythrocytes in maternal blood during pregnancy established using flow cytometry. *Am J Clin Pathol* 2011, **136**(4): 631–6.

61 Subira D, *et al*. Significance of the volume of fetomaternal hemorrhage after performing prenatal invasive tests. *Cytometry B Clin Cytom* 2011, **80**(1): 38–42.

62 Austin E. Guidelines for the estimation of fetomaternal haemorrhage. BCSH website www.bcshguidelines.com/documents/BCSH_FMH_bcsh_sept2009.pdf 2009 2009.

63 Radel DJ, *et al*. A combined flow cytometry-based method for fetomaternal hemorrhage and maternal D. *Transfusion* 2008, **48**(9): 1886–91.

64 Mandy FF, Nicholson JK, McDougal JS. Guidelines for performing single-platform absolute CD4+ T-cell determinations with CD45 gating for persons infected with human immunodeficiency virus. Centers for Disease Control and Prevention. *MMWR Recomm Rep* 2003, **52**(RR-2): 1–13.

65 Henon P, *et al*. Primordial role of CD34+ 38- cells in early and late trilineage haemopoietic engraftment after autolo-gous blood cell transplantation. *Br J Haematol* 1998, **103**(2): 568–81.

66 Gajkowska A, *et al*. Flow cytometric enumeration of CD34+ hematopoietic stem and progenitor cells in leukapheresis product and bone marrow for clinical transplantation: a comparison of three methods. *Folia Histochem Cytobiol* 2006, **44**(1): 53–60.

67 Gratama JW, *et al*. Flow cytometric enumeration of CD34+ hematopoietic stem and progenitor cells. European Working Group on Clinical Cell Analysis. *Cytometry* 1998, **34**(3): 128–42.

68 Crockard AD. Diagnosis and carrier detection of chronic granulomatous disease in five families by flow cytometry. *Int Arch Allergy Immunol* 1997, **114**(2): 144–52.

69 Holland SM. Chronic granulomatous disease. *Clin Rev Allergy Immunol* 2010, **38**(1): 3–10.

70 van Vliet DN, Brandsma AE, Hartwig NG. (Leukocyte-adhesion deficiency: a rare disorder of inflammation). *Ned Tijdschr Geneeskd* 2004, **148**(50): 2496–500.

71 Yakubenia S, *et al*. Leukocyte trafficking in a mouse model for leukocyte adhesion deficiency II/congenital disorder of glycosylation IIc. *Blood* 2008, **112**(4): 1472–81.

72 Gombart AF, *et al*. Neutrophil-specific granule deficiency: homozygous recessive inheritance of a frameshift mutation in the gene encoding transcription factor CCAAT/enhancer binding protein – epsilon. *Blood* 2001, **97**(9): 2561–7.

73 Shiohara M, *et al*. Phenotypic and functional alterations of peripheral blood monocytes in neutrophil-specific granule deficiency. *J Leukoc Biol* 2004, **75**(2): 190–7.

74 Lanza F. Clinical manifestation of myeloperoxidase deficiency. *J Mol Med (Berl)* 1998, **76**(10): 676–81.

75 Kutter D. Prevalence of myeloperoxidase deficiency: population studies using Bayer-Technicon automated hematology. *J Mol Med (Berl)* 1998, **76**(10): 669–75.

76 Hoy A, *et al*. Growing significance of myeloperoxidase in non-infectious diseases. *Clin Chem Lab Med* 2002, **40**(1): 2–8.

77 Linden MD, *et al*. Application of flow cytometry to platelet disorders. *Semin Thromb Hemost* 2004, **30**(5): 501–11.

78 Schmidt V, Hilberg T. ThromboFix platelet stabilizer: advances in clinical platelet analyses by flow cytometry? *Platelets* 2006, **17**(4): 266–73.

79 Lindahl TL, Fagerberg IH, Larsson A. A new flow cytometric method for measurement of von Willebrand factor activity. *Scand J Clin Lab Invest* 2003, **63**(3): 217–23.

80 Jennings LK, *et al*. Analysis of human platelet glycoproteins IIb-IIIa and Glanzmann's thrombasthenia in whole blood by flow cytometry. *Blood* 1986, **68**(1): 173–9.

81 Kannan M, *et al*. Carrier detection in Glanzmann thrombasthenia: comparison of flow cytometry and Western blot with respect to DNA mutation. *Am J Clin Pathol* 2008, **130**(1): 93–8.

82 Beltrame MP, *et al*. Flow cytometry as a tool in the diagnosis of Bernard-Soulier syndrome in Brazilian patients. *Platelets* 2009, **20**(4): 229–34.

83 Maurer-Spurej E, Pittendreigh C, Wu JK. Diagnosing platelet delta-storage pool disease in children by flow cytometry. *Am J Clin Pathol* 2007, **127**(4): 626–32.

84 Noris P, *et al*. Autosomal dominant thrombocytopenias with reduced expression of glycoprotein Ia. *Thromb Haemost* 2006, **95**(3): 483–9.

85 Schafer A, Bauersachs J. Endothelial dysfunction, impaired endogenous platelet inhibition and platelet activation in diabetes and atherosclerosis. *Curr Vasc Pharmacol* 2008, **6**(1): 52–60.

86 Wang ZY, *et al*. Comparative study of platelet activation markers in diabetes mellitus patients complicated by cerebrovascular disease. *Blood Coagul Fibrinolysis* 2001, **12**(7): 531–7.

87 Yi ZS, *et al*. Detection of platelet activation by flow cytometry in patients with pre-eclampsia. *Di Yi Jun Yi Da Xue Xue Bao* 2003, **23**(10): 1095–6.

88 Burdess A, *et al*. Platelet activation in patients with peripheral vascular disease: Reproducibility and comparability of platelet markers. *Thromb Res* 2012, **129**(1): 50–5.

89 Cha JK, *et al*. Surface expression of P-selectin on platelets is related with clinical worsening in acute ischemic stroke. *J Korean Med Sci* 2002, **17**(6): 811–6.

90 Mohan IV, Mikhailidis DP, Stansby GP. Platelet activation in bypass surgery for critical limb ischemia. *Vasc Endovascular Surg* 2007, **41**(4): 322–9.

91 Morse DS, Adams D, Magnani B. Platelet and neutrophil activation during cardiac surgical procedures: impact of cardiopulmonary bypass. *Ann Thorac Surg* 1998, **65**(3): 691–5.

92 Ogata N, *et al*. Increased levels of platelet-derived microparticles in patients with diabetic retinopathy. *Diabetes Res Clin Pract* 2005, **68**(3): 193–201.

93 Nomura S. Function and clinical significance of platelet-derived microparticles. *Int J Hematol* 2001, **74**(4): 397–404.

94 Nomura S, Ozaki Y, Ikeda Y. Function and role of microparticles in various clinical settings. *Thromb Res* 2008, **123**(1): 8–23.

95 Cui W, *et al*. Detection of platelet-derived microparticles using flow cytometry and its clinical application. *Chin Med Sci J* 2003, **18**(1): 26–30.

96 Xiong G, *et al*. Analysis of individual platelet-derived microparticles, comparing flow cytometry and capillary electrophoresis with laser-induced fluorescence detection. *Analyst* 2003, **128**(6): 581–8.

97 Solanilla A, *et al*. Platelet-associated CD154 in immune thrombocytopenic purpura. *Blood* 2005, **105**(1): 215–8.

98 Okano K, *et al*. Development of an improved assay system for activated platelet counts and evaluation by aspirin monitoring. *Transl Res* 2010, **155**(2): 89–96.

99 Sane DC, *et al*. Frequency of aspirin resistance in patients with congestive heart failure treated with antecedent aspirin. *Am J Cardiol* 2002, **90**(8): 893–5.

100 Ferraris VA, *et al*. Aspirin and postoperative bleeding after coronary artery bypass grafting. *Ann Surg* 2002, **235**(6): 820–7.

101 Dropinski J, *et al*. The additive antiplatelet action of clopidogrel in patients with coronary artery disease treated with aspirin. *Thromb Haemost* 2007, **98**(1): 201–9.

102 Serebruany VL, *et al*. Effects of clopidogrel and aspirin in combination versus aspirin alone on platelet activation and major receptor expression in diabetic patients: the PLavix Use for Treatment Of Diabetes (PLUTO-Diabetes) trial. *Am Heart J* 2008, **155**(1): 93 e1–7.

103 Peter K, *et al*. Flow cytometric monitoring of glycoprotein IIb/IIIa blockade and platelet function in patients with acute myocardial infarction receiving reteplase, abciximab, and ticlopidine: continuous platelet inhibition by the combination of abciximab and ticlopidine. *Circulation* 2000, **102**(13): 1490–6.

CHAPTER 11
Reactive and Non-neoplastic Phenomena

Reactive changes in peripheral blood leucocyte indices are frequently encountered in the haematology laboratory. In many situations the cause of these changes is immediately apparent for example, where useful clinical information is provided with the request for analysis. We are all familiar with post-operative or steroid induced neutrophilia, for example, or the myeloid left shift which appears as a response to sepsis. The clinician will be far more familiar with the patient's clinical circumstances than the laboratory scientist or haematologist. An all important telephone call can often clarify matters by correlating laboratory findings with the clinical history, often obviating the need for further specific investigation. It is important to be familiar with the wide variety of reactive and non-neoplastic haematology laboratory phenomena that can arise as a result of lifestyle factors, inflammatory disease, immunodeficiency, stress, infection, neoplasia, medication and surgery.

The term 'non-neoplastic' in the chapter title refers to haematological neoplasms: the reactions and the haematological sequelae of solid tumours are perhaps best covered here, for want of a better home. Reactions to solid tumours are common in clinical and laboratory practice so it is important to be aware of the consequences they generate and how best to interpret these pathological phenomena.

Haematological disturbances are most frequently encountered in peripheral blood but reactive changes can also be evaluated using flow cytometry not only on bone marrow but also on bronchoalveolar lavage specimens and pleural, pericardial and cerebrospinal fluids.

Peripheral blood

Lymphocytosis

Stress lymphocytosis

Transient stress induced lymphocytosis is a common phenomenon that is under recognized. It typically occurs in patients with emergency medical conditions, including myocardial infarction, epilepsy, trauma, bleeding, sickle cell crises and obstetric complications [1–4]. It is acute in onset, often resolves within 24–48 hours, and may at least in part result from lymphocytic mobilization in response to supra-normal levels of adrenaline. The pre-morbid lymphocyte count is usually normal, unlike patients with clonal LPD where the lymphocytosis evolves slowly with time. The magnitude of the lymphocytosis varies widely but is usually in the order of $4-10.4 \times 10^9$/L [5]. Morphologically there are no particular features which might help predict this entity, but it is often accompanied by a neutrophilia and sometimes a stress induced leucoerythroblastosis. The lymphocytosis results from an absolute increase in T-cells, B-cells and NK cells. Both the CD4$^+$ and CD8$^+$ T-cell populations are increased, with no disturbance of the normal CD4/CD8 ratio, though there is a significant increase in memory T-cells and the CD8$^+$ compartment appears enriched by CD57$^+$ cytotoxic T-cells [5]. This may indicate a physiological means of augmenting the anamnestic immune response.

Practical Flow Cytometry in Haematology Diagnosis, First Edition. Mike Leach, Mark Drummond and Allyson Doig.
© 2013 John Wiley & Sons, Ltd. Published 2013 by John Wiley & Sons, Ltd.

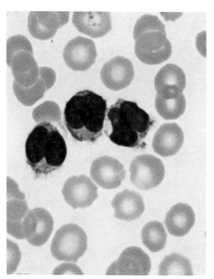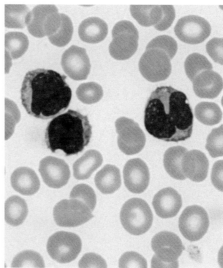

Figure 11.1 Typical lymphoid morphology in polyclonal B lymphocytosis.

Exercise induced lymphocytosis

In keeping with the stress lymphocytosis noted above it is not surprising that strenuous exercise can induce a similar phenomenon [6]. Both are, of course, associated with increased levels of adrenalin and the cell adhesion molecule ICAM-1 with subsequent modulation of lymphocyte adhesion to vascular endothelium [7]. Furthermore, beta-adrenergic antagonist treatment can mitigate this phenomenon. The lymphocytosis is closely associated with the timing of the exercise activity and in the majority of cases it will resolve within a few hours. Lymphocyte subsets are again not significantly altered, but there is a relative increase in CD8$^+$ CD56$^+$ T-cells [8].

Smoking

Cigarette smoking is sometimes associated with a lymphocytosis due to a polyclonal B-cell proliferation. The peripheral blood lymphocytosis is mild to moderate, with a median count of 7.35×10^9/L [9]. Although the pathophysiology of this condition is poorly understood it is considered a benign phenomenon. There is a frequent associated cytogenetic abnormality, with isochromosome 3q being a common finding. This is an intriguing scenario in that an apparently reactive polyclonal proliferation has acquired a cytogenetic abnormality. This challenges our current understanding of the relevance of cytogenetic findings in the differentiation of neoplastic from reactive proliferations.

Considering the prevalence of cigarette smoking this entity is rare, though individuals who are HLA-DR7 positive may have a much increased susceptibility [10]. Morphologically, these polyclonal B-cells are unusual as they have a tendency to exhibit binucleate or bilobated nuclei (Figure 11.1).

As the description implies there is polyclonal expression of B-cell surface light chains and a tendency to a polyclonal increase in serum IgM. A minority of patients can develop mild splenomegaly and lymphadenopathy but this condition tends to resolve in most patients on cessation of smoking and it is an important condition to recognize as it rarely, if ever, requires treatment [9, 11].

Viral lymphocytosis

An atypical peripheral blood lymphocytosis is a common response to viral infection. The best characterized response is that seen following Epstein Barr virus (EBV) infection, where the generic term 'infectious mononucleosis' (IM) actually describes the pleomorphic peripheral blood mononuclear cell response. Epstein Barr virus is the commonest cause of a virus induced reactive lymphocytosis, particularly in adolescents and young adults, accounting for 85% of cases [12].

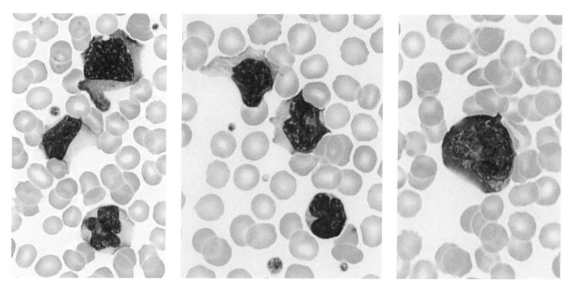

Figure 11.2 Pleomorphic activated large lymphocytes (atypical mononuclear cells) typically seen as a response to EBV infection.

A number of other viral infections, including adenovirus, rubella, herpes, varicella, hepatitis C, HIV and cytomegalovirus are able to trigger a similar IM reaction. Epstein Barr virus infection is notable for the florid lymphocytosis it induces [12], often in association with a mild thrombocytopenia and/or neutropenia and raised serum transaminases, alongside a history of fever, fatigue, sore throat and lymphadenopathy. The presence of heterophile antibodies (anti-species antibodies reactive against ovine, equine and bovine red cells) is strongly associated with IM due to EBV; they are usually absent in the non-EBV IM patients. The lymphocytosis is due to a proliferation of activated cytotoxic T-cells, even though the virus primarily infects B-lineage lymphoid cells. Morphologically these cells are medium to large, with plentiful convoluted cytoplasm and pleomorphic nuclei. Some of the larger cells show a deep blue cytoplasm; the presence of these cells alongside the other changes and the clinical history are a useful pointer to the diagnosis (Figure 11.2). On an FSC versus SSC plot these cells appear in the large lymphocyte or blast gate, with some cells encroaching on the monocyte zone.

Flow cytometry shows the lymphocytosis to be due to an activated cytotoxic T-cell population which has a CD3+ CD8+ CD38+ HLA-DR+ phenotype. A very common finding is the loss of/or dim expression of CD7; other pan T antigens, such as CD5 are sometimes lost, but CD7 is by far the most frequently affected [13]. The presence of HLA-DR is a very useful indicator to the reactive nature of these cells as DR expression is, with the exception of cutaneous T-cell lymphoma, not a regular feature seen in any of the clonal mature T-cell lymphoproliferative disorders [14]. Infectious mononucleosis due to EBV infection is more likely to show a higher absolute lymphocyte count with higher percentages of atypical lymphocytes on the blood film. The immunophenotypic characteristics, however, are largely similar in EBV versus non-EBV cases [12].

Post-splenectomy lymphocytosis

A leucocytosis and thrombocytosis is a common finding in patients with a history of splenectomy or in those with hyposplenic states. The leucocytosis is generated by a mild increase in all parameters; a lymphocytosis is often seen alongside a mild neutrophilia, monocytosis and eosinophilia. The blood film will show Howell-Jolly bodies and this constellation of features, together with the relevant history, if provided, should be enough to conclude the situation. It is not uncommon, however, for immunophenotyping studies to be requested by scientists or clinicians not aware of this scenario, particularly if the blood film has not been carefully examined.

The immunophenotypic profile of the lymphocytosis tends to show a relative increase in all components, with no

WORKED EXAMPLE 11.1

A 15-year-old female presented with a short history of sore throat, headache and lethargy. She was noted to have tender cervical lymphadenopathy. An FBC showed Hb130g/L, WBC 15×10⁹/L, neutrophils 1.4×10⁹/L, lymphocytes 11×10⁹/L, platelets 130×10⁹/L. The blood film showed activated large lymphocytes. Flow cytometry studies, gating on lymphocytes, generated the following data:

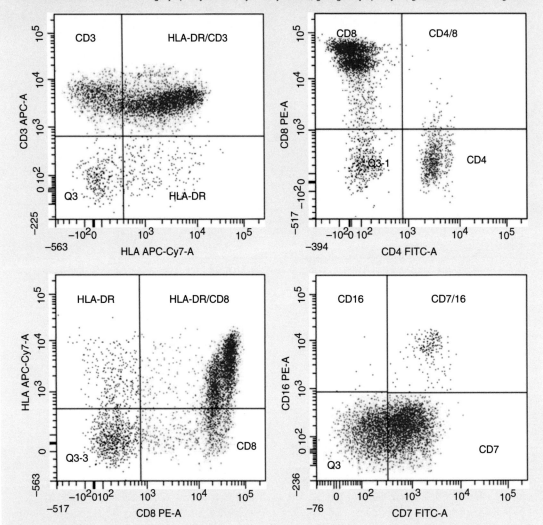

Note the prominent CD8 lymphocytosis, the heterogenous expression of HLA-DR and partial loss/dim expression of CD7. This is all typical of the response to EBV infection. Loss of antigen expression, particularly CD7 alone, does not indicate a neoplastic proliferation.

major deviations in T or B-cell populations [15]. A higher relative contribution may be generated by NK cells [16] and γδ T-cells [17] so the cytometrist should be aware of this and not be tempted to consider a clonal disorder. It appears that splenectomy allows the resetting of peripheral blood homeostasis in terms of leucocyte levels similar to that seen with platelet counts. Of interest, exercise induced lymphocytosis appears to be abrogated by splenectomy, suggesting that splenic sinus endothelium marginated lymphocytes might contribute to this phenomenon [18].

Neoplasia induced lymphoid reactions

T and NK cell reactions are not infrequently seen in the presence of, and as a reaction to, a neoplastic condition. We have all experienced cases where a prominent cytotoxic T-cell response is seen in patients with haemopoietic neoplasms in peripheral blood: these prominent LGL type responses are often seen alongside the neoplastic cells in peripheral blood smears.

These responses have been documented as a response to a variety of haematological neoplasms, including acute and chronic myeloid leukaemia, chronic lymphocytic leukaemia, lymphoma and multiple myeloma [19]. These patients show significantly higher proportions of activated T-cells, with a particular increase in the following subsets: CD3+ CD57+, CD3+ HLA-DR+, CD3+ CD16/56+, CD4+ CD57+ CD8+ CD57+, CD8+ CD28−. Loss of CD28 is a feature of chronic T-cell activation and CD8+ CD28− activated T-cells are capable of intense cytotoxic activity [20]. These cells are prominent in patients experiencing chronic immune stimulation from neoplasia, inflammatory disorders, autoimmune disease and graft versus host disease [21]. It is notable that CD4+ CD57+ proliferations are also seen in reactive states and when seen as a response to haematological neoplasms they occur in patients with B-cell derived but not myeloid neoplasms, suggesting a possible causal relationship with tumour HLA-DR expression [22]. Overall, reactive T-cell proliferations are more commonly seen in, but not restricted to, the CD8+ T-cell compartment.

A recent phenomenon of lymphocytosis due to LGL proliferations in patients with chronic myeloid leukaemia or Ph+acute lymphoblastic leukaemia undergoing treatment with dasatinib, has been described [23, 24]. This can affect up to one quarter of patients, can become a chronic phenomenon and interestingly is correlated with a rapid early response to treatment, so in fact appears to be a favourable characteristic. However, the same patients were more likely to report other treatment related side effects such as fever and effusions. The cells usually have a CD2+ CD3+ CD8+ CD16+ CD56+ CD57+ phenotype and apparent clonality as shown by TCR gene rearrangement which has been demonstrated in some cases. This phenomenon appears unique to dasatinib and has not been noted during use of the other tyrosine kinase inhibitors.

Inflammatory disorders

Disturbance of T-cell subsets, sometimes in association with a mild peripheral blood lymphocytosis have been described in a number of non-neoplastic inflammatory disorders [17, 21, 25]. It is important to note that these T-cell reactions not only involve both the CD4+ and CD8+ T-cell populations but also that most will express antigens indicating T-cell activation, notably CD 57, CD16, CD56, HLA-DR, CD25 and CD69, with conversely, loss of CD28 [21, 25, 26].

Lymphopenia

Peripheral blood lymphopenia is a relatively common finding in routine laboratory haematology practice. In the majority of cases, particularly in the absence of relevant background information, this entity in isolation does not need further investigation. Absolute lymphopenia has been described in a wide variety of clinical scenarios [27–29]; the most familiar is that associated with human immunodeficiency virus (HIV) infection where a lymphopenia is often used as a surrogate indicator of established infection. We regard this as poor practice; if HIV infection is suspected, because of symptoms and potential risk factors, then an HIV test with appropriate counselling is the investigation of choice. CD4 lymphopenia has multiple potential aetiologies; this finding should not be misinterpreted in the absence of relevant specific virological investigation.

Autoimmunity

Lymphopenia has long been associated with a variety of autoimmune diseases. It has been documented in a variety of conditions, including rheumatoid arthritis, systemic lupus erythematosus, polymyositis, sarcoidosis, coeliac disease and Crohn's disease [28, 30–33]. In addition, it is also important to note that many of these conditions are actually treated with lymphocytotoxic medications which act by depleting autoreactive T lymphoid populations and in doing so generate a lymphopenia (see section below) as part of their therapeutic effect. A lymphopenia noted in these circumstances, therefore, should not prompt unnecessary and inappropriate investigations.

Medications

A number of immunomodulatory medications frequently induce a lymphopenia; in fact their immunosuppressive activity is in part mediated through their

Table 11.1 An abbreviated summary of inherited immunodeficiency disorders causing a marked quantitative disturbance in T and B lymphocyte populations.

Disorder	T-cells	B-cells	NK cells	Immuno globulins	Other
Reticular dysgenesis	–	–	–	–	Pancytopenia Very rare
Combined immunodeficiency syndromes	–	+/–	–	–	Very rare
Di George syndrome	–	+	+	+/–	Thymic aplasia
Ataxia telangiectasia	↓CD4	+	+	+/–	Lymphoid tumours
CD3 deficiency	↓CD3	+	+	–	
Bruton agammaglobulinaemia	+	–	+	–	
Common variable immunodeficiency	+	+/–	+	–	Not uncommon

Key: + present – absent +/– variable.

lymphocytotoxic effects. Drugs such as corticosteroids, methotrexate, mercaptopurine and azathioprine all commonly induce a lymphopenia. Purine analogue cytotoxic agents such as fludarabine and cladribine and the monoclonal anti-CD52 antibody alemtuzumab are all capable of generating a severe lymphopenia. A history of exposure to any of these medications is therefore important in assessing any patient with a severe lymphopenia. This is important not only in explaining the lymphopenia but also in terms of risk of opportunistic infections and viral reactivations which these patients can encounter.

Inherited immune deficiency disorders

A full discussion of this extensive topic is outside of the scope of this text. This small section is appropriate in the context of immunophenotypic peripheral blood lymphoid analysis. It is important to recognize that a number of inherited disorders can generate significant alterations in peripheral blood B and T lymphocyte and sometimes NK populations. Many of these patients will be encountered in paediatric practice, but some escape undiagnosed into adulthood, particularly common variable immunodeficiency (CVID). As the name implies the latter disorder is the most prevalent and represents a heterogenous group of genetic conditions which show impairment of normal B-cell maturation and differentiation. It is characterized by

onset in the second and third decades, by recurrent bacterial respiratory infections, hypogammaglobulinaemia and a poor response to vaccination. Some patients develop lymphadenopathy and splenomegaly so these findings might prompt investigations and in particular flow cytometry studies, looking for clonal lymphoid proliferations. The majority of CVID patients show normal peripheral blood B-cell numbers, but have increased proportions of CD19+ SIg-cells. Flow cytometry, using specific lymphocyte subset panels, is important in diagnosis and classification of CVID by defining relative numbers of CD19+ CD21+sIgM- sIgD- class switched memory B-cells [34].

Some outline knowledge of these disorders is necessary in diagnostic flow cytometry as the depletion of one lineage might erroneously be interpreted as showing an excess of the other and if T-cells or B-cells are absent this needs to be explained. Furthermore, some of these conditions demonstrate an increased susceptibility to neoplastic lymphoid proliferations and immune dysregulatory phenomena. Immunophenotypic analysis might therefore be enhanced by some awareness of these possibilities. The main conditions capable of causing significant quantitative alterations in lymphoid subsets are summarized in an abbreviated form in Table 11.1 [35]. Please refer to comprehensive literature, if you suspect from the clinical history and immunophenotypic profile, that an inherited disorder of immune function ought to be considered.

Bone marrow

As noted in Chapter 4 the normal bone marrow is a complex tissue composed of multiple haemopoietic lineages at various stages of maturation. These populations are differentially affected by various disease states and non-neoplastic reactions are common. Such reactions can influence one or more lineages. For example, the reaction to bacterial infection is one of pure myeloid expansion, whereas the reactive bone marrow seen in patients with Hodgkin lymphoma often shows an expansion of myeloid (particularly eosinophils driven by IL-5), lymphoid and plasma cell populations. In addition, monocytes and macrophages may be stimulated to respond and haemophagocytosis of cells and cell debris is another common reactive phenomenon. It is therefore essential to be aware of the patient circumstances and any established diagnoses before a bone marrow can be comprehensively assessed. It is also important to have reference ranges for bone marrow populations in normal individuals. This data is not easily acquired but the work of Brooimans et al. [36], summarized in Table 11.2, has significantly assisted our understanding.

Myeloid expansions

Significant expansion of the myeloid component is commonly seen as a result of infection, corticosteroid therapy, vasculitic disorders, use of granulocyte colony

Table 11.2 The distribution of major leucocyte subpopulations present in 78 selected bone marrow aspirates with >80% purity taken from healthy individuals [36].

Cell type	5th centile	Median	95th centile
CD34+ cells	0.7	1.8	2.8
Immature cells	2.5	5.9	9.2
Maturing myeloid	59.5	73.7	85.5
Monocytes	2.0	3.5	5.8
Lymphocytes	5.7	13.4	25.0
Remaining cells	1.4	2.5	4.5

stimulating factor (G-CSF) and as a reaction to tumours. If the underlying condition is known there should be no diagnostic difficulty, in particular as all components of the myeloid series are expanded and there should be no significant dysplasia or excess of blasts. Immunophenotyping, therefore, should not be either necessary or informative but it is worthwhile to note that some immunophenotypic changes can result from infection and exposure to granulocyte colony stimulating factors. These changes should be recognized in appropriate circumstances and not be confused with disease states.

Infection is the commonest cause of a neutrophilia and myeloid left shift seen in peripheral blood reactions, whether it be in hospital based or community patients. Often the diagnosis is obvious in the presence of specific infective symptoms, physical signs and fever in parallel to laboratory tests showing increases in acute phase reactants. The clinical suspicion is often later confirmed when the infecting organism is isolated using appropriate cultures. In other situations a diagnosis of infection may not be straightforward: patients on high dose steroids, the immuno-compromised, patients in intensive care units and neonates are just a few examples of the type of patient that may not show typical responses. Early diagnosis with initiation of antibiotic therapy might be particularly valuable in these vulnerable groups.

Up-regulation of surface CD64 on neutrophils is a well recognized response to infection and is driven by inflammatory cytokines, endogenous GCSF and interferon γ. Increases in CD64 begin within 4–6 hours of onset of infection and appearance of this antigen appears to correlate with an increase in neutrophil bactericidal and fungicidal activity. As CD64 expression is negligible in normal resting neutrophils the assessment of CD64 expression has been assessed as an early indicator of infective phenomena [37–42]. It shows a high sensitivity and specificity and outperforms C reactive protein, absolute neutrophil count, myeloid left shift and ESR in predicting sepsis [38]. It is useful in adults, children and neonates [41, 42] and is able to differentiate between true infection and systemic inflammatory response to auto-immune disease such as rheumatoid arthritis and systemic lupus erythematosus [40]. Its utility in differentiating bacterial from viral infection, however, remains to be determined.

G-CSF therapy is frequently used in haematological practice as a means of mobilizing therapeutic precursor cell populations. It is also used in patients as a means of minimizing cytotoxic drug induced neutropenia or as a way of potentiating chemotherapeutic effect. The utility of G-CSF therapy in stem cell mobilization is well documented and covered in more detail in Chapter 10. In general terms G-CSF treatment induces a more primitive activated myeloid immunophenotype with increased expression of CD34, HLA-DR, CD71 and CD14, whilst reducing the intensity of CD15, CD16 and CD10 accordingly [43]. The expression of HLA-DR on lymphocytes, however, was not affected [43]. In the short term, measured in hours, granulocytes show increased expression of CD16, CD11b and CD66. These changes all recover to normal after G-CSF exposure is discontinued.

Peripheral blood and bone marrow monocytes can also take on immunophenotypic changes in reactive scenarios. Treatment with G-CSF, stem cell factor and interferon alpha can all induce expression of CD56 [44, 45]. Reactive monocytes expressing CD16 and CD56 are potent antigen presenting cells which secrete TNFα and are expanded in patients with active Crohn's disease [46]; CD16 and HLA-DR expression is also well recognized as a response to HIV infection [47]. Monocytes are also an important cell lineage which becomes activated in response to bacterial infection. The expression of HLA-DR has been the focus of some studies, but there is no clear consensus as to its value in the early diagnosis of sepsis.

Otherwise the immunophenotype of reactive marrow cells should not be significantly altered from normal. The presence of multiple phenotypic changes on monocytes is more in keeping with myelodysplastic syndromes, particularly CMML [48]. The finding of a reactive blood and bone marrow profile may in itself, if unexplained, be an indication for further specific systematic investigation to exclude underlying inflammatory, infective or neoplastic disorders.

Maturation arrest

This is a phenomenon where myeloid precursor maturation is arrested, usually at the promyelocyte/myelocyte stage. Segmented bone marrow neutrophils are scarce and there is a paucity of neutrophils in peripheral blood. Maturation arrest can be induced by a variety of conditions, including medications, inflammatory diseases like rheumatoid arthritis and as a response to sepsis and toxic states. Most frequently the maturation arrest occurs at the myelocyte/band cell stage. On rare occasions the accumulation of arrested myeloid precursors, particularly promyelocytes, may even mimic acute promyelocytic leukaemia (Figure 11.3).

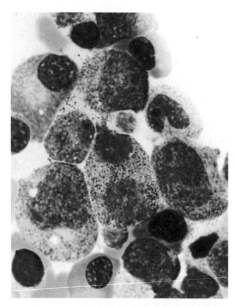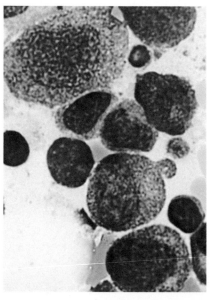

Figure 11.3 Bone marrow aspirate showing maturation arrest with prominent promyelocytes in a patient with folate deficiency and alcohol toxicity.

If in doubt, flow cytometry should resolve the situation as malignant and reactive promyelocytes have subtly different immunophenotypes.

Haematogones

Haematogones are normal bone marrow B-cell precursors which can be expanded in recovering bone marrow and reactive states. Their assessment and differentiation from B lymphoblasts is covered in detail in Chapter 4.

Marrow aplasia

The hypoplastic myelodysplastic syndromes (MDS) can at times be difficult to differentiate from idiopathic hypoplastic/aplastic anaemias. Rather than completely separate entities these disorders might be considered as two related stem cell disorders situated at either end of a heterogenous spectrum. The myelodysplasias commonly show dysplastic morphology and cytogenetic aberrations, whilst in aplastic anaemia dysplasia is absent or mild and cytogenetic studies are typically normal. Some patients present with an indeterminate condition somewhere between the two and an accurate diagnosis is very important in terms of deciding appropriate therapy [49, 50]. Furthermore some patients with cytopenias due to an apparent myelodysplasia seem to respond to immunosuppressive therapy [50]. Finally, both conditions can be associated with an increase of PNH like clones which show relative expansion and survival advantage due to the depletion of normal precursor populations. The flow cytometric analysis of red cell and granulocyte GPI anchors in PNH is discussed fully in Chapter 10.

The main difficulty in defining these two conditions is due the relative paucity of cells for examination. Bone marrow aspirates are often particulate but grossly hypocellular so if metaphase preparations fail to yield cytogenetic information we are often unclear as to the significance. Are there not enough cells for a viable result or are these cells cytogenetically normal? An apparent hypo/acellular specimen is very difficult to assess morphologically and the residual lymphocytes and plasma cells often apparent in hypoplastic marrows might be given inappropriate significance. CD34+ haemopoietic progenitors are central to the pathogenesis of both these disorders, being the target of autoimmune attack in aplastic anaemia and the neoplastic transformation in MDS. Flow cytometry is valuable in assessing CD34+ CD45^{dim} progenitors in both these conditions and might assist considerably in differentiating between the two. A

Table 11.3 Discrimination between hypoplastic MDS and aplastic anaemia according to CD34+ CD45^{dim}bone marrow population percentages. Hypoplastic MDS was defined according to clonal cytogenetic abnormalities or eventual progression to refractory anaemia with excess blasts or AML. Aplastic anaemia was defined by standard criteria for diagnosis and the absence of neoplastic evolution on follow-up.

Diagonsis	CD34 mean % (range)
Aplastic anaemia	0.13 (+/– 0.02)
Hypoplastic MDS	3.5 (+/– 0.5)

normal marrow CD34+ percentage is in the order of 0.82 +/– 0.24% [51] or 1.4% [36]. A number of studies have shown that aplastic anaemia is associated with normal or decreased CD34+ CD45^{dim} marrow percentages, whilst MDS shows normal or increased levels [51–53]. Furthermore, the proportion of CD34+ populations in MDS appears to gradually increase as the disease evolves and progresses [51].

The findings of Matsui et al. [53] showed significant differences in CD34+ populations, (p < 0.0001) and are summarized in Table 11.3. This study allowed excellent discrimination between the two conditions, a threshold of 1% CD34+ cells shows 100% sensitivity and specificity. CD34 percentage enumeration may therefore offer significant diagnostic potential in the evaluation of hypoplastic marrows with paucicellular aspirates. Finally, when employing such estimations it is important to avoid peripheral blood contamination of the aspirate (mostly in MDS), as discussed in Chapter 3, otherwise the percentages might potentially be reduced due to peripheral blood leucocyte contamination.

Bone marrow involvement by non-haemopoietic tumours

The bone marrow is a relatively frequent site of involvement by metastasis from a variety of non-haemopoietic tumours. Primary tumours of lung, breast, thyroid, kidney and prostate are the entities most frequently encountered in bone marrow samples. As discussed in Chapter 3, the quality of bone marrow aspirate specimens is often affected by metastatic tumour because of the tendency to induce marrow fibrosis, so making an aspirate unobtainable in many cases. These tumours are sometimes demonstrable in aspirate samples using morphological and flow

WORKED EXAMPLE 11.2

A three-year-old girl presented with anorexia, irritability and abdominal pain. She had a palpable abdominal mass and a mild pancytopenia. A peripheral blood film was non-informative. A bone marrow aspirate was submitted for investigation of a possible acute lymphoblastic leukaemia. The marrow aspirate was hypoparticulate, but cellular, with clumps of abnormal cells. The presence of a large abdominal mass in the context of likely bone marrow involvement should always lead to the consideration of a diagnosis of neuroblastoma. This is a neuroectodermal neoplasm that arises from adrenal tissue in children. It has an affinity for bone metastasis particularly to the maxilla, mandible and skull, with early bone marrow involvement.

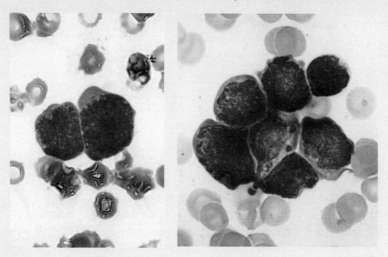

The immunophenotyping studies, summarised below, show the CD45 negative cells to express CD56 and CD15.

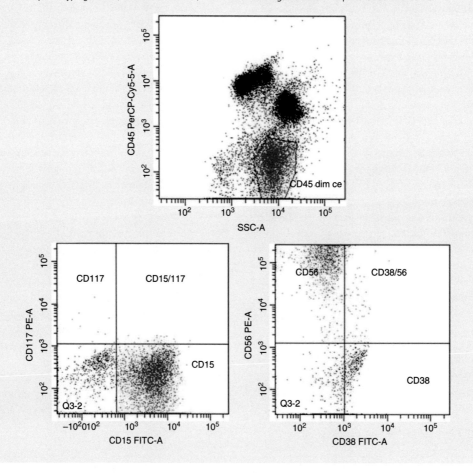

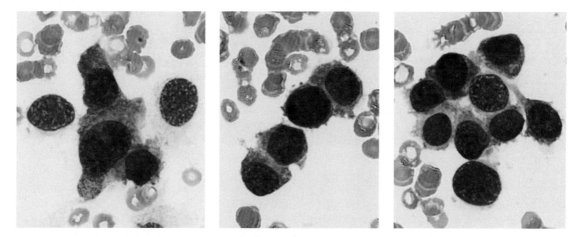

Figure 11.4 Carcinoma cells in a bone marrow aspirate specimen. Note the tendency for cells to remain adherent, their size, lack of resemblance to normal marrow cells, irregular cytoplasm and blue nucleoli.

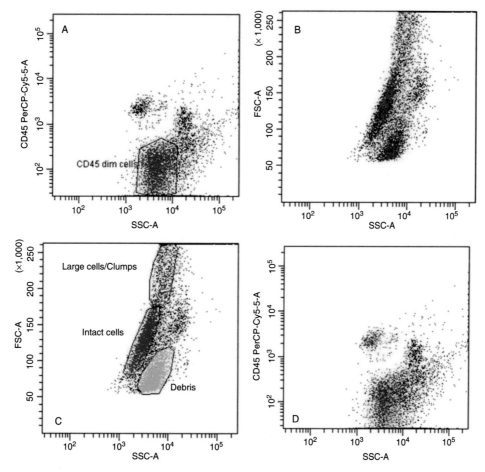

Figure 11.5 Plot A shows an abnormal CD45 versus SSC plot with a large population of CD45⁻ cells (red events). Plot B shows the behaviour of these cells in a FSC versus SSC plot with apparent tumour cells appearing in a number of different zones. Plot C shows how this phenomenon can be explained in terms of intact single cells, cell debris and cell clumps. Plot D confirms this principle showing the cell clumps and debris to generate more side scatter than single intact tumour cells. Note the small CD45⁺ lymphocyte population (red) (plot D) caught within the lower aspect of the intact cell gate (plot C) and the residual granulocytes and monocytes (black events) in both.

cytometry analysis. As these patients often present with pancytopenia, flow cytometry studies on marrow aspirate samples may be requested in order to exclude acute leukaemia.

The morphological assessment of these aspirates is important as this often gives the first clue that a non-haemopoietic tumour may be present. These samples rarely contain marrow particles, are often hypocellular and may just show small aggregates of tumour cells. These cell populations ought to be identified on the CD45 versus SSC plot, appearing as a CD45 negative (not dim) population often with abnormal side scatter properties due to the cell aggregates. These aggregates may fail to disperse when handled in flow studies and so single cells may not be analysable in the cytometer flow channel. Morphologically, non-haemopoietic cells tend to have prominent blue staining nucleoli, but have very variable size and nuclear and cytoplasmic characteristics according to the cell of origin (Figure 11.4).

In terms of flow assessment it is important to be aware of the characteristics of non-haemopoietic cells. The particular affinity of solid tumours to form clumps is all important in deciphering flow assessments of the involved tissues. Figure 11.5 illustrates many of the issues encountered.

Flow cytometry is informative here in a number of respects. First, note the abnormal scatter on the CD45 versus SSC, with a significant CD45 negative population, the absence of CD45 dim cells alongside some preservation of residual lymphocytes, monocytes and myeloid cells (black CD45$^+$ events separated according to side scatter). Second, the gated (CD45$^-$) population exhibits limited expression of antigens normally encountered on haemopoietic cells: in fact all the standard precursor antigens of myeloid and lymphoid lineages were absent. The cells expressed CD56 (very brightly) which is well recognized in non-haemopoietic tumours, but also CD15. CD15 is known to be expressed in neuroblastoma. The diagnosis therefore is metastatic neuroblastoma. A tissue biopsy of the abdominal mass ensured an independent confirmation of this diagnosis.

Pleural and pericardial fluids

Pleural and pericardial fluid specimens are often submitted for examination from patients who have undergone therapeutic or diagnostic drainage procedures. These specimens can have valuable diagnostic potential in haematological practice as we noted in the relevant sections, particularly the precursor lymphoblastic leukaemias/lymphomas and the varied lymphoproliferative disorders. They are a very useful resource for the diagnosis of follicular, marginal zone and diffuse large B-cell lymphomas and particularly for cortical type T lymphoblastic lymphoma, where a mediastinal presentation with pleural or pericardial involvement is frequent. Please refer to the relevant sections in Chapters 5 and 6 for a discussion of the applications of flow cytometry to the examination of effusions where these conditions are being considered.

Reactive phenomena of the cellular populations in effusions are also important in a diagnostic capacity. In the absence of involvement by a primary haematological disorder, the nature and type of lymphocyte, macrophage, neutrophil and eosinophil response can be informative as to the ultimate likely diagnosis responsible for the effusion. These effusions can be encountered as a response to a variety of solid tumours or as reactive response in inflammatory and infective conditions.

Certain rules apply:
• In the majority of cases a reactive T-cell response is seen, regardless of the underlying pathology.
• The reactive T-cell population forms the bulk of the cellularity in such specimens and neoplastic cells, if present, may constitute a minor population in absolute cell numbers.
• CD8$^+$ T-cells with an activated immunophenotype HLA-DR$^+$ CD57$^+$ CD25$^+$ CD28$^-$ are common in pleural reactions.

Morphologically the cells in effusions appear distorted from the cytospin process and frequently show cytoplasmic vacuolation and artefactual nuclear conformational change. Certain characteristics, such as cell size and the presence of nucleoli, however, are not affected and remain reliable features in the distinction between reactive and neoplastic populations.

Any patient with a pleural or pericardial effusion needs a comprehensive systemic evaluation and the cytologic and immunophenotypic findings can only be correctly interpreted in light of a full clinical history. A full assessment of a patient with a pleural effusion requires details of the clinical history, physical findings, radiological findings, laboratory data and characteristics of the effusion. In broad terms, transudates (total protein

<30 g/L) are due to mechanical/cardiac disorders, whereas exudates (total protein >30 g/L) are usually due to infective, inflammatory and neoplastic diseases. Flow cytometry is particularly of value in the evaluation of the latter type of effusion.

As might be anticipated, proteinaceous effusions with a high cell count and predominant neutrophilia are seen in infective and post-infective disorders. As a general rule, neutrophilic infiltrates appear as an acute phenomenon in many scenarios, but these cells are gradually replaced by monocytes and macrophages as the disorder takes on a more chronic course [54]. Pleural fluid macrophages, however, derived from peripheral blood monocytes, have no diagnostic value [55]. In chronic pleural effusions, lymphocytes become the predominant cell population. A lymphocytic effusion is seen in a number of chronic clinical scenarios, including connective tissue diseases, tuberculosis, sarcoidosis, post surgery, lymphoma and metastatic carcinoma. The reactive lymphocytes in many of these conditions show an activated phenotype affecting CD4+ and CD8+ cells. The proportions of CD4+ and CD8+ T-cells and percentages of B-cells should largely resemble those in peripheral blood. In some situations, the best characterized being neuroborreliosis, reactive CD4+ CD8+ cells are noted in small numbers [56]. These should not be interpreted as being neoplastic. As discussed above, sarcoidosis is noted for its association with reactive CD4+ cells and similar patterns to those seen in BAL fluid are seen in sarcoid related pleural effusions.

In any lymphocytic effusion it is important to search for neoplastic cells, either carcinoma or lymphoma cells. There is often much cell debris in these specimens, which has to be gated out of any analysis. Carcinoma cells are pleomorphic on side scatter, but are CD45 negative. It is important to pay attention to minor non-lymphocytic populations in pleural and pericardial fluid, particularly if they appear to be non-haemic and CD45 negative. Careful morphologic assessment of pleural fluid smears may help in this respect, but it is important to be aware of the precautions noted above. In addition benign mesothelial cells are commonly encountered in effusions and should not be mistaken for tumour cells on morphological grounds alone. Flow cytometry on serous effusions is a useful diagnostic procedure capable of identifying a variety of metastatic carcinomas using a panel of carefully selected epithelial antigen directed fluorochrome linked

Table 11.4 Summary of fluorochrome linked antibodies useful in characterization of tumour cells in serous effusions.

Antibody	Tissue target	Tumour
Anti-CD45	Haemopoietic cells	Leukaemia and lymphoma
Anti-EpCAM	Epithelial cells	Carcinomas of: Breast Lung Colon Prostate NB: Not squamous tumours
Anti-CD99	Neuroectodermal cells	Ewing tumour Neuroectodermal tumours Sarcomas Lymphoblastic lymphoma
Anti-myogenin	Muscle cells	Rhabdomyosarcoma
Anti-CD56	NCAM expressing cells	Small cell carcinoma Neuroectodermal tumours Neuroblastoma Leukaemia and lymphoma

Reproduced from Chang et al. [59], with permission from American Society for Clinical Pathology.

antibodies [57, 58]. It is important to use multiple epithelial directed antibodies [58] as each behaves variably with different tumours and in the knowledge that the flow findings have to be accurate and carry great clinical importance in terms of decisions on therapy and the prognosis for the patient. Epithelial cells of endometrial origin, from normal menstruation reflux or endometriosis, could be misidentified as malignant cells in peritoneal fluid/effusions, particularly as malignant ascitic involvement is often from cells forming a minor population in absolute percentage terms [57]. By using a selection of antibodies, summarized in Table 11.4, it is possible to identify the likely derivation of the non-haemopoietic neoplasm [59]. Clearly, these immunophenotypic findings need to be interpreted in the light of the patient's history and current clinical circumstances. Some antigens, CD56 for example, are promiscuous and are expressed by a wide spectrum of neoplastic and non-neoplastic cells.

In summary, flow cytometry has great potential in the evaluation of serous effusions for malignant involvement. Each laboratory needs to gather their own expertise and experience using the antibodies commercially available and to evaluate optimal gating strategies when searching for neoplastic contamination from a variety of tumours with a very disparate immunophenotype.

Pleural fluid eosinophilia is defined as a pleural fluid eosinophil count >10% of the total nucleated cell count. These cells are attracted to the pleural space as a response to the cytokine interleukin 5. Eosinophils are prominent in effusions due to reactions to drugs, fungi, helminths, vasculitis, some carcinomas, Hodgkin and T-cell lymphomas [60]. It should also be noted that eosinophilic effusions are commonly seen post trauma, for example following thoracic surgery or traumatic haemothorax.

Plasma cells are commonly present in small numbers in effusions: the presence of large populations should raise suspicion of involvement by a neoplastic plasma cell disorder where flow cytometry will identify an aberrant immunophenotype.

Bronchoalveolar lavage specimens

The lung is a complex organ which is constantly exposed to a multitude of antigens in the air that we breathe. In addition to the natural anatomical barriers and muco-ciliary clearance there are cell mediated protective mechanisms in place. Macrophages are the most prevalent cell encountered along the bronchoalveolar epithelium, alongside effector T lymphocytes. These T lymphocyte populations are not only important in maintaining health of the host but might also be implicated in the pathogenesis of a number of inflammatory lung diseases. The simplest way to recover and study such lymphocytes is through the use of bronchoalveolar lavage (BAL). BAL is the sampling of the lower respiratory tract through the instillation and subsequent recovery of sterile saline solution at the time of bronchoscopy. It is an important procedure which frequently assists in the diagnosis of pulmonary infection, particularly in the immunocom-promised host. It also has diagnostic and prognostic value in the assessment of a number of inflammatory lung diseases.

BAL fluid is eminently suitable for examination using flow cytometry. It does, however, in addition to mac-rophages and lymphocytes, often recover a host of other cells including neutrophils, eosinophils, mast cells and epithelial cells, together with cell debris generated by the procedure. In addition, a number of non-pulmonary

materials such as carbon, starch, talc, pollen, hair and mineral fibres are often encountered. The cytometrist needs to be aware of this extraneous material and debris which needs to be gated out by using a CD45 versus side scatter or CD2 versus side scatter approach in identifying intact T lymphocytes. The lymphocytes present in nor-mal BAL fluid constitute about 10% of cells, whilst over 80% are macrophages. The T-cell subsets roughly parallel those seen in peripheral blood, with a 2:1 CD4:CD8 ratio. B-cells are scarce, forming less than 5% of all lymphocytes [61].

A large number of diseases have been investigated using flow cytometry on BAL [62] fluid but its most useful current application appears to be in the diagnosis of sarcoidosis, a disorder where standard clinical and laboratory diagnostic tests can often give indeterminate results. The number and proportion of CD4 and CD8 cells is abnormal in sarcoidosis and interstitial pneu-monitis. The lymphocyte percentage can be increased to between 30% and 70% in both conditions [63]. Sarcoidosis is associated with a marked increase in the CD4:CD8 ratio and can be as high as 10:1 to 20:1. In hypersensitivity pneumonitis the CD4:CD8 ratio is often reversed. Other diseases including pulmonary tuberculosis do not disturb the CD4:CD8 ratio. CD103 is an integrin expressed on a population of normal bron-choepithelial T-cells and may be involved in trans-epithelial migration. By examining CD4+ T-cells for loss of concurrent CD103 expression, CD103:CD4 <0.31, the sensitivity and specificity for a diagnosis of sarcoidosis can be further improved [64].

This continues to be an area for development and it seems likely that in the future immunophenotypic studies might be applicable to other cell populations of BAL fluid to aid understanding and diagnosis in patients with a variety of lung diseases.

Cerebrospinal fluid

Cerebrospinal fluid (CSF) is normally paucicellular with a total cell count (mainly lymphocytes) of less than 10 cells/mm^3, a total protein of less than 0.4 g/L and a glucose level 1–2 mL less than peripheral blood. As noted with other body fluids CSF cells can show reactions to infection, inflammation and neoplasia. A knowledge of the clinical history is, therefore, again essential. Diagnosis of CSF involvement with acute leukaemia and lymphoproliferative disorders is covered in those chapters.

A major limitation in applying flow cytometry to CSF specimens is the relatively small volume of fluid normally available, usually 2–3 mL, and the relative scarcity of cells in these samples. It is therefore important to use a well-defined panel of antibodies with the greatest discriminatory value.

Bacterial meningitis is well recognized for inducing high CSF cell counts composed predominantly of neutrophils. The clinical presentation alongside typical reactive laboratory phenomena and modern microbiological diagnostic techniques, should not lead to difficulty in diagnosis. Apart from bacterial infection, CSF pleiocytosis is virtually always due to CD3+ lymphocytic reactions.

WORKED EXAMPLE 11.3

A 45-year-old man presented with facial weakness, difficulty swallowing and diplopia. Magnetic resonance imaging studies of the brain and brain stem were normal. A CSF examination showed a lymphocytosis (0.01x10⁹/L) and significantly raised protein level of 4.5 g/L. Flow cytometry on CSF demonstrated that all cells were CD45 positive (not shown). Lymphocyte gating and sub-analysis identified a population of cells with an activated CD8+, pan T phenotype, HLA-DR expression and partial loss of CD7 (selected plots shown below). The final diagnosis was Miller-Fischer syndrome, a variant of Guillain-Barré syndrome.

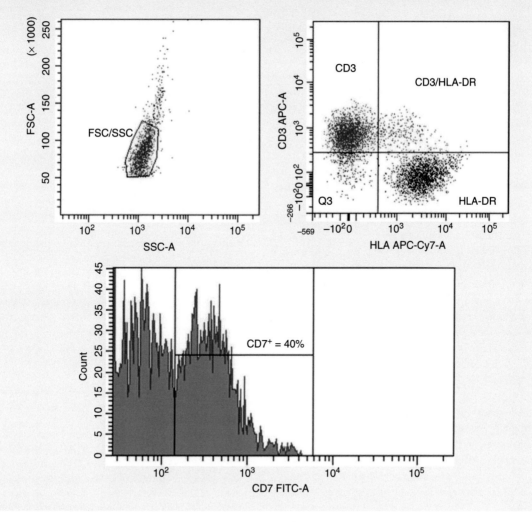

Such reactions are seen in viral meningitis, multiple sclerosis and neuroborreliosis [56], and the reactive T-cells, with varying ratios of CD4:CD8, frequently show evidence of activation in the form of HLA-DR and CD25 expression.

Leptomeningeal carcinomatosis (LC) is a devastating metastatic complication of a variety of solid tumours. There is often a high index of suspicion of LC in patients presenting with headache and cranial nerve palsies, particularly if MRI studies show meningeal enhancement and CSF shows increased protein levels. A cytological diagnosis, though, can be difficult to confirm and may need multiple CSF samplings over time. The CSF cell count and protein level can be normal, even in patients with confirmed LC.

Flow cytometry using carefully selected antibody panels can make a very real contribution to diagnosis and is able to detect neoplastic cells when cytology is negative. The use of an antibody directed at EpCAM, an epithelial adhesion molecule [65] appears particularly useful. It is expressed by most adenocarcinomas, but with different intensity according to organ of origin; hepatocellular, renal and squamous carcinomas are least likely to express this antigen [66]. We should note that in the majority of patients with LC, the malignant cell population constitutes less than 5% of CSF cells or <1 malignant cell per mm³ [67]. False negative results are more likely with small samples, delayed processing, sampling from a site not clearly involved on MRI (lumbar puncture versus ommaya reservoir sampling) and sampling fewer than two times [68]. They can be minimized, therefore, by withdrawing at least 10.5 mL for analysis, processing the sample immediately, obtaining CSF from a site of suspected disease and repeating the procedure if the initial cytology is negative [68]. Clearly, the assessment of CSF requires experience, expertise and familiarity in antibody profiles when dealing with such specimens and the challenges they present. Each laboratory needs to be assured and confident in their approach to CSF examination.

In summary, we can see that reactive cell changes are commonly encountered in the cell populations of blood, bone marrow and tissue fluids. It is important to be aware of these phenomena so that immunophenotypic data can be optimally utilized for accurate diagnosis in the assessment of cellular reactions to a wide variety of systemic diseases.

References

1 Groom DA, et al. Transient stress lymphocytosis during crisis of sickle cell anemia and emergency trauma and medical conditions. An immunophenotyping study. Arch Pathol Lab Med 1990, 114(6): 570–6.
2 Siddiqui MA, Esmaili JH. Transient reactive lymphocytosis associated with acute middle cerebral artery aneurysmal rupture. J Natl Med Assoc 1997, 89(4): 283–4.
3 Teggatz JR, Parkin J, Peterson L. Transient atypical lymphocytosis in patients with emergency medical conditions. Arch Pathol Lab Med 1987, 111(8): 712–4.
4 Pinkerton PH, et al. Acute lymphocytosis after trauma – early recognition of the high-risk patient? J Trauma 1989, 29(6): 749–51.
5 Karandikar NJ, et al. Transient stress lymphocytosis: an immunophenotypic characterization of the most common cause of newly identified adult lymphocytosis in a tertiary hospital. Am J Clin Pathol 2002, 117(5): 819–25.
6 Martina B, et al. Physiologic exercise-induced lymphocytosis. Blut 1990, 60(4): 255–6.
7 Rehman J, et al. Dynamic exercise leads to an increase in circulating ICAM-1: Further evidence for adrenergic modulation of cell adhesion. Brain Behav Immun 1997, 11(4): 343–51.
8 Singh, A, et al. Lymphocyte subset responses to exercise and glucocorticoid suppression in healthy men. Med Sci Sports Exerc 1996, 28(7): 822–8.
9 Mossafa H, et al. Persistent polyclonal B lymphocytosis with binucleated lymphocytes: a study of 25 cases. Groupe Francais d'Hematologie Cellulaire. Br J Haematol 1999, 104(3): 486–93.
10 Gordon DS, et al. Persistent polyclonal lymphocytosis of B lymphocytes. N Engl J Med 1982, 307(4): 232–6.
11 Troussard X, Mossafa H, Salaun V. Persistent polyclonal lymphocytosis (PPLB). Leukemia 1999, 13(3): 497–8.
12 Hudnall SD, et al. Comparative immunophenotypic features of EBV-positive and EBV-negative atypical lymphocytosis. Cytometry B Clin Cytom 2003, 55(1): 22–8.
13 Weisberger J. et al. Down-regulation of pan-T-cell antigens, particularly CD7, in acute infectious mononucleosis. Am J Clin Pathol 2003, 120(1): 49–55.
14 Chadburn A, Inghirami G,. Knowles DM. T-cell activation-associated antigen expression by neoplastic T-cells. Hematol Pathol 1992, 6(3): 131–41.
15 Juneja S, et al. Post-splenectomy lymphocytosis. Clin Lab Haematol 1995, 17(4): 335–7.
16 Demeter J. Persistent lymphocytosis of natural killer cells after splenectomy. Br J Haematol 1995, 91(1): 253–4.
17 Roden AC, Morice WG, Hanson CA. Immunophenotypic attributes of benign peripheral blood gammadelta T cells and

conditions associated with their increase. *Arch Pathol Lab Med* 2008, **132**(11): 1774–80.

18 Nielsen HB, *et al.* Splenectomy impairs lymphocytosis during maximal exercise. *Am J Physiol* 1997, **272**(6 Pt 2): R1847–52.

19 Van den Hove LE, *et al.*, Peripheral blood lymphocyte subset shifts in patients with untreated hematological tumors: evidence for systemic activation of the T cell compartment. *Leuk Res* 1998, **22**(2): 175–84.

20 Azuma M,. Phillips JH, Lanier LL. CD28- T lymphocytes. Antigenic and functional properties. *J Immunol* 1993, **150**(4): 1147–59.

21 Strioga M, PasukonieneV, Characiejus D. CD8+ CD28- and CD8+ CD57+ T cells and their role in health and disease. *Immunology* 2011, **134**(1): 17–32.

22 Van den Hove LE, *et al.* CD57+/CD28- T cells in untreated hemato-oncological patients are expanded and display a Th1-type cytokine secretion profile, ex vivo cytolytic activity and enhanced tendency to apoptosis. *Leukemia* 1998. **12**(10): 1573–82.

23 Valent JN, Schiffer CA, Prevalence of large granular lymphocytosis in patients with chronic myelogenous leukemia (CML) treated with dasatinib. *Leuk Res* 2011, **35**(1): e1–3.

24 Mustjoki S, *et al.* Clonal expansion of T/NK-cells during tyrosine kinase inhibitor dasatinib therapy. *Leukemia* 2009, **23**(8): 1398–405.

25 Cagnoli L, *et al.* T cell subset alterations in idiopathic glomerulonephritis. *Clin Exp Immunol* 1982, **50**(1): 70–6.

26 Ferenczi K, *et al.* CD69, HLA-DR and the IL-2R identify persistently activated T cells in psoriasis vulgaris lesional skin: blood and skin comparisons by flow cytometry. *J Autoimmun* 2000, **14**(1): 63–78.

27 Al-Aska A, *et al.* CD4+ T-lymphopenia in HIV negative tuberculous patients at King Khalid University Hospital in Riyadh, Saudi Arabia. *Eur J Med Res* 2011, **16**(6): 285–8.

28 Calzascia T, *et al.* CD4 T cells, lymphopenia, and IL-7 in a multistep pathway to autoimmunity. *Proc Natl Acad Sci USA* 2008, **105**(8): 2999–3004.

29 Craig SB, *et al.* Lymphopenia in leptospirosis. *Ann Trop Med Parasitol* 2009, **103**(3): 279–82.

30 Kirtava Z, *et al.* CD4+ T-lymphocytopenia without HIV infection: increased prevalence among patients with primary Sjogren's syndrome. *Clin Exp Rheumatol* 1995, **13**(5): 609–16.

31 Rivero SJ, Diaz-Jouanen E, Alarcon-Segovia D. Lymphopenia in systemic lupus erythematosus. Clinical, diagnostic, and prognostic significance. *Arthritis Rheum* 1978, **21**(3): 295–305.

32 Heimann TM, Bolnick K, Aufses AH, Jr. Prognostic significance of severe preoperative lymphopenia in patients with Crohn's disease. *Ann Surg* 1986, **203**(2): 132–5.

33 Sweiss NJ, *et al.* Significant CD4, CD8, and CD19 lymphopenia in peripheral blood of sarcoidosis patients correlates

with severe disease manifestations. *PLoS One* 2010, **5**(2): e9088.

34 Warnatz K, Schlesier M. Flowcytometric phenotyping of common variable immunodeficiency. *Cytometry B Clin Cytom* 2008, **74**(5): 261–71.

35 Illoh OC. Current applications of flow cytometry in the diagnosis of primary immunodeficiency diseases. *Arch Pathol Lab Med* 2004, **128**(1): 23–31.

36 Brooimans RA, *et al.* Flow cytometric differential of leukocyte populations in normal bone marrow: Influence of peripheral blood contamination1. *Cytometry B Clin Cytom* 2008, **76B**(1): 18–26.

37 Cid J, *et al.* Neutrophil CD64 expression as marker of bacterial infection: a systematic review and meta-analysis. *J Infect* 2010, **60**(5): 313–9.

38 Davis BH, *et al.* Neutrophil CD64 is an improved indicator of infection or sepsis in emergency department patients. *Arch Pathol Lab Med* 2006, **130**(5): 654–61.

39 Hoffmann JJ. Neutrophil CD64: a diagnostic marker for infection and sepsis. *Clin Chem Lab Med* 2009, **47**(8): 903–16.

40 Hussein OA, El-Toukhy MA, El-Rahman HS. Neutrophil CD64 expression in inflammatory autoimmune diseases: its value in distinguishing infection from disease flare. *Immunol Invest* 2010, **39**(7): 699–712.

41 Ng PC, *et al.* Neutrophil CD64 is a sensitive diagnostic marker for early-onset neonatal infection. *Pediatr Res* 2004, **56**(5): 796–803.

42 Rudensky B, *et al.* Neutrophil CD64 expression as a diagnostic marker of bacterial infection in febrile children presenting to a hospital emergency department. *Pediatr Emerg Care* 2008, **24**(11): 745–8.

43 Zarco MA, *et al.* Phenotypic changes in neutrophil granulocytes of healthy donors after G-CSF administration. *Haematologica* 1999, **84**(10): 874–8.

44 Papewalis C, *et al.* IFN-alpha skews monocytes into CD56+-expressing dendritic cells with potent functional activities in vitro and in vivo. *J Immunol* 2008, **180**(3): 1462–70.

45 Sconocchia G, *et al.* G-CSF-mobilized CD34+ cells cultured in interleukin-2 and stem cell factor generate a phenotypically novel monocyte. *J Leukoc Biol* 2004, **76**(6): 1214–9.

46 Grip O, *et al.* Increased subpopulations of CD16(+) and CD56(+) blood monocytes in patients with active Crohn's disease. *Inflamm Bowel Dis* 2007, **13**(5): 566–72.

47 Thieblemont N, *et al.* CD14lowCD16high: a cytokine-producing monocyte subset which expands during human immunodeficiency virus infection. *Eur J Immunol* 1995, **25**(12): 3418–24.

48 Xu Y, *et al.* Flow cytometric analysis of monocytes as a tool for distinguishing chronic myelomonocytic leukemia from reactive monocytosis. *Am J Clin Pathol* 2005, **124**(5): 799–806.

49 Tichelli A, *et al.* Morphology in patients with severe aplastic anemia treated with antilymphocyte globulin. *Blood* 1992, **80**(2): 337–45.

50 Brodsky RA, Jones RJ. Aplastic anaemia. *Lancet* 2005, **365**(9471): 1647–56.

51 Otawa M, *et al.* Comparative multi-color flow cytometric analysis of cell surface antigens in bone marrow hematopoietic progenitors between refractory anemia and aplastic anemia. *Leuk Res* 2000, **24**(4): 359–66.

52 Rizzo S, *et al.* Stem cell defect in aplastic anemia: reduced long term culture-initiating cells (LTC-IC) in CD34+ cells isolated from aplastic anemia patient bone marrow. *Hematol J* 2002, **3**(5): 230–6.

53 Matsui WH, *et al.* Quantitative analysis of bone marrow CD34 cells in aplastic anemia and hypoplastic myelodysplastic syndromes. *Leukemia* 2006, **20**(3): 458–62.

54 Antony VB, *et al.* Recruitment of inflammatory cells to the pleural space. Chemotactic cytokines, IL-8, and monocyte chemotactic peptide-1 in human pleural fluids. *J Immunol* 1993, **151**(12): 7216–23.

55 Risberg B, *et al.* Detection of monocyte/macrophage cell populations in effusions: a comparative study using flow cytometric immunophenotyping and immunocytochemistry. *Diagn Cytopathol* 2001, **25**(4): 214–9.

56 Adam P, *et al.* Immunophenotypic analysis of cerebrospinal fluid cell populations with the Cell-Dyn Sapphire haematology analyser: method feasibility and preliminary observations. *Int J Lab Hematol* 2010, **32**(1 Pt 2): 22–32.

57 Risberg B, *et al.* Flow cytometric immunophenotyping of serous effusions and peritoneal washings: comparison with immunocytochemistry and morphological findings. *J Clin Pathol* 2000, **53**(7): 513–7.

58 Davidson B, *et al.* Detection of malignant epithelial cells in effusions using flow cytometric immunophenotyping: an analysis of 92 cases. *Am J Clin Pathol* 2002, **118**(1): 85–92.

59 Chang A. *et al.* Lineage-specific identification of nonhematopoietic neoplasms by flow cytometry. *Am J Clin Pathol* 2003, **119**(5): 643–55.

60 Rubins JB, Rubins HB. Etiology and prognostic significance of eosinophilic pleural effusions. A prospective study. *Chest* 1996, **110**(5): 1271–4.

61 Burastero SE, *et al.* The repertoire of T lymphocytes recovered by bronchoalveolar lavage from healthy nonsmokers. *Eur Respir J* 1996, **9**(2): 319–27.

62 Agostini C, *et al.* Pulmonary immune cells in health and disease: lymphocytes. *Eur Respir J* 1993, **6**(9): 1378–401.

63 Costabel U. The alveolitis of hypersensitivity pneumonitis. *Eur Respir J* 1988, **1**(1): 5–9.

64 Kolopp-Sarda MN, *et al.* Discriminative immunophenotype of bronchoalveolar lavage CD4 lymphocytes in sarcoidosis. *Lab Invest* 2000, **80**(7): 1065–9.

65 Subira D, *et al.* Role of flow cytometry immunophenotyping in the diagnosis of leptomeningeal carcinomatosis. *Neuro Oncol* 2012, **14**(1): 43–52.

66 Spizzo G, *et al.* EpCAM expression in primary tumour tissues and metastases: an immunohistochemical analysis. *J Clin Pathol* 2011, **64**(5): 415–20.

67 Strik H, Prommel P. Diagnosis and individualized therapy of neoplastic meningitis. *Expert Rev Anticancer Ther* 2010, **10**(7): 1137–48.

68 Glantz MJ, *et al.* Cerebrospinal fluid cytology in patients with cancer: minimizing false-negative results. *Cancer* 1998, **82**(4): 733–9.

Index

Note: page numbers in italics refer to figures; page numbers in bold refer to tables.

Practical Flow Cytometry in Haematology Diagnosis, First Edition. Mike Leach, Mark Drummond and Allyson Doig.
© 2013 John Wiley & Sons, Ltd. Published 2013 by John Wiley & Sons, Ltd.

Printed and bound by CPI Group (UK) Ltd, Croydon, CR0 4YY

05/02/2025

14638453-0001